ESSENTIALS OF
BODY FLUIDS

Gabriel Duarte

ALLIED
HEALTH
PRESS

Essentials of Body Fluids

Author: **Gabriel Duarte**

Allied Health Press
4164 Lakeshore Road
Burlington ON L7L 1A4
Canada
www.alliedhealthpress.com
Email: orders@arclereducation.com

ISBN: 978-1-77956-273-9

ABOUT THE AUTHOR

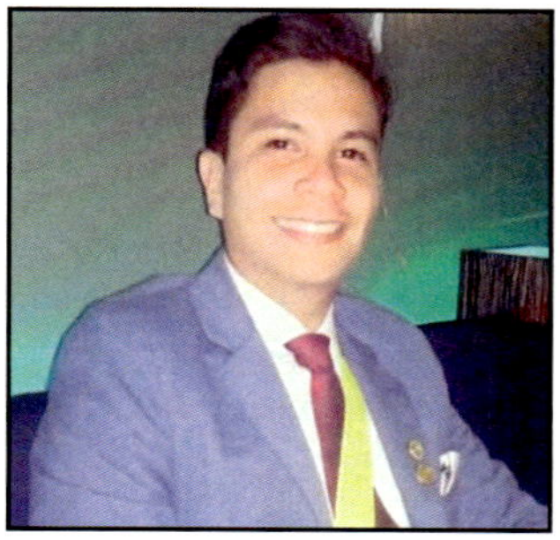

Gabriel is a doctor, passionate about radiology and diagnostic imaging with a solid clinical background. He completed his medical studies at the Universidad de Los Andes, Venezuela; and later he dedicated himself to the approach in anatomy, ultrasound, diagnosis and tomography studies. Besides, he has special training in teaching for undergraduate studies, human anatomy chairs and educational consulting. His passion for writing, editing and scientific research has led him to create experience as an author of many publications. Gabriel is a highly trained professional committed with teaching and high-quality professional medical practice.

Word Roots, Prefixes, and Suffixes by Chapter

Chapter 1 Introduction to body Fluids/Analysis

angi-: blood vessels

hemat-: blood

thromb-: blood clot

vas-, vasculo-: blood vessels

ven-, (phlebo): venous blood

Chapter 2 The Kidney

adren/o: adrenal gland

arteriol/o: arteriole

nephr(o)-: kidney

pelv(i/o): pelvis

phleb/o: vein

pyel/o: renal pelvis

ren(o): renal

ur/o: urine, urinary tract

ure(a/o): urine, urinary tract

ureter/o: ureter

Chapter 3 Renal Function

albumin/o: A protein produced by the liver is albumin

azot/o: A combining form that refers to "urea" or "nitrogen"

calic/o, cali/o: A combining form that refers to "calyx (plural: calyces)"

cyst/o, vesic/o: Combining forms used to describe the "urinary bladder"

glomerul/o: A combining form used to describe the "glomerulus (plural: glomeruli)"

hydr/o: The combining form hydr/o refers to "water"

lith/o: A combining form that pertains to "stone" or "calculus"

Chapter 4 Urine Examination

cyst/o: bladder

hypo: hypothermia

meta: metabolism

-oma: tumor

hemat/o, hem/o: blood

hepat/o: liver

-uria: urine, urination

urin/o: urine, urinary tract

Chapter 5 Renal and Metabolic Disease

-it is: inflammation

nephro-: relating to the kidneys

-opathy: a disease or disorder

-osis: a condition or a process

-uria: denoting a condition of the urine

Hypo-: below normal or deficient

bacteri-: pertaining to bacteria

cardi-: kardía, of or pertaining to the heart

-iasis: condition, formation, or presence of

Chapter 6 Cerebrospinal Fluid Analysis

abdom-: the abdomen

aden-: glands

angi-: blood vessels

arteri-: arteries

arthr-, articul-: joints

cardi-, coron-: the heart

Chapter 7 Pleural, Pericardial, and Peritoneal Fluid Analysis

carp-: the wrist

cerebr-, encephal-: the brain

cervic-: the neck

chondr-: cartilage

cyst-: bladder

cran-: the skull

cut-, derm-: the skin

cyt-: cell

enter-: the intestines

glut-: buttocks

hemat-, hemato-: blood

hepat-: the liver

Chapter 8 Synovial Fluid Analysis

arthr-, articul-: joints

carp-: the wrist

tal-:ankle:

-centesis: urgical puncture to remove fluidw

syn-: together, with [prefix]

synov/o: synovial membrane

-desis:surgical fixation of bone or joint

Chapter 9 Analysis of Vaginal Secretions

Vagin-: Root referring to the vagina.

-al: Suffix indicating "pertaining to."

Dis-: Prefix meaning "apart" or "away."

-charge: Suffix indicating a flow or release.

Vaginitis: Combining form indicating inflammation

Chapter 10 Fecal Analysis

Fec-: (related to feces)

Gastro-: (related to the stomach or gastrointestinal tract)

Micro-: (small, minute)

Macro-: (large, visible to the naked eye)

Bio-: (related to life or living organisms)

-Chemical: (pertaining to chemicals)

-scopy: Denotes a visual examination or inspection

Table of Contents

3 Renal Function 67

4 Urine Examination 107

5 Renal and Metabolic Disease 143

6 Cerebrospinal Fluid Analysis 185

LIST OF FIGURES

LIST OF TABLES

PREFACE

Biofluids, also known as body fluids, are vital liquids found in the human body that are essential for maintaining bodily functions. These fluids help regulate body temperature, circulate blood, transport nutrients, and produce protective substances to fight off diseases, ensuring optimal bodily function.

The main component of body fluids is water, which makes up about 75% of the human body's cells. Body fluids are divided into extracellular, intracellular, and transcellular categories, each serving specific functions to support cellular activities.

Blood and plasma are important body fluids that protect against infections, exchange nutrients and waste products, and regulate blood circulation. Electrolytes found in body fluids help balance fluid levels and support the movement and function of various body parts.

In forensic science, body fluids are valuable sources of evidence in criminal investigations. Analysis of these fluids can provide critical information about crime scenes, victims, and perpetrators. DNA extracted from body fluids can be compared to samples from suspects or victims to establish their involvement in a crime.

The book "Essentials of Body Fluids" aims to provide a comprehensive overview of the types and functions of body fluids. It is a valuable resource for students, researchers, and healthcare professionals interested in understanding the importance of body fluids in maintaining health.

The book covers the composition, functions, and regulation of body fluids, as well as their role in various disease states. It also discusses practical aspects of collecting, handling, and analyzing body fluids in clinical settings, as well as emerging research trends and technologies in the field.

Overall, "Essentials of Body Fluids" serves as a guide to understanding the critical role of biofluids in maintaining health and well-being, empowering readers to appreciate the importance of fluid balance for overall health.

Chapter

INTRODUCTION TO BODY FLUIDS/ANALYSIS

1

Contents

Introduction

Bodily fluids play a crucial role in maintaining balance within the human body by transporting essential nutrients, electrolytes, hormones, and waste products. Understanding and analyzing bodily fluids is vital for clinical diagnostics as it helps identify and treat various medical conditions, providing valuable insights into a person's health. Blood, which circulates throughout the body, carries nutrients and oxygen to tissues while removing waste products. Blood analysis, including tests like coagulation profiles, blood chemistry, CBC, and blood typing, is fundamental in medical diagnostics to detect abnormalities indicating illnesses like organ dysfunction, blood disorders, and infections.

Urine, produced by the kidneys through filtering blood, is another important bodily fluid. Urinalysis involves examining the physical, chemical, and microscopic characteristics of urine, such as color, pH, protein, and glucose levels. Deviations from normal urine composition can indicate systemic diseases, metabolic disorders, renal issues, or infections. Cerebrospinal fluid, surrounding and nourishing the brain and spinal cord, is analyzed through lumbar punctures to evaluate pressure, appearance, cell counts, and presence of pathogens for diagnosing neurological diseases like meningitis and encephalitis.

Synovial fluid in joints acts as a lubricant and shock absorber for smooth movement. Analyzing synovial fluid helps diagnose conditions like infections, gout, and arthritis by evaluating viscosity, protein concentration, cell counts, and crystal presence. Other bodily fluids like pericardial, pleural, and peritoneal fluids are also essential for maintaining homeostasis and diagnosing conditions like peritonitis and pleural effusions.

The examination of bodily fluids aids in diagnosing and forecasting illnesses by detecting changes in biochemical constituents that may indicate physiological or pathological conditions. Monitoring specific elements in bodily fluids can serve as markers for disease identification, leading to timely diagnosis and treatment planning. Body fluid analysis is also used for therapeutic screenings and health assessments, providing valuable information on treatment efficacy. Clinical laboratories rely on advanced analytical techniques to measure chemical species in biological fluids for accurate diagnostic purposes.

Orientation and Directional Terms

Term	Definition	Illustration
Complete blood count	A complete blood is a study that provides information about the quantity and distribution of different types of blood cells, including red blood cells, white blood cells, and platelets.	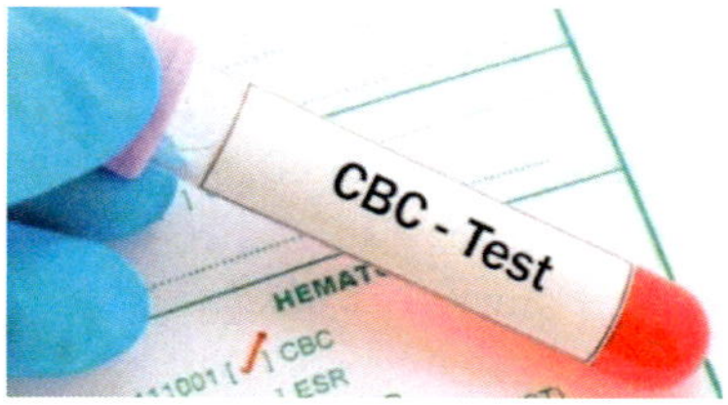
Cerebrospinal fluid	Cerebrospinal fluid is a clear, colorless body fluid found within the tissue that surrounds the brain and spinal cord of all vertebrates.	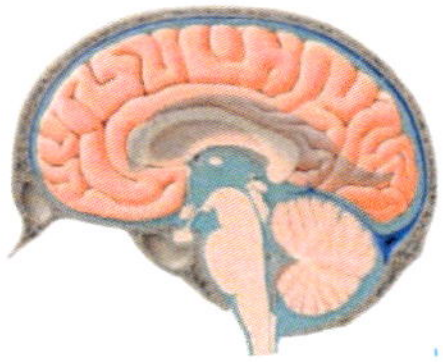
Extracellular fluid	Extracellular fluid (ECF) denotes all body fluid outside the cells of any multicellular organism.	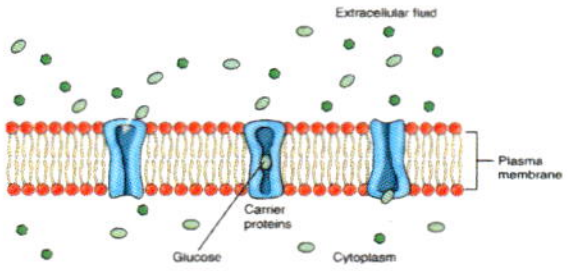
Central Nervous system	The central nervous system is the brain and spinal cord, while the peripheral nervous system consists of everything else.	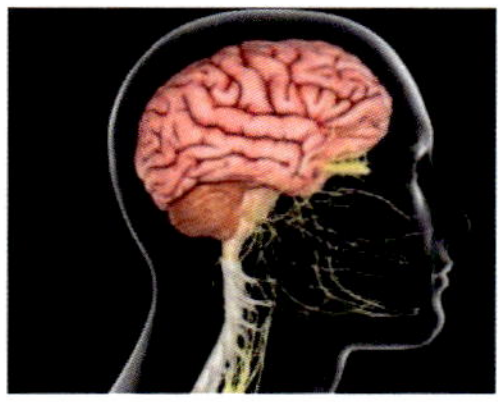
Synovial Fluid	Synovial fluid, also called synovia, is a viscous, non-Newtonian fluid found in the cavities of synovial joints.	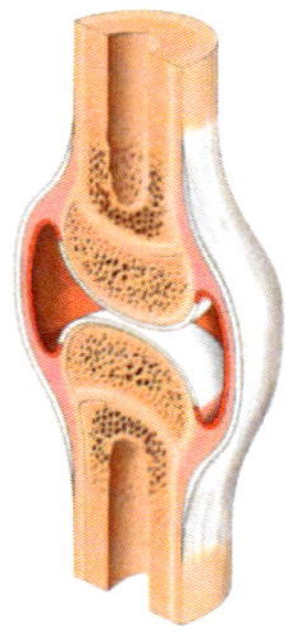

1.1. Basic Concepts

Body fluids are aqueous liquids that carry a wide range of solutes and metabolic products and also contain the cellular and ionic components required for healthy bodily operation. The most common way to classify body fluids is based on whether they are found inside or outside of the cell membrane.

Two-thirds of all bodily fluid is called intracellular fluid (ICF), sometimes known as cytosol. It is found inside cells and is divided into compartments by different organelle membranes. The majority of this fluid is water, but it also contains a variety of other materials and dissolved and suspended proteins. Ionic concentrations (such as sodium and potassium) are critical to proper ICF function, as it is the difference between these levels and ion concentrations found outside the cell that drives several essential cellular processes, including:

- Osmoregulation
- Cell signaling
- Creation of action potentials in endocrine, muscle and nerve cells

Extracellular fluid (ECF), which makes up approximately one-third of the body's total fluid content, surrounds cells and acts as a conduit for the body's natural flow of nutrients and waste products from metabolism. ECF can be sub-categorized according to composition, function and body location, and includes:

- Plasma
- Lymph
- Cerebrospinal fluid (CSF)
- Saliva
- Interstitial fluid
- Other body-generated fluids such as milk, sweat and urine

Some common body fluids that are analyzed include blood, urine, saliva, cerebrospinal fluid, synovial fluid, and sweat. Each of these fluids can provide valuable information about a person's health and can help to diagnose and monitor various medical conditions.

For example, blood tests can detect infections, anemia, and conditions such as diabetes and kidney disease. Urine tests can provide information about kidney function, urinary tract infections, and drug use. Cerebrospinal fluid analysis can help to diagnose conditions affecting the brain and spinal cord, such as meningitis and multiple sclerosis.

In addition to diagnosing medical conditions, analysis of body fluids can also be used to monitor the effectiveness of treatments and to track disease progression. For example, cancer patients may undergo regular blood tests to monitor tumor markers and assess their response to chemotherapy.

Overall, the analysis of body fluids is an important tool in modern medicine and can provide valuable insights into a person's health and well-being. It is essential for healthcare professionals to understand the significance of these tests and to interpret the results accurately in order to provide the best possible care for their patients.

Examples of body fluids are:

- Blood plasma (carries blood cells, nutrients, hormones and others)
- Urine (waste product secreted by the kidney)
- Interstitial fluid (the fluid that are located in between cells)
- Cerebrospinal fluid (fluid surrounding the brain and spinal cord)
- Saliva and intestinal fluid (aid the process of digestion)

Blood and urine samples are the most

common types of routine samples collected for laboratory testing in the biochemistry lab. Compared to blood and urine samples, other fluids such as synovial, peritoneal, ascitic, and cerebrospinal fluid are less common. This is because extracting these fluids from the body necessitates difficult steps. It is advised to run paired samples—fluid and blood samples—for the majority of bodily fluid biochemistry analyses to verify the diagnosis of illnesses. A basic understanding of the various bodily fluid types is essential because these fluids play a role in the development and manifestation of life-threatening conditions like cancer and heart failure. (Cotran et al., 2005; Strasinger and Lorenzo, 2008; Liachovitzky Carlos, 2015; Pearson, 2018)

1.1.1. Cerebrospinal Fluid (CSF)

Cerebrospinal fluid (CSF) is a clear, colorless, and vital bodily fluid that circulates throughout the brain's ventricular system as well as the subarachnoid space surrounding the brain and spinal cord. It serves as a protective cushion, a conduit for nutrients, a means of eliminating waste, and a controller of intracranial pressure, among other vital functions that are essential to preserving the health and functionality of the central nervous system (CNS).

Within the brain's ventricles, specifically the lateral, third, and fourth ventricles, specialized cells known as choroid plexus produce the majority of CSF. The process by which the choroid plexus epithelium filters, secretes, and modifies plasma results in this production. Although the total volume present at any given time is much smaller, approximately 125-150 milliliters in adults, the fluid is continuously generated at a rate of about 500 milliliters per day in humans.

Carefully controlled CSF composition provides the best possible environment for the central nervous system. It is composed of water, proteins, glucose, electrolytes (like sodium, potassium, and chloride), and trace amounts of other materials. These elements are kept within specific ranges, and any departures may point to neurological disorders. For example, decreased glucose levels may point to metabolic problems, whereas increased protein levels may point to inflammation or infection. The provision of mechanical support and cushioning to the brain and spinal cord is one of the main purposes of CSF. By serving as a shock absorber, it protects these fragile structures from harm or abrupt movements. This cushioning effect is especially important because even small physical disturbances can cause damage to the brain.

Additionally, CSF acts as a conduit for waste products and nutrients to be transferred from the blood to the central nervous system. It ensures that neurons and other brain cells have the necessary materials for proper function and that their metabolic needs are satisfied by delivering vital substances like glucose, oxygen, and hormones. In addition, CSF removes toxins and waste products from metabolism, which contributes to the CNS's ability to remain stable and clean.

The flow of cerebrospinal fluid, known as CSF circulation, is a well-defined pathway that CSF takes within the brain. CSF is produced in the ventricles and then travels through the ventricular system and subarachnoid space to envelop the brain and spinal cord. It then exits into the bloodstream through specialized structures within the dural sinuses called arachnoid granulations, also known as villi. The continuous circulation of CSF helps maintain its volume and pressure within the central nervous system.

Disturbances in the composition or circulation of CSF can lead to various neurological disorders. Conditions like hydrocephalus, characterized by an excess of CSF in the brain, can increase intracranial pressure and potentially damage brain tissue if left untreated. On the other hand, diseases such as meningitis or subarachnoid hemorrhage can alter the composition of CSF, leading to inflammation, infection, or other pathological changes within the central nervous system.

As a crucial component of the central nervous system, cerebrospinal fluid plays a key role in waste removal, transporting nutrients, providing support, and regulating intracranial pressure. The precise control of its composition and circulation is essential for maintaining CNS health and function, as any disruptions in the dynamics of CSF can have significant neurological consequences. It is crucial to comprehend CSF's function in the body to diagnose and treat a variety of neurological disorders (Figure 1.1).

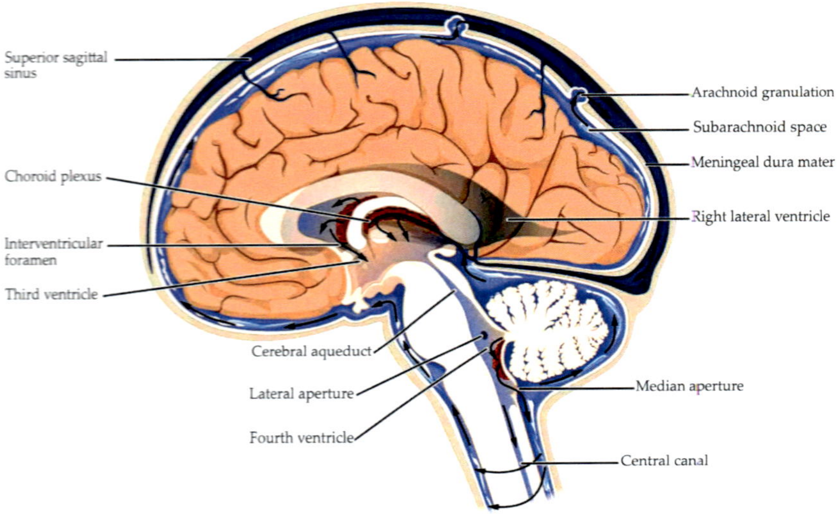

Figure 1.1. *CSF.*

Source: By OpenStax - https://cnx.org/contents/FPtK1zmh@8.25:fEI3C8Ot@10/Preface, CC BY 4.0, https://commons.wikimedia.org/w/index.php?curid=30147960.

Cerebrospinal fluid (CSF) originates from the brain and spinal cord.

The functions of CSF are:

- Protect the brain within the skull and the spinal cord against any impact on the Central Nervous System (CNS).
- Circulates chemicals and nutrients that are filtered from the blood.
- Removes waste products and harmful metabolites from the brain.

1. **CSF Biochemistry Test:** CSF biochemistry test is requested by the doctor when the patient is having symptoms involving the Central Nervous System (CNS). For instance, severe headache, difficulty with speech, seizure, etc. Mainly, two analytes will be analyzed by the laboratory technician which are protein and glucose.

Cerebrospinal Protein

- **Elevated Protein Value:** As protein is a large molecule, this molecule does not easily cross the blood-brain barrier. Therefore, when CSF protein is elevated, this suggests that the blood-brain barrier is damaged and the patient might suffer from meningitis, hemorrhage (excessive bleeding) or multiple sclerosis.
- **Reduced Protein Value:** Fluid is leaking from CNS.
- Cerebrospinal Fluid Glucose

2. Normal Glucose Value for CSF is Typically 2/3 of the Blood Glucose:

- **Elevated Glucose Value:** As a result of plasma elevations.
- **Low Glucose Value:** Indication of bacterial or viral infection which also depends on the full blood count test results. CSF glucose is usually reduced when foreign cells such as bacteria or elevation of white blood cells (WBC), mainly neutrophils, consume glucose. The diagnosis would favor bacterial meningitis. Likewise, if the CSF glucose value is normal, but WBC is elevated mainly in monocytes and lymphocytes, the patient is suspected of having viral, fungal, or parasitic origin infection.

1.1.2. Synovial Fluid

One important bodily fluid that is essential to the health and functionality of joints in the musculoskeletal system is synovial fluid. It is a transparent, thick liquid that is present in the synovial cavity, which is the space around joints like the hip, shoulder, and knee. Lubrication, shock absorption, nutrient distribution, and waste removal are just a few of the vital roles synovial fluid plays in keeping joints healthy and mobile.

Lubricating joint surfaces to lower friction and promote smooth movement between articulating bones is one of synovial fluid's main purposes. Hyaluronic acid and lubricin, two molecules found in the fluid, create a lubricating layer over the surfaces of the articular cartilage. This lubricant is necessary to minimize cartilage deterioration, stop damage, and maintain joint function over time. Joints may suffer from increased friction due to inadequate synovial fluid and lubrication, which can cause pain, inflammation, and eventually degenerative changes like osteoarthritis.

In addition to cushioning joints and protecting them from the impact of mechanical forces during movement, synovial fluid serves as a shock absorber. Because of the fluid's viscoelastic characteristics, there is a lower chance of damage to the cartilage and other joint structures because the fluid can absorb and distribute forces evenly across the joint surfaces. This shock-absorbing feature is especially crucial when engaging in repetitive motions or high-impact exercises like running or jumping.

Synovial fluid is essential for supplying the avascular articular cartilage with nutrients. The fluid is full of vital nutrients that are required to keep chondrocytes, the cells that makeup cartilage tissue, healthy and metabolically active. These nutrients include oxygen, glucose, and amino acids. Through diffusion from the synovial fluid, these nutrients are delivered to the cartilage, guaranteeing that the cartilage gets the nourishment it requires to stay healthy and functional. Waste products are released into the synovial fluid by the chondrocytes and other cells in the joint during regular metabolic processes. Eventually, the waste products are removed from the joint by drainage or circulation. Inflammation, tissue damage, and degenerative joint diseases can be exacerbated by the buildup of hazardous materials inside the joint, which can be avoided by effectively eliminating waste products.

To keep synovial fluid lubricating and shock-absorbing, its composition is carefully controlled. Water makes up the majority of it, with trace amounts of proteins, electrolytes, and glycosaminoglycans (GAGs) like proteoglycans and hyaluronic acid. These molecules help the fluid maintain its viscosity and lubricating properties, which promote easy mobility and healthy joint function. The lubricating qualities of synovial fluid can be disrupted and joint pain and dysfunction can result from changes in its composition, such as an increase in inflammatory cytokines or a decrease in hyaluronic acid concentration.

The dynamics of synovial fluid can be disturbed by several things, such as trauma, inflammation, infection, or underlying medical disorders. Changes in synovial fluid composition and volume can cause joint pain, stiffness, and functional impairment. These conditions include gout, osteoarthritis, and rheumatoid arthritis. To effectively prevent and treat musculoskeletal disorders, it is imperative to comprehend the function of synovial fluid in joint health and disease.

Synovial fluid which is also known as joint fluid originates from the cavities of joints (space between bones) (Figure 1.2).

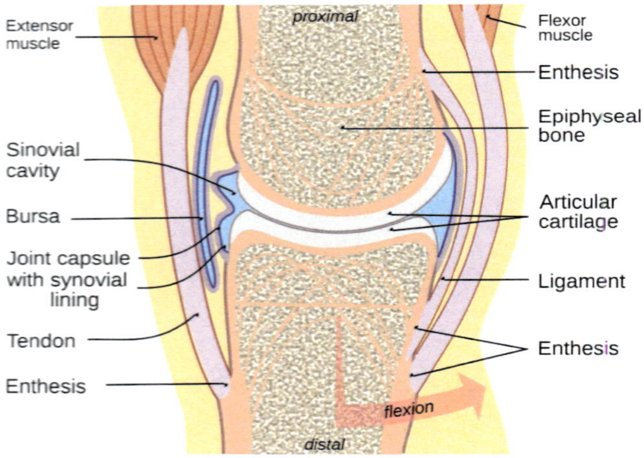

Figure 1.2. *Synovial joint.*

Source: By Madhero88 - Own work, CC BY-SA 3.0, https://commons.wikimedia.org/w/index.php?curid=10158699.

1.1.2.1. Synovial Fluid Analysis

An examination known as synovial fluid analysis is utilized to evaluate the characteristics and composition of synovial fluid extracted from a joint. This process is crucial in diagnosing and treating various joint-related diseases like infectious arthritis, inflammatory arthritis, and crystal arthropathies. By providing valuable information about the root cause of joint symptoms, the analysis aids in the accurate diagnosis and formulation of an appropriate treatment plan.

During the synovial fluid analysis procedure, synovial fluid is typically withdrawn from the affected joint using a sterile needle and syringe. Although the knee, shoulder, hip, and wrist are the most commonly aspirated joints, other joints may also be sampled if necessary. Local anesthesia is often administered to minimize the patient's discomfort during the procedure.

After the synovial fluid is collected, it is sent to a laboratory for examination. Depending on the suspected underlying condition and clinical presentation of the patient, a variety of tests may be conducted as part of the analysis.

Some of the key components of synovial fluid analysis include:

1. **Gross Appearance:** The visual inspection of synovial fluid can provide initial clues about its characteristics. Normal synovial fluid is clear and straw-colored, whereas abnormal fluid may appear cloudy, bloody, or turbid, indicating the presence of inflammation, infection, or other pathological changes.
2. **Cell Count and Differential:** A cell count is performed to determine the total number of cells present in the synovial fluid, including white blood cells (WBCs) and red blood cells (RBCs). The differential count distinguishes between different types of WBCs, such as neutrophils, lymphocytes, and monocytes. Elevated WBC counts, particularly neutrophils, are suggestive of inflammation or infection within the joint.
3. **Microscopic Examination:** Synovial fluid is examined under a microscope to assess for the presence of crystals, bacteria, or other microorganisms. Crystals, such as monosodium urate (associated with gout) or calcium pyrophosphate dihydrate (associated with pseudogout), can help diagnose crystal arthropathies. Identification of bacteria or other pathogens can confirm the diagnosis of infectious arthritis.
4. **Biochemical Analysis:** Various biochemical tests may be performed on synovial fluid to assess its composition. This may include measurements of glucose, protein, lactate dehydrogenase (LDH), and inflammatory markers such as C-reactive protein (CRP) and erythrocyte sedimentation rate (ESR). Abnormal levels of these substances can provide additional diagnostic information and help monitor disease activity.
5. **Culture and Sensitivity Testing:** Synovial fluid culture is performed to identify the presence of bacteria or fungi and determine their antibiotic susceptibility. This information is crucial for guiding antimicrobial therapy in cases of septic arthritis or other infectious joint conditions.

The patient's clinical history, physical examination findings, and results from additional diagnostic tests must all be taken into account when interpreting the synovial fluid analysis results. To make an accurate diagnosis and create a treatment plan that is specific to each patient's needs, a thorough approach is required. When evaluating joint disorders, synovial fluid analysis is a useful tool that can help guide clinical decision-making and improve patient outcomes. This test is usually requested by doctors in medical cases like joint inflammation or joint injury. Biochemistry analytes such as total protein, glucose, albumin, lactate dehydrogenase (LDH) and uric acid are considered clinically important.

- **Glucose:** Typically, under fasting conditions, the concentration of glucose in the synovial fluid should not be more than 0.55 mmol/L lower than the blood value level. A low value of synovial fluid suggests infection or joint inflammation due to the glycolytic activities of bacteria of white blood cells.

- **Protein:** As protein is a large molecule, these molecules are not filtered through the synovial membrane. Normal synovial fluid protein is approximately 1/3 of blood plasma value. Synovial membrane permeability is altered by inflammation. Thus, the elevation synovial protein value indicates that patients might suffer from hemorrhagic or inflammatory joint.
- **Lactate Dehydrogenase (LDH):** LDH is usually raised in conditions like rheumatoid arthritis.
- **Uric acid:** A synovial fluid uric acid test is performed to verify the diagnosis of gout apart from the result obtained from the serum uric acid test.

1.1.3. Peritoneal/Ascitic Fluid

Ascitic fluid, or peritoneal fluid when present in the peritoneal cavity, is a vital bodily fluid that is important for the health and function of abdominal organs and the peritoneum. The accumulation of fluid in the peritoneal cavity, known as ascites, can be caused by conditions such as liver cirrhosis, heart failure, malignancies, and infections. Knowledge of the composition and properties of ascitic fluid is necessary for diagnosing the root cause of ascites and determining the best treatment approach.

Ascitic fluid is a clear, straw-colored fluid with a composition similar to plasma but with a higher concentration of electrolytes and lower levels of protein. With contributions from lymphatic drainage and local production within the peritoneal cavity, it is primarily derived from plasma ultrafiltration across the peritoneal membrane. The fluid facilitates the exchange of nutrients, lubricates the peritoneal surfaces, and helps remove waste from the abdominal organs, among other crucial roles.

Liver cirrhosis is a main factor in the development of ascites, a condition where fluid builds up in the abdominal cavity. This chronic liver disease is marked by fibrosis, impacting liver function. Patients with cirrhosis experience portal hypertension, causing increased resistance to blood flow through the liver. This leads to the creation of collateral circulation and elevated hydrostatic pressure in the splanchnic circulation. The increased pressure gradient causes fluid to leak from the hepatic sinusoids into the peritoneal cavity, resulting in ascitic fluid accumulation.

The ascitic fluid composition can offer important diagnostic insights into the underlying cause of ascites. Evaluation of the fluid's appearance, cell count, differential, protein concentration, and serum-ascites albumin gradient (SAAG) are common components of ascitic fluid analysis. The SAAG, calculated by subtracting the ascitic fluid albumin concentration from the serum albumin concentration, is a useful marker for distinguishing between portal hypertension-related ascites (SAAG $\geq$ 1.1 g/dL) and non-portal hypertension-related ascites (SAAG $<$ 1.1 g/dL).

Apart from liver cirrhosis, other frequent reasons for ascites are infections, cancers (like peritoneal carcinomatosis), and congestive heart failure (like spontaneous bacterial peritonitis). In ascitic fluid analysis, each of these conditions may show distinctive results, such as elevated WBC counts and bacterial cultures in spontaneous bacterial peritonitis, malignant cells in peritoneal carcinomatosis, and elevated protein levels in ascites linked to nephrotic syndrome. Treatment of the underlying cause of ascites and relief from symptoms associated with fluid accumulation are the main goals of ascitic fluid management. Dietary sodium restriction, diuretic medication (such as furosemide and spironolactone), paracentesis (removing extra fluid from the peritoneal cavity), and, in extreme situations, liver transplantation or the implantation of a transjugular intrahepatic portosystemic shunt (TIPS) for refractory ascites brought on by liver cirrhosis are examples of therapeutic interventions. All things considered, peritoneal fluid analysis is a useful tool for the assessment and care of ascites patients, offering crucial diagnostic data and directing treatment choices. Healthcare professionals can improve patient outcomes and quality of life by implementing appropriate interventions after learning about the underlying pathophysiology and etiology of ascites. Our capacity to treat this difficult clinical condition will be further improved by ongoing research into the mechanisms underlying the formation of ascites and the creation of innovative treatment modalities.

Abdominal Cavity Showing Peritoneum

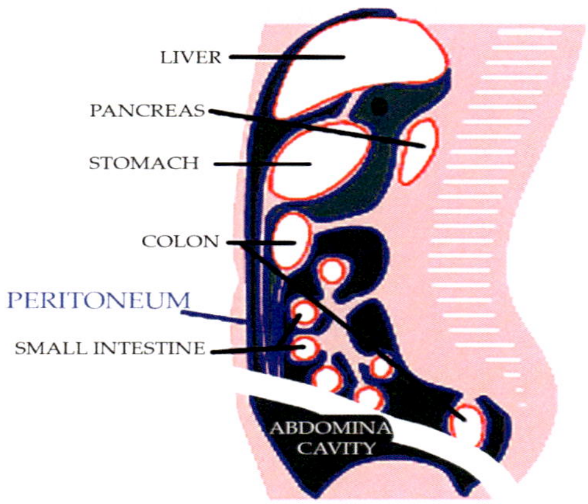

Source: http://myhealth.moh.gov.my/images/kimiahayat/fluid-peritoneal.png.

The accumulation of peritoneal fluid usually happens due to:

- **Transudate:** An imbalance in pressure within blood vessels due to conditions like liver diseases.
- **Exudates:** Injury or inflammation of the peritoneum that causes an excess amount of fluid inside abdominal space such as malignancies.

1.1.3.1. Peritoneal Fluid Analysis

Albumin is the most crucial biochemistry test to run when analyzing peritoneal fluid. Both serum albumin and peritoneal fluid albumin levels will be examined to distinguish between transudate and exudate conditions. The difference (serum-ascites albumin gradient, or SAAG) will be assessed to ascertain whether transudates or exudates are present in the abdominal cavity.

- **Transudate**
  - o Value of SAAG above 1.1 g/dL is considered evidence of a transudate condition.
  - o The level of total protein will be low (approximately <30 g/L)
- **Exudate**
  - o Value of SAAG below 1.1 g/dL is considered evidence of the occurrence of exudates.
  - o The level of total protein will be high (approximately >30g/L)

Other biochemistry tests that may be performed in addition to albumin may include:

- **Glucose:** For normal patients, glucose value should be almost equal to the blood glucose levels. However, if infection does occur, peritoneal fluid glucose value will be low due to the glycolytic activities of bacteria or white cells.

The diagnostic process known as "peritoneal fluid analysis" is used to assess the properties and makeup of fluid that has been drawn from the abdomen's peritoneal cavity, which houses organs like the spleen, stomach, liver, and intestines. When there is a possibility of abdominal pathology, such as infection, inflammation, or cancer, this analysis is usually carried out. It can offer important information to support diagnosis and direct treatment choices.

The process of collecting fluid for peritoneal fluid analysis is known as paracentesis, and it is typically carried out in a sterile setting with a needle and syringe. After that, the fluid is sent to a lab for examination, where a range of tests can be run to determine its composition and other characteristics. Assessing the appearance of the fluid, including its color and clarity, is one of the main steps in the peritoneal fluid analysis process. While turbidity, cloudiness, or discoloration are abnormal findings, they can also signal the presence of infection, bleeding, or other pathological processes. Normal peritoneal fluid is clear and straw-colored.

Important components of peritoneal fluid analysis include cell count and differential. To find out how many cells overall—including white blood cells (WBCs) and red blood cells (RBCs)—are in the fluid, a cell count is done. An increased WBC count, especially when neutrophils are the predominant cell type, could be a sign of infection or inflammation in the peritoneal cavity, as in peritonitis cases. Microscopical analysis of peritoneal fluid can identify a range of cellular components, such as bacteria, fungi, and cancerous cells. The confirmation of the diagnosis of peritoneal malignancy or infectious peritonitis, respectively, can be aided by the identification of these organisms or abnormal cells. Measurements of lactate dehydrogenase (LDH), protein, glucose, and amylase levels are among the biochemical parameters of peritoneal fluid that can be analyzed. Disturbances in these metrics can offer supplementary diagnostic insights and may indicate specific ailments, like bacterial peritonitis (lower glucose), cancer (higher LDH), or pancreatitis (higher amylase).

Cultures of peritoneal fluid are frequently used to detect the existence of bacteria or fungi and assess how susceptible they are to antibiotics. Antimicrobial therapy in cases of infectious peritonitis must be guided by this information to avoid treatment failure or the emergence of antibiotic resistance. Depending on the clinical situation and suspected underlying pathology, additional specialized tests may also be performed on peritoneal fluid. These could include tests for specific markers of inflammation, such as interleukin-6 (IL-6), tumor necrosis factor-alpha (TNF-alpha), or other cytokines, as well as tests for the presence of ascitic fluid albumin gradient (SAAG), which can be used to distinguish between ascites related to portal hypertension and ascites unrelated to portal hypertension.

An invaluable diagnostic technique for determining the fundamental cause of abdominal pathology is peritoneal fluid analysis. Health care professionals can improve patient outcomes by accurately diagnosing conditions and developing treatment plans based on the makeup and properties of peritoneal fluid.

1.1.4. Pleural Fluid

The fluid that surrounds the lungs and lines the inside surface of the chest wall is called pleural fluid, and it is an essential part of the respiratory system. It is a transparent, straw-colored substance. It is necessary for immune defense, lubrication, and respiratory mechanics, as well as for the integrity and proper operation of the lungs and pleura. Comprehending the makeup and properties of pleural fluid is essential for diagnosing and treating a range of respiratory ailments, such as cancers, infections, and pleural effusions.

The pleura produces and absorbs pleural fluid continuously by carefully balancing the hydrostatic and oncotic pressures. Normal physiological conditions result in a small volume of fluid that serves as a lubricant, enabling the lungs to move freely within the chest cavity during respiration. This is because the production and absorption of pleural fluid are tightly regulated. Disturbances in this equilibrium, however, may cause an excess of fluid to build up in the pleural space and cause a pleural effusion.

Pleural fluid has a similar composition to plasma, but it contains less protein and cells. It is mostly composed of glucose, water, electrolytes (such as potassium, sodium, and chloride), and trace amounts of proteins (such as albumin and immunoglobulins). Mesothelial cells, which line the pleural cavity and aid in the creation and absorption of pleural fluid, are also present in the fluid.

The diagnostic process of pleural fluid analysis involves analyzing the properties and makeup of fluid extracted from the pleural cavity, usually via a thoracentesis procedure. The analysis offers insightful knowledge regarding the underlying cause of pleural effusions, which aids in directing future diagnostic assessments and treatment choices. The evaluation of fluid appearance, cell count, differential, and biochemical parameters are important aspects of pleural fluid analysis. The gross appearance of pleural fluid can offer preliminary hints regarding its etiology; features like color, clarity, and viscosity can reveal possible underlying conditions. For instance, turbid or bloody fluid may indicate trauma, infection, or cancer, whereas clear fluid is more frequently observed in transudative effusions brought on by diseases like liver cirrhosis or heart failure.

The distinction between exudative and transudative effusions can be made with the aid of pleural fluid differential analysis and cell count. Increased capillary permeability and inflammation-induced exudative effusions are characterized by elevated total cell counts, predominantly neutrophils or lymphocytes, depending on the underlying cause. On the other hand, transudative effusions, which result from an imbalance between hydrostatic and oncotic pressures, usually have a higher concentration of monocytes and a lower cell count.

Protein, glucose, lactate dehydrogenase (LDH), and pH measurements are a few examples of biochemical tests that can be performed on pleural fluid. Deviations from these parameters can help distinguish between different pleural effusion etiologies and offer more diagnostic information. For instance, low blood sugar levels (.<60 mg/dL) are suggestive of empyema or rheumatoid pleuritis, while elevated LDH levels (> 200 IU/L) could be a sign of bacterial infection or cancer. Microscopical analysis of pleural fluid enables the identification of abnormal cellular elements such as malignant cells, fungi, bacteria, or other elements.

The identification of these organisms or cells can direct appropriate treatment strategies and aid in the confirmation of the diagnosis of malignancy, infectious pleuritis, or other underlying conditions.

An invaluable diagnostic technique for determining the underlying cause of pleural effusions is the pleural fluid analysis. Healthcare professionals can improve patient outcomes and quality of life by accurately diagnosing patients and developing treatment plans based on the characteristics and composition of pleural fluid. Further investigation into the pathophysiology of pleural effusions, along with the creation of innovative diagnostic methods, will improve our capacity to identify and treat these complex respiratory disorders (Figure 1.3).

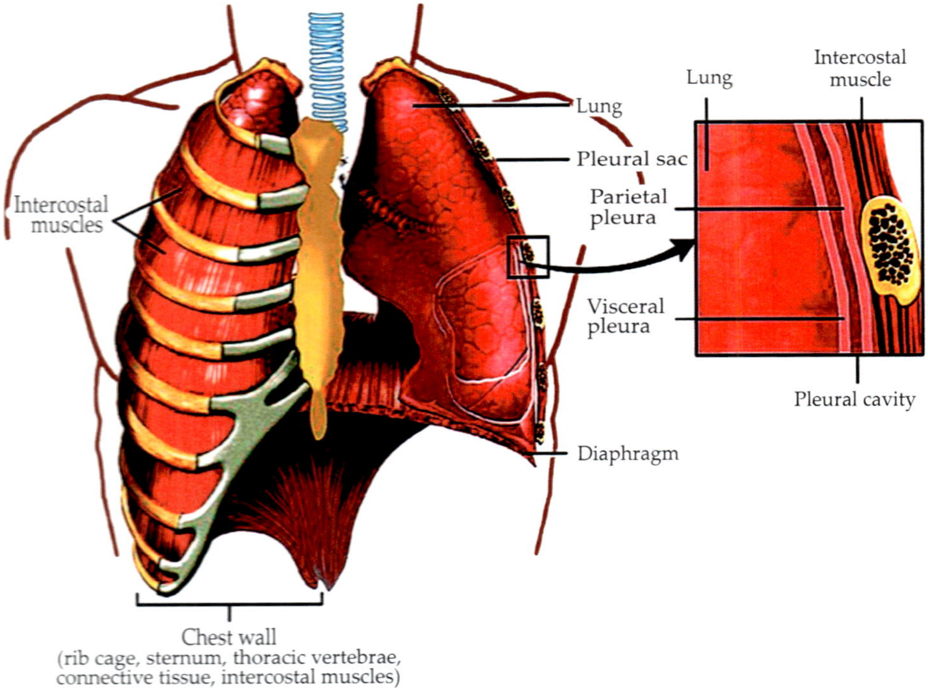

Figure 1.3. *Pleural cavity.*

Source: By OpenStax College - Anatomy & Physiology, Connexions Web site. http://cnx.org/content/col11496/1.6/, Jun 19, 2013., CC BY 3.0, https://commons.wikimedia.org/w/index.php?curid=30148380

The fluid that surrounds the lung and is produced inside the chest cavity is called pleural fluid. The purpose of the pleural fluid is to lubricate the respiratory system. Pleural effusion is the term used to describe the buildup of fluid inside the pleural space. Pneumonia and heart failure are two ailments that can cause pleural effusion.

The accumulation of fluid usually happens due to:

- **Transudate:** An imbalance pressure within blood vessels or low blood protein concentration which causes fluid to leak inside the pleural space. This condition is normally due to heart failure or cirrhosis.
- **Exudates:** Injury or inflammation of the pleurae that causes excess amount of fluid inside pleural space. Exudate effusion usually occurs in cases like pneumonia, tuberculosis and cancer.

1.1.4.1. Pleural Fluid Analysis

A diagnostic procedure called pleural fluid analysis is used to assess the properties and makeup of fluid that has accumulated in the pleural cavity, which is the area between the two layers of pleura that surround the lungs. When there is a possibility of a pleural effusion—which can be caused by several underlying illnesses, including infection, inflammation, cancer, or heart failure—this analysis is usually carried out.

Thoracentesis is the process of extracting pleural fluid for analysis, which entails inserting a needle through the chest wall into the pleural space to gather a sample of fluid.

Once obtained, the pleural fluid is sent to a laboratory for comprehensive analysis, which includes several key components:

1. **Appearance:** The gross appearance of pleural fluid can provide initial clues about its etiology. Normal pleural fluid is usually clear and pale yellow in color. Turbidity, blood-tinged appearance, or milky appearance may suggest infection, bleeding, or chylothorax, respectively.
2. **Volume:** The volume of pleural fluid obtained during thoracentesis can vary widely and may be indicative of the severity or chronicity of the underlying condition. Large-volume pleural effusions may exert pressure on the lungs, leading to symptoms such as dyspnea (shortness of breath) or respiratory distress.
3. **Cell Count (Differential):** A cell count is performed to determine the total number of cells present in the pleural fluid, including white blood cells (WBCs) and red blood cells (RBCs). The differential count distinguishes between different types of WBCs, such as neutrophils, lymphocytes, eosinophils, and macrophages. Elevated WBC counts, particularly neutrophils, may indicate infection or inflammation, whereas lymphocytic predominance may suggest tuberculosis or malignancy.
4. **Biochemical Analysis:** Various biochemical tests are performed on pleural fluid to assess its composition. This includes measurements of glucose, protein, lactate dehydrogenase (LDH), pH, and levels of specific markers such as adenosine deaminase (ADA) or carcinoembryonic antigen (CEA). Abnormalities in these parameters can provide valuable diagnostic information and help differentiate between various etiologies of pleural effusions.
5. **Microscopic Examination:** Pleural fluid is examined under a microscope to detect the presence of microorganisms, malignant cells, or other abnormal cellular elements. Identification of bacteria, fungi, or malignant cells can confirm the diagnosis of infectious pleuritis, malignancy, or other underlying conditions.
6. **Cytology:** Cytological examination of pleural fluid involves evaluating the cellular composition and morphology of the cells present in the sample. This can help identify malignant cells and establish a diagnosis of primary or metastatic malignancy involving the pleura.

It is necessary to take into account the patient's clinical history, physical examination results, imaging studies, and additional laboratory testing when interpreting pleural fluid analysis. To correctly identify the underlying cause of the pleural effusion and direct suitable treatment plans, which may entail chemotherapy, antibiotics, drainage techniques, or supportive care, a thorough approach is required. Pleural fluid analysis is a crucial component in improving patient outcomes and management of patients with pleural effusions. It is a useful tool in this regard.

To diagnose patients experiencing breathing difficulties and chest pain, a sample of pleural fluid will be aspirated from the lung. The measurements of total protein, albumin, and LDH levels in biochemistry are associated with pleural fluid analysis.

- **Transudate**
  - Total protein, albumin and LDH levels will be low.
  - Value of SAAG above 1.1 g/dL is considered evidence of a transudate condition.
- **Exudate**
  - Total protein, albumin and LDH levels will be high.
  - Value of SAAG below 1.1 g/dL is considered evidence of the occurrence of exudates.
  - Glucose level will be low.

1.1.5. Types of Body Fluids

Different types of fluids, each with unique compositions and functions, are found throughout the human body. These liquids are essential for supporting biological processes, preserving physiological balance, and moving nutrients and waste materials.

The different types of body fluids include:

1.1.5.1. Blood

Blood is a specialized bodily fluid that circulates through the cardiovascular system, delivering oxygen and nutrients to cells and tissues while removing waste products. It consists of plasma, which is a fluid portion containing water, electrolytes, proteins (such as albumin and globulins), hormones, and nutrients, as well as cellular components such as red blood cells (erythrocytes), white blood cells (leukocytes), and platelets.

The main components of blood include:

1. **Plasma:** Plasma is the liquid component of blood. It is a thick fluid that makes up 55% of the total blood volume with the rest of the volume made by blood components such as RBC, WBC and platelets. Plasma is 91% water and the rest of the total volume is made up of dissolved ions, suspended proteins, dissolved gases, nutrient molecules and waste products.. Albumin is the major protein in plasma. Other proteins include immunoglobulins and clotting factors.
2. **Red Blood Cells:** 40% of the blood contains red blood cells. RBCs contain the protein hemoglobin which gives a red color to the blood.
3. **White Blood Cells:** The white blood cells are very few in number. The WBC to RBC ratio is 1:600. They mainly protect the body against infections. Many WBCs cross the walls of the vessels and penetrate other tissues.
4. **Platelets:** These are fewer in number than the red blood cells. The platelets help in the clotting of blood at the site of a wound.

1.1.5.2. Lymph

The colorless fluid found in the interstitial tissues is called lymph. It moves via the entire lymphatic system. It is known as blood without red blood cells. Through this fluid, gases, hormones, and nutrients are exchanged. It is made up of lymphocytes, which are important for the body's immunological reactions. Lymph is a colorless, clear fluid that flows through the lymphatic system, an intricate web of organs, vessels, and nodes that regulates immune response, fluid homeostasis, and lipid absorption. It comes from the fluid called interstitial fluid, which envelops cells in tissues. It is essential for preserving homeostasis and protecting the body from illnesses and infections. The lymphatic system is a supplementary circulatory system that works in tandem with the cardiovascular system to carry substances such as immune cells and lymphatic fluid throughout the body.

Immune defense and surveillance are one of the main roles of the lymph. Numerous immune cells, including macrophages, dendritic cells, and lymphocytes (such as T, B, and natural killer cells) are found in the lymph. These cells are important in identifying and getting rid of infections, foreign antigens, and aberrant cells. The bone marrow generates lymphocytes, which then develop into mature T cells and B cells, or lymphoid organs like the spleen and lymph nodes, where they are activated and differentiated into specific effector cells.

Immune cells and antibodies can more easily travel to areas of inflammation and infection thanks to the lymphatic system, which enables them to mount an immune response that neutralizes pathogens and eradicates infections. Small, bean-shaped structures called lymph nodes are found along lymphatic vessels. They act as filtering points where immune cells come into contact with antigens in lymphatic fluid and react to them. Specialized areas found in lymph nodes called germinal centers are where immune cells multiply and differentiate in response to antigenic stimulation, producing memory cells and antibodies that are specific to the antigen.

The lymphatic system plays a vital role in maintaining fluid balance in the body, in addition to supporting immune function. Acting as a drainage system, lymphatic vessels collect excess interstitial fluid and return it to the bloodstream to prevent tissue swelling and edema. These vessels absorb fluid, proteins, lipids, and other substances from the interstitial space and transport them through various lymphatic structures to lymph nodes, ultimately returning them to the bloodstream.

Furthermore, the lymphatic system is responsible for the absorption and transport of dietary fats and fat-soluble vitamins through specialized vessels called lacteals in the small intestine. These nutrients are then transported via lymphatic fluid to the bloodstream for distribution throughout the body, supporting lipid metabolism and energy balance. This process is crucial for the absorption of essential dietary nutrients and overall health.

Many conditions and illnesses, such as lymphedema, lymphangitis, and lymphoma, can result from disruption of lymphatic function. The accumulation of lymphatic fluid and tissue swelling that characterizes lymphedema is frequently brought on by compromised lymphatic drainage as a result of surgery, trauma, infection, or congenital abnormalities. Inflammation of the lymphatic vessels, or lymphhangitis, is usually brought on by a bacterial infection that has spread from a nearby wound or skin infection. One kind of cancer that affects lymphocytes or lymphoid tissues is called lymphoma, and it causes unchecked growth and tumor formation in the lymphatic system.

The lymph is an important fluid that is involved in fluid balance, lipid metabolism, and immune response. It facilitates immune surveillance and defense against infections and diseases by acting as a conduit for immune cells and antibodies. Furthermore, the lymphatic system transfers dietary fats and fat-soluble vitamins from the gastrointestinal tract to the bloodstream and eliminates surplus interstitial fluid to maintain fluid balance. Comprehending the roles and importance of lymph is essential to understanding fluid dynamics, the immune system, and the general health and wellness of the body.

1.1.5.3. Composition of Body Fluids

Body fluids are made up of a wide range of substances, each with a distinct composition and purpose. These liquids are essential for supporting physiological homeostasis, promoting cellular activity, and preserving physiological equilibrium. The location, function, and unique requirements of the body determine the composition of bodily fluids.

The composition of the body fluids is explained below:

Body Fluids	Composition
Intracellular Body Fluids	70% water, ions, and molecules
Extracellular Body Fluids	Cations and Anions
Transcellular Fluid	Electrolytes such as sodium, bicarbonate and chloride ions.

1.1.5.4. Functions of Body Fluids

The important functions of body fluids include:

1. The body fluids facilitate the transportation of oxygen and nutrients throughout the body and remove waste from the body.
2. They help in regulating body temperature.
3. They maintain an efficient metabolism of the body.

1.1.6. Circulation

The flow of blood through the body's vessels, known as circulation, transports gases and nutrients to and eliminates waste from the various body parts. The blood carries chemicals, gases, nutrients, waste products, and other materials.

This process is termed circulation. The human circulatory system serves the following functions:

1. Transport of respiratory gases.
2. Transport of nutrients to the cells.
3. Transport of hormones from the endocrine glands to the respective organs.
4. Destruction of pathogens.
5. Transport of metabolic waste to the excretory organs for removal.

- **Types of Circulatory Systems:** The circulatory system is of two types:
    - o Open circulatory system
    - o Closed circulatory system

Blood does not circulate in closed vessels but rather through portions of the body cavity in the open circulatory system. In insects, this system is frequently observed. Closed Circulatory System: Blood is pumped through tubes that are closed and pressurized to a suitable degree. Everything that is vertebrate has this system.

- **Mechanism of Circulation:** The primary organ involved in blood circulation is the heart. The human heart is made up of two lower chambers known as ventricles and two upper chambers known as atria or auricles. While veins return deoxygenated blood from various body parts to the heart for purification, arteries transport oxygenated blood from the heart to the body. An exception are the pulmonary veins and arteries. Blood that has lost oxygen is removed from the heart by the pulmonary artery and returned to it by the pulmonary vein.

A bicuspid or mitral valve divides the left auricle from the left ventricle, while a tricuspid valve separates the right auricle from the right ventricle. The blood cannot return to the auricles because of these valves.

Two semilunar valves are present, each between the right ventricle and pulmonary artery, and the left ventricle and aorta. These valves prevent the blood from flowing back into the heart.

- o The deoxygenated blood is pumped into the right ventricle through the superior vena cava (which carries deoxygenated blood from the upper regions of the body) and inferior vena cava (which carries deoxygenated blood from the lower parts of the body). The oxygenated blood is carried by the pulmonary veins from the lungs to the left auricle. This is called auricular circulation.
- o Most of the auricular blood passes into the ventricles during diastole and the process is known as diastasis.
- o The rest of the blood passes into the ventricles during auricular systole.
- o The blood from the left ventricle passes from the left ventricle into the systemic aorta and deoxygenated blood passes from the right ventricle into the pulmonary aorta during ventricular systole.
- o The oxygenated blood is distributed to all the body parts by the systemic arch while the pulmonary aorta carries deoxygenated blood to the lungs.

During circulation, some fluid is forced out of the bloodstream and is filtered by the lymph nodes to get rid of bacteria and other debris. Through lymph vessels, the filtered fluid is returned to the bloodstream.

1.1.7. Circulatory Disorders

To ensure that blood reaches every part of the body healthily, the circulatory system runs around the clock. However, blood vessel blockages may have an impact on how well the heart functions. This can result in stroke and other heart conditions. The following illnesses may have an impact on how well the heart functions.

- **Hypertension:** High blood pressure does not show any symptoms. It damages the heart and important organs. With high blood pressure, the blood is pumped out with very high pressure.
- **Coronary Heart Disease:** This affects the arteries primarily. The deposition of fats, cholesterol, cell debris, and clotting agents hardens the arteries. After a period of time, the blow flow is completely blocked.
- **Heart Attack:** Myocardial infarction is the medical term for heart attacks. A heart attack is brought on by blockages that prevent blood from reaching the heart. The heart muscles are entirely harmed by this. A heart attack can be caused by several risk factors, including smoking, high blood pressure, obesity, stress, and high cholesterol and fats.
- **Angina:** Angina or chest pain occurs due to coronary heart disease. The blockage of the arteries reduces the blood flow to the heart. Pain and

pressure are experienced in the center of the chest.

- **Heart Failure:** When the heart stops pumping enough blood to meet the requirements of the body, it is known as heart failure. Chest pain, rapid breathing, and fainting are the symptoms of heart failure (Cotran et al., 2005; Strasinger and Lorenzo, 2008; Liachovitzky Carlos, 2015; Pearson, 2018).

1.2. Physiology of Body Fluids

The physiology of body fluids plays a crucial role in maintaining the homeostasis of the body. Body fluids are primarily composed of water, electrolytes, and proteins, and they are distributed throughout the body in various compartments such as intracellular and extracellular fluid. The balance of these fluids is essential for the proper functioning of cells and organs.

One of the key functions of body fluids is to transport nutrients, oxygen, and waste products throughout the body. Blood, which is a major body fluid, carries oxygen from the lungs to the tissues and removes carbon dioxide and other waste products from the cells. This process is essential for the survival of cells and for maintaining overall health.

The regulation of body fluids is controlled by a complex system involving hormones, the kidneys, and the cardiovascular system. Hormones such as aldosterone and antidiuretic hormone play a crucial role in regulating the balance of water and electrolytes in the body. The kidneys also play a vital role in maintaining the balance of body fluids by filtering out waste products and reabsorbing essential substances.

Imbalances in body fluids can lead to serious health problems. Dehydration, for example, occurs when the body loses more fluid than it takes in, leading to symptoms such as dry mouth, fatigue, and dizziness. On the other hand, overhydration can lead to water intoxication, which can cause symptoms such as headaches, nausea, and confusion.

Maintaining the balance of body fluids is crucial for overall health and wellbeing. It is important to stay hydrated by drinking an adequate amount of water and electrolytes, especially during hot weather or after intense physical activity. Monitoring changes in body fluids and seeking medical attention if imbalances occur can help prevent serious health complications.

In conclusion, the physiology of body fluids is essential for the proper functioning of cells and organs in the body. Maintaining the balance of these fluids is crucial for overall health and wellbeing, and imbalances can lead to serious health problems. By understanding the role of body fluids and taking steps to ensure their balance, we can support our health and prevent potential complications.

The intricate processes involved in the control, distribution, and upkeep of the many fluid compartments within the human body are collectively referred to as the physiology of body fluids. These fluids, which include interstitial fluid, lymph, blood, pleural fluid, synovial fluid, lymph node fluid, and peritoneal fluid, are essential for sustaining homeostasis, promoting nutrition exchange, and supporting cellular function.

Osmosis, the flow of water across semipermeable membranes in response to variations in solute concentration, is one of the basic ideas of body fluid physiology. This procedure aids in controlling the fluid balance between various compartments, guaranteeing that cells stay adequately hydrated while avoiding undue edema or shrinkage. The selective permeability of cell membranes to water and the active transport of ions (e.g., sodium, potassium, and chloride) across cell membranes sustain the osmotic pressure gradient between intracellular and extracellular fluid compartments.

An essential part of the body's fluid distribution and circulation is the cardiovascular system. The heart pumps blood, the main fluid of the circulatory system, through blood vessels to supply hormones, nutrition, and oxygen to tissues and organs all over the body. Additionally, blood acts as a transport medium for carbon dioxide, other materials that must be eliminated from tissues, and waste products from metabolism. To ensure proper tissue perfusion and oxygen delivery, blood volume, blood pressure, and cardiac output must be regulated.

The intricate relationships between different fluid compartments, regulatory systems, and physiological processes are all part of the physiology of bodily fluids. For optimum health and function, it is crucial to maintain tissue perfusion, osmotic equilibrium, and fluid balance. Dehydration, edema, electrolyte imbalances, and other health issues can result from disruptions in fluid distribution or balance, underscoring the significance of comprehending and preserving the physiological dynamics of body fluids.

The body is formed by solids and fluids. The fluid part is more than two third of the whole body. Water forms most of the fluid part of the body.

- In humans, the total body water varies from 45% to 75% of body weight.
- In a normal young adult male, the body contains 60% to 65% of water and 35% to 40% of solids.
- In a normal young adult female, the water is 50% to 55% and solids are 45% to 50%.
- In females, water is less because of more amount of subcutaneous adipose tissue.
- In thin persons, water content is more than that in obese persons.
- In old age, water content is decreased due to an increase in adipose tissue.
- The total quantity of body water in an average human that weighs about 70 kg is about 40 L.

1.2.1. Importance of Body Fluids

- **In Homeostasis:** The internal environment is the fluid medium in which body cells continue to exist. Substances including glucose, oxygen, ions, lipids, vitamins, and amino acids are all part of the internal environment. which are necessary for the cell's growth and operation. In addition to being a primary component of the internal environment, water is crucial for maintaining homeostasis.
- **In Transport Mechanism:** The transport medium that allows unwanted substances to exit the cells and nutrients and other necessary substances to enter them is body water. Water serves as a vital conduit for the transportation of numerous chemicals, including vitamins, hormones, enzymes, and electrolytes, throughout the body.
- **In Metabolic Reactions:** Water inside the cells forms the medium for various metabolic reactions, which are necessary for the growth

and functional activities of the cells.

- **In Texture of Tissues:** Water inside the cells is necessary for the characteristic form and texture of various tissues.
- **In Temperature Regulation:** Water plays a vital role in the maintenance of normal body temperature.

1.2.2. Distribution of Body Fluids

The total water in the body is about 40 L. It is distributed into two major compartments

1. **Intracellular fluid (ICF):** Its volume is 22 L and it forms 55% of the total body water
2. **Extracellular fluid (ECF):** Its volume is 18 L and it forms 45% of the total body water. ECF is divided into 5 subunits:
    - Interstitial fluid and lymph (20%)
    - Plasma (7.5%)
    - Fluid in bones (7.5%)

Fluid in dense connective tissues like cartilage (7.5%) and transcellular fluid (2.5%) that includes:

- Cerebrospinal fluid
- Intraocular fluid
- Digestive juices
- Serous fluid – intrapleural fluid and pericardial fluid
- Synovial fluid in joints f. Fluid in the urinary tract.

1.2.3. Composition of Body Fluids

Body fluids contain water and solids. Solids are organic and inorganic substances.

- **Organic Substances:** Organic substances are glucose, amino acids and other proteins, fatty acids and other lipids, hormones and enzymes.
- **Inorganic Substances:** Inorganic substances present in body fluids are sodium, potassium, calcium, magnesium, chloride, bicarbonate, phosphate and sulfate.

ECF contains large quantities of sodium, chloride, bicarbonate, glucose, fatty acids and oxygen.

ICF contains large quantities of potassium, magnesium, phosphates, sulfates and proteins.

- The pH of ECF is 7.4.
- The pH of ICF is 7.0.

1.2.4. Water Content

The amount of water in the human body is referred to as body water in physiology. It constitutes a sizeable portion of the body's overall composition. Water is essential to life for a variety of reasons. The majority of the material in every human cell is water found in the cytoplasm. Additionally, water offers a fluid environment that facilitates molecular transport throughout the body and extracellular communication. In addition, water plays a crucial role in biochemical processes like hydrolysis which are essential to physiology. The physical characteristics of water, such as the surface tension of the water in the lungs' alveoli, are essential to many organ systems.

1.2.5. Overall Water Content

A human weighing 70 kg on average has about 40 liters of water in total, or 57% of his total body weight, in his body. This can account for as much as 79% of the body weight in a newborn, but it gradually declines from birth to old age, with the majority of the decline happening in the first ten years of life. Additionally, obesity lowers the body's water content, sometimes to as low as 45%. Different tissue types allow the body's fluid compartments, which are scattered throughout its cavities, to contain different amounts of water. The altered fluid compartments in diseased states where body water is impacted can provide hints about the nature of the issue.

1.2.6. Water Content Regulation and Measurement

The renal and neuro-endocrine systems play a major role in controlling body water. Because water content regulates blood pressure and cardiac output, it is one of the most crucial aspects of homeostasis. Hormones such as atrial natriuretic peptide (ANP), renin, angiotensin II, anti-diuretic hormone (ADH), and aldosterone mediate a large portion of this regulation.

Some of these hormones, like angiotensin-converting enzyme (ACE) and angiotensin-converting protein (ANP), are also secreted by the heart and lungs. These hormones function as messengers between the kidneys and the hypothalamus. There are numerous clinical techniques for figuring out body water. Calculations based on body weight and urine output can be used to obtain an estimate that is not entirely accurate. Dilution and equilibration using mass spectrometry, which gauges the amount of water in a subject's breath samples, is an additional method of measuring body water content.

A person's degree of hydration is determined through bioelectrical impedance analysis using highly accurate measurements of the resistance to an electric current passing through bodily tissues. A lower level of hydration will result in more resistance to electrical flow through the body because water conducts electricity (Cotran et al., 2005; Strasinger and Lorenzo, 2008; Liachovitzky Carlos, 2015; Pearson, 2018).

1.3. Body Fluids and Their Compartments

The human body is composed of fluid compartments that contain the fluids from the various tissues. Comparing a fluid's position and properties to those of other fluids within compartments is typically done using fluid compartments. Although there may be some similarities between fluid compartments and the divisions made by the body's anatomical compartments, these terms are not interchangeable. The location of fluid compartments with respect to the cellular membrane of the cells that comprise the body's tissues defines them.

The extracellular fluid and the intracellular fluid make up the two main compartments that contain all of the bodily fluid. Blood plasma and interstitial fluid make up the extracellular fluid. There is an additional tiny fluid compartment known as transcellular fluid. This compartment contains the cerebrospinal fluid as well as the fluid found in the synovial, peritoneal, pericardial, and intraocular spaces. Although its composition occasionally varies significantly from that of the plasma or interstitial fluid, it is typically regarded as a specific kind of extracellular fluid. The total volume of transcellular fluids is between one and two liters.

In a 70-kilogram adult man, the total body water is about 60% of the body weight or about 42 liters. This percentage depends on age, gender, and degree of obesity.

The proportion of total body weight that is made up of fluids steadily declines with age. This decline is partly explained by the fact that aging is typically linked to an increase in body fat percentage, which lowers the body's proportion of water. Women typically have a higher percentage of body fat than men do, therefore their total body water makes up roughly 50% of their body weight on average.

The percentage of total body water in premature and neonatal babies varies between 70 and 75% of their body weight. As a result, we should be aware that there are differences in "average" body fluid compartments based on factors like age, gender, and body fat percentage.

In many other countries, the average body weight (and fat mass) has increased rapidly during the past 30 years. Currently, the average body weight for men older than 20 years in the United States is estimated to be approximately 86.4 kg, and for women, it is 74.1 kg.

- **Intracellular Fluid Compartment:** The 42 liters of fluid in the body are made up of approximately 28 liters of intracellular fluid, which is found inside each of the 100 trillion cells. Therefore, in a "average" person, intracellular fluid makes up roughly 40% of total body weight. Each cell's fluid is made up of a unique mixture of various components, but these substances' concentrations are consistent throughout the cell. In actuality, from the simplest microbes to humans, the makeup of cell fluids is strikingly similar across a wide range of animals. This is the reason why the intracellular fluid of every single cell is regarded as a single, enormous fluid compartment.
- **Extracellular Fluid Compartment:** Extracellular fluid is the term used to describe all fluids that are not inside of cells. When combined, these liquids make up around 20% of the body weight or 14 liters in the case of a 70-kg man. The interstitial fluid, which comprises over three-quarters (11 liters) of the extracellular fluid, and the plasma, which comprises nearly one-fourth, or approximately 3 liters, of the extracellular fluid, are the two largest compartments. The non-cellular component of blood, known as plasma, constantly exchanges materials with the interstitial fluid through the capillary membranes' pores. Proteins are the only solutes in the extracellular fluid that are not highly permeable through these pores. Because of this continuous mixing of extracellular fluids, the composition of the interstitial and plasma fluids is similar, except for proteins, which are more concentrated in the plasma.

1.3.1. Disturbance of Volume Concentration of Body Fluid

Changes in the volume and concentration of bodily fluids can have a profound impact on general health and physiological function. Numerous factors, such as variations in fluid intake and output, modifications to electrolyte balance, hormonal imbalances, and pathological conditions impacting fluid-regulating mechanisms, can cause these disruptions.

Here are some common disturbances of volume and concentration of body fluids:

1. **Dehydration:** When the body does not have as much water as it needs, dehydration results. It may arise from insufficient fluid consumption, excessive fluid loss (e.g., sweating, diarrhea, vomiting, or a mix of the two. Reduced blood volume, elevated plasma osmolality, and compromised cellular function are the results of dehydration. Thirst, dry mouth, dark urine, lightheadedness, and exhaustion are possible symptoms. Rehydration therapy must be

administered quickly in cases of severe dehydration since it can be fatal.

2. **Overhydration (Fluid Overload):** Overhydration, or fluid overload, occurs when there is an excess of body water relative to the body's needs. It can result from excessive fluid intake, impaired renal function (e.g., renal failure), or conditions such as heart failure or liver cirrhosis, which lead to fluid retention. Overhydration can cause fluid accumulation in tissues (edema), increased blood volume, dilutional hyponatremia (low sodium levels), and impaired cardiac and respiratory function.

3. **Electrolyte Imbalances:** Electrolytes, such as sodium, potassium, chloride, calcium, and magnesium, play crucial roles in maintaining fluid balance, nerve function, muscle contraction, and acid-base balance. Disturbances in electrolyte levels can occur due to various factors, including inadequate dietary intake, excessive losses (e.g., diarrhea, vomiting, sweating), hormonal imbalances (e.g., aldosterone, antidiuretic hormone), or renal dysfunction. Electrolyte imbalances can lead to symptoms such as muscle weakness, cardiac arrhythmias, neurological changes, and fluid shifts between compartments.

4. **Hypoosmolality and Hyperosmolality:** Osmolality refers to the concentration of solutes in body fluids, primarily sodium, glucose, and urea. Hypoosmolality occurs when the osmolality of body fluids is lower than normal, leading to water retention and dilutional hyponatremia. This can result from excessive water intake, syndrome of inappropriate antidiuretic hormone secretion (SIADH), or certain medications. Hyperosmolality, on the other hand, occurs when the osmolality of body fluids is higher than normal, leading to dehydration and hypernatremia. Causes include inadequate water intake, diabetes insipidus, or hyperglycemia.

5. **Edema:** Edema is the abnormal accumulation of fluid in interstitial spaces, leading to tissue swelling and increased extracellular fluid volume. It can result from increased capillary hydrostatic pressure (e.g., heart failure), decreased plasma oncotic pressure (e.g., hypoalbuminemia), lymphatic obstruction (e.g., lymphedema), or inflammation. Edema can occur locally (e.g., peripheral edema) or systemically (e.g., pulmonary edema) and may be associated with symptoms such as swelling, pain, and impaired mobility.

It is necessary to determine the underlying cause of disturbances in the volume and concentration of bodily fluids and to implement appropriate interventions to manage them. This could involve the use of diuretics, fluid replacement therapy, electrolyte supplements, dietary changes, and the management of underlying medical issues. To minimize risks and improve patient outcomes, close observation of electrolyte levels, fluid status, and therapeutic response is necessary.

1.3.2. Volume Contraction

Loss of total body sodium causes volume depletion, also known as extracellular fluid (ECF) volume contraction. Kidney failure, burns, diuretics, vomiting, and excessive perspiration are among the causes. Reduced skin turgor, dry mucous membranes, tachycardia, and orthostatic hypotension are some of the clinical symptoms. Clinical diagnosis is made. Water and sodium are administered as part of the treatment.

Water is lost from the ECF space rapidly when the major extracellular cation (sodium) is lost because water crosses plasma membranes in the body by passive osmosis. Thus, loss of sodium invariably results in loss of water. Nevertheless, serum sodium concentration in volume-depleted patients can be high, low, or normal depending on a variety of factors (despite the decreased total body sodium content). Effective Circulating Volume (ECF) and volume are related. Hypovolemia, or low ECF, typically results in a drop in effective circulating volume, which lowers organ perfusion and produces clinical consequences.

1.3.2.1. Symptoms and Signs of Volume Contraction

When there is a fluid loss, < 5% of ECF volume (mild volume depletion), the only sign may be diminished skin turgor (best assessed at the upper torso). Skin turgor may be low in older patients regardless of volume status. Patients may complain of thirst. Dry mucous membranes do not always correlate with volume depletion, especially in older patients and in mouth-breathers. Oliguria is typical. When ECF volume has diminished by 5 to 10% (moderate volume depletion), orthostatic tachycardia, hypotension, or both are usually, but not always, present. Also, orthostatic changes can occur in patients without ECF volume depletion, particularly patients deconditioned or bedridden. Skin turgor may decrease further. When fluid loss is > 10% of the ECF volume (severe volume depletion), shock indicators (e.g., tachycardia, tachypnea, hypotension, disorientation, and inadequate capillary refill) may transpire.

1.3.2.2. Diagnosis of Volume Contraction

- Clinical findings
- Sometimes serum electrolytes, BUN (blood urea nitrogen), and creatinine
- Rarely plasma osmolality and urine chemistries

Patients at risk are thought to be at risk for volume depletion; these patients are typically those who have a history of increased fluid losses, diuretic therapy, renal or adrenal disorders, or inadequate fluid intake (particularly in comatose or disoriented patients). Clinical diagnosis is the norm. Pre- and post-workout weights are sometimes used to monitor athletes' dehydration; if precise patient weights are known both before and after fluid loss, the difference can be used to estimate volume loss accurately.

When the reason is clear-cut and simple to fix (e.g., Serum electrolytes, BUN, and creatinine are measured; otherwise, laboratory testing is not required (e.g., acute gastroenteritis in otherwise healthy patients). Urine sodium, creatinine, and osmolality as well as plasma osmolality are measured in patients with cardiac or renal disease and when there is a suspicion of a clinically significant electrolyte abnormality that is not evident from serum test results. Urine chloride is also measured in the presence of metabolic alkalosis.

Although measurement is rarely necessary, volume depletion results in decreased central venous pressure and pulmonary artery occlusion pressure. Measurement, an invasive procedure, is sometimes required for patients—such as those with advanced chronic kidney disease or unstable heart failure—for whom even small increases in volume may be harmful.

The following concepts are helpful when interpreting urine electrolyte and osmolality values:

- During volume depletion, normally functioning kidneys conserve sodium. Thus, the urine sodium concentration is usually < 15 mEq/L (< 15 mmol/L); the fractional excretion of sodium (urine sodium/ serum sodium divided by urine creatinine/serum creatinine) is usually < 1%; also, urine osmolality is often > 450 mOsm/kg (> 450 mmol/kg).
- When metabolic alkalosis is combined with volume depletion, urine sodium concentration may be high because large amounts of bicarbonate are spilled in the urine, obligating the excretion of sodium to maintain electrical neutrality. In this instance, a urine chloride concentration of < 10 mEq/L(< 10 mmol/L) more reliably indicates volume depletion.
- Misleadingly high urinary sodium (generally > 20 mEq/L [> 20 mmol/L]) or low urine osmolality can also occur due to renal sodium losses resulting from renal disease, diuretics, or adrenal insufficiency.

Volume depletion frequently increases the BUN and serum creatinine concentrations; the ratio of BUN to creatinine is often >20:1. Values such as hematocrit often increase in volume depletion but are difficult to interpret unless baseline values are known.

1.3.2.3. Treatment of Volume Contraction

- **Replacement of Sodium and Water:** Once the source of the volume depletion is identified and addressed, fluids are administered to replenish any lost fluid and to meet daily fluid needs. When patients are conscious and not vomiting, mild-to-moderate volume deficits may be compensated with increased oral intake of sodium and water; oral rehydration regimens for children are covered elsewhere. In cases where oral intake is restricted or unsafe, tube feedings may also be utilized.

  If oral fluid replacement is not feasible or the volume deficits are severe, IV 0.9% saline or a buffered electrolyte solution (e.g., Ringer's lactate) is administered. Although Ringer's lactate and other buffered solutions have lower chloride concentrations and may lessen the development of hyperchloremic metabolic acidosis, both are safe and well tolerated. Although there is conflicting evidence, it appears that Ringer's lactate should be used instead of saline. Three to four times the intravascular volume deficit is made up by these two solutions because they both distribute equally into the extracellular space (Stephen Jones, Inderbir Gill, Raymond Rackley, 2006).

A Closer Look

Body fluids

Body fluids play crucial roles in maintaining the physiological balance necessary for human health. These fluids encompass a diverse array of substances found within the body, each serving distinct functions essential for survival and overall well-being. Blood, the primary circulatory fluid, carries oxygen and nutrients to tissues while removing waste products like carbon dioxide. It also contains immune cells and proteins that defend against infections and regulate bodily functions. Cerebrospinal fluid (CSF), found within the brain and spinal cord, provides cushioning and support to these vital organs, acting as a shock absorber. It also facilitates the exchange of nutrients and waste products between the brain and bloodstream.

Synovial fluid, present in joints, reduces friction and wear between cartilage-covered surfaces, ensuring smooth movement and flexibility. Its composition allows for nutrient delivery to cartilage and the removal of metabolic waste. Other body fluids, such as saliva, digestive juices, sweat, and tears, contribute to various physiological processes, including digestion, temperature regulation, and protection against pathogens.

The composition and regulation of these fluids are tightly controlled by the body's homeostatic mechanisms. Imbalances or abnormalities in fluid levels or composition can lead to significant health issues, ranging from dehydration to electrolyte imbalances and impaired organ function. Understanding the roles and dynamics of body fluids is essential for diagnosing and treating medical conditions effectively. Advances in medical science continue to unravel the complexities of these fluids, paving the way for improved diagnostic techniques and therapeutic interventions in healthcare practices.

Summary

- The analysis of body fluids plays a critical role in the diagnosis and prognosis of a disease. A change in concentration or composition of a particular biochemical constituent in body fluids is used as an indicator of a physiological or pathological condition.
- Body fluids are aqueous liquids containing the cellular and ionic components necessary for proper body function while also providing transport for a vast array of solutes and products of metabolism.
- Cerebrospinal fluid (CSF) is a vital, clear, and colorless bodily fluid found in the brain and spinal cord, circulating within the ventricular system of the brain, and the subarachnoid space around the brain and spinal cord.
- Cerebrospinal fluid is a vital component of the central nervous system, providing mechanical support, nutrient transport, waste removal, and regulation of intracranial pressure.
- Synovial fluid is a crucial bodily fluid that plays a fundamental role in the health and function of joints within the musculoskeletal system.
- Peritoneal fluid, also known as ascitic fluid when it accumulates in the peritoneal cavity, is a crucial bodily fluid that plays a significant role in maintaining the health and function of the abdominal organs and the peritoneum, the membrane that lines the abdominal cavity.
- Pleural fluid, a vital component of the respiratory system, is a clear, straw-colored fluid found within the pleural cavity, which surrounds the lungs and lines the inner surface of the chest wall.
- Blood is a specialized bodily fluid that circulates through the cardiovascular system, delivering oxygen and nutrients to cells and tissues while removing waste products.
- The physiology of body fluids encompasses the intricate processes involved in the regulation, distribution, and maintenance of various fluid compartments within the human body.
- The fluids of the various tissues of the human body are divided into fluid compartments. Fluid compartments are generally used to compare the position and characteristics of the fluid in relation to the fluid within other compartments.
- Volume depletion is suspected in patients at risk, most often in patients with a history of inadequate fluid intake (especially in comatose or disoriented patients), increased fluid losses, diuretic therapy, and renal or adrenal disorders.

References

1. Al-Kahtani, M. A., Zuleta, C., Caviedes-Vidal, E., & Garland Jr., T. (2004). Kidney mass and relative medullary thickness of rodents in relation to habitat, body size, and phylogeny. *Physiological and Biochemical Zoology, 77*(3), 346–365.
2. Barrett, K. E., Barman, S. M., Yuan, J. X. -J., & Brooks, H. (2019). *Ganong's Review of Medical Physiology* (26th ed.). New York: McGraw Hill Education.

3. Cotran, R. S. S., Kumar, V., Fausto, N., Robbins, S. L., & Abbas, A. K. (2005). *Robbins and Cotran Pathologic Basis of Disease*. St. Louis, MO: Elsevier Saunders.

4. De Luca, L. A., Menani, J. V., & Johnson, A. K. (2014). *Neurobiology of Body Fluid Homeostasis: Transduction and Integration*. Boca Raton (FL): CRC Press/Taylor & Francis; 2014. PMID: 24829987.

5. Garcia-Tsao, G. (2007). Cirrhosis and its sequelae. In L. Goldman & D. Ausiello (Eds.), *Cecil Medicine* (23rd ed., chap. 157). Philadelphia, PA: Saunders Elsevier.

6. Jones, J. S., Gill, I. S., & Rackley, R. (2006). Operative Urology at the Cleveland Clinic. In A. C. Novick, I. S. Gill, E. A. Klein, & J. H. Ross (Eds.), *Urology Annals, 8*, S102–S108. Totowa, NJ: Humana Press.

7. Kalantar-Zadeh, K., Jafar, T. H., Nitsch, D., Neuen, B. L., & Perkovic, V. (2021). Chronic Kidney Disease. *The Lancet, 398*(10302), 786–802.

8. Liachovitzky, C. (2015). *Human Anatomy and Physiology Preparatory Course*. CUNY Bronx Community College. CUNY Academic Works.

9. Nahon, I., Waddington, G., Dorey, G., & Adams, R. (2011). The history of urologic surgery: from reeds to robotics. *Urologic Nursing, 31*(3), 173–180.

10. Porcel, J. M., & Light, R. W. (2006). Diagnostic approach to pleural effusions in adults. *American Family Physician, 2006 Apr 1;73(7):1211-20.*

11. Santambrogio, L. (2018). The Lymphatic Fluid. *International Review of Cell and Molecular Biology, 337*, 111–133.

12. Strasinger, S. K., & Lorenzo, M. S. (2008). *Urinalysis and Body Fluids*. 5th Edition, F. A. Davis Company, Philadelphia

13. Carlström M, Wilcox CS, Welch WJ (2010). Adenosine A(2) receptors modulate tubuloglomerular feedback. Am J Physiol Renal Physiol. 2010 Aug;299(2):F412-7.

Chapter

THE KIDNEY

2

Contents

Introduction

The kidneys are two reddish-brown, bean-shaped organs that filter blood. In adult humans, they are situated in the retroperitoneal space on the left and right, and their length is approximately 12 centimeters (4+1/2 inches). Blood enters them through the paired renal arteries and leaves through the paired renal veins. The ureters, which are tubes that convey excreted urine to the bladder, are connected to each kidney.

The kidney is involved in the regulation of different body fluid volumes, fluid osmolality, acid-base balance, different electrolyte concentrations, and toxin elimination. One-fifth of the blood volume that enters the kidneys is filtered at the glomerulus. Amino acids, sodium, bicarbonate, glucose, and solute-free water are a few examples of materials that are reabsorbed. A few examples of substances secreted are uric acid, hydrogen, ammonium, and potassium. The kidney's anatomical and functional unit is the nephron. A mouse kidney has only about 12,500 nephrons, compared to approximately 1 million nephrons in an adult human kidney. In addition, the kidneys perform tasks without the assistance of the nephrons. For instance, they synthesize the hormones erythropoietin and renin and transform a precursor of vitamin D into its active form, calcitriol.

One of the most important public health issues in the world today is chronic kidney disease (CKD). Between 5 and 7 million people worldwide are thought to require renal replacement therapy due to kidney failure, with the estimated prevalence of CKD being 13.4%. The assessment of kidney function by estimating the glomerular filtration rate (eGFR) using serum creatinine, kidney biopsy, and CT scan to check for abnormal anatomy are among the procedures used in the management of kidney disease. Kidney failure can be treated with dialysis or a kidney transplant; when renal function falls below 15%, one or both of these treatments are almost always conducted in order. To treat renal cell carcinoma, nephrectomy is commonly employed.

Kidney function is the subject of renal physiology. The medical specialty of nephrology deals with disorders of the kidneys, such as pyelonephritis, acute kidney injury, nephrotic and nephritic syndromes, and chronic kidney disease (CKD). Diseases affecting the anatomy of the kidneys and urinary tract are the focus of urology. These include renal cysts, kidney and ureteral stones, cancer, and obstructions of the urinary tract.

The word "renal" is an adjective meaning "relating to the kidneys", and its roots are French or late Latin. Whereas according to some opinions, "renal" should be replaced with "kidney" in scientific writings such as "kidney artery", other experts have advocated preserving the use of renal as appropriate including in "renal artery".

Orientation and Directional Terms

Term	Definition	Illustration
Nephron	A nephron is the basic structural and functional unit of the kidney. They are microscopic structures composed of a renal corpuscle and a renal tubule.	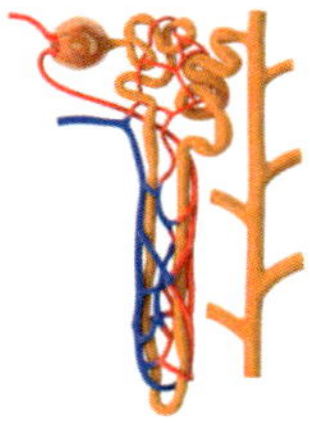
Renal columns	The renal columns are described as medullary extensions of the renal cortex that extend between renal pyramids towards the renal sinus. The renal columns delineate individual lobes of the kidney, aiding in their distinction.	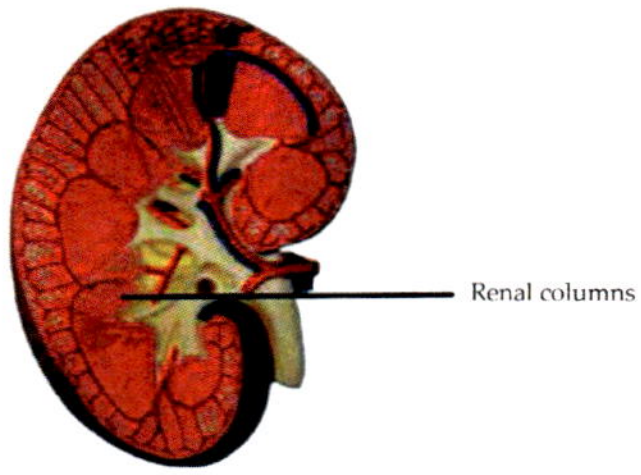
Papillary duct	Papillary ducts are anatomical structures of the kidneys, previously known as the ducts of Bellini. Papillary ducts represent the most distal portion of the collecting duct. They receive renal filtrate (precursor to urine) from several medullary collecting ducts and empty into a minor calyx.	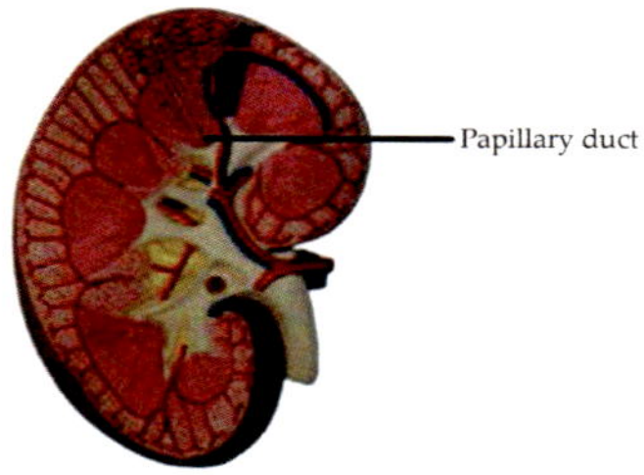
Renal artery	The renal artery is a branch of the abdominal aorta that carries blood from the heart to be filtered in the kidneys.	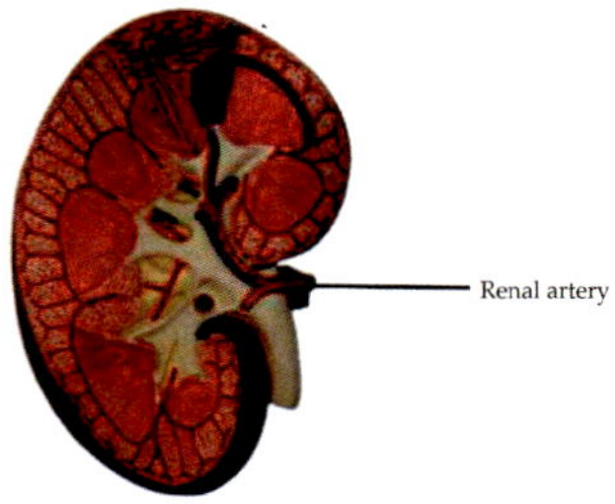
Renal corpuscle	A renal corpuscle is the blood-filtering component of the nephron of the kidney. It consists of a glomerulus - a tuft of capillaries composed of endothelial cells, and a glomerular capsule known as Bowman's capsule.	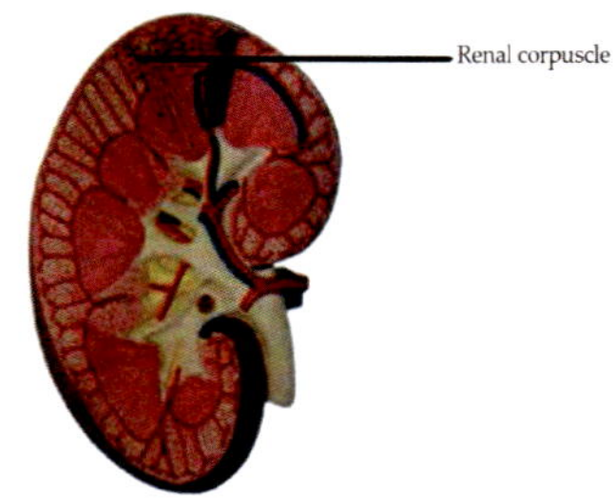

2.1. Kidney Structure

The kidneys are two bean-shaped structures in the peritoneal cavity that are situated posterior to and below the liver (Figure 2.1). Known also as the suprarenal glands, the adrenal glands are located atop each kidney. The kidneys filter all of the blood in the human body several times a day; in the process, these organs consume nearly 25% of the oxygen that is taken in through the lungs. Through aerobic respiration, oxygen enables the kidney cells to produce chemical energy in the form of ATP efficiently. Urine is the filtrate that the kidneys excrete.

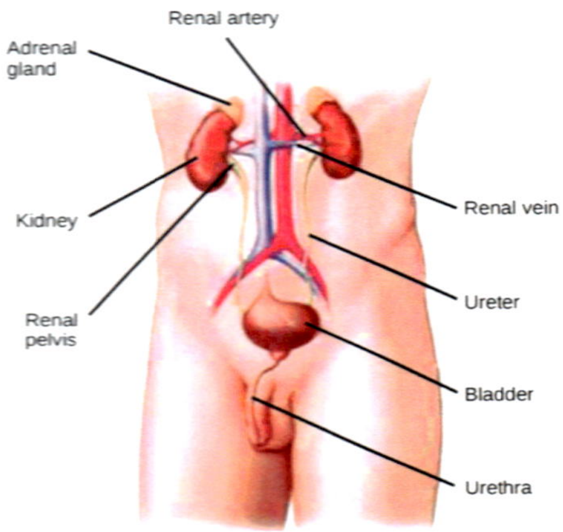

Figure 2.1. *Kidneys filter the blood, producing urine that is stored in the bladder prior to elimination through the urethra.*

Source: https://courses.lumenlearning.com/wm-biology2/chapter/kidneys/.

As seen in Figure 2.2, the kidneys are surrounded by three layers on the outside. The renal fascia, a strong layer of connective tissue, is the outermost layer. The perirenal fat capsule, which makes up the second layer, aids in stabilizing the kidneys. The renal capsule is the third and innermost layer. The kidney's interior is divided into three sections: the renal pelvis in the area known as the hilum of the kidney, the medulla in the center, and the outer cortex. The kidney's concave hilum is where blood vessels and nerves enter and exit, and it's also where the ureters exit the body. The kidney resembles a bean. Nephrons, the functional unit of the kidney, are present in the renal cortex, which makes it granular. The renal pyramids are several pyramid-shaped tissue masses that make up the medulla. Renal columns are the spaces between the pyramids where the blood vessels pass. Renal papillae, or the tips of the pyramids, are directed toward the renal pelvis. Each kidney contains eight renal pyramids on average. The term "lobes of the kidney" refers to the cortical region that borders the renal pyramids. The ureter exiting the kidney is reached by the renal pelvis. The renal pelvis splits into two or three internal extensions known as the major calyces, which then split into the minor calyces on the inside of the kidney. Urine-bearing tubes called ureters leave the kidney and empty into the bladder.

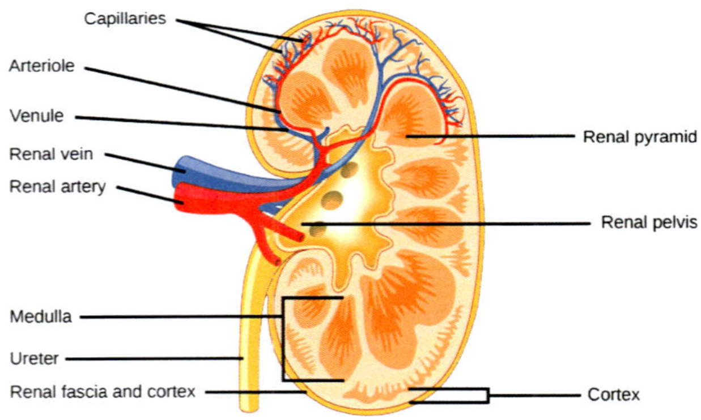

Figure 2.2. *The internal structure of the kidney is shown.*

Source: https://courses.lumenlearning.com/wm-biology2/chapter/kidneys/.

The kidney's network of blood vessels is crucial to both its structure and function because it filters blood. The renal hilum is the point of entry and exit for the veins, arteries, and nerves that supply the kidney. The aorta splits into the renal arteries, which are named after the part of the kidney they pass through, and the renal veins exit to join the inferior vena cava at the end of the renal blood supply. As the renal arteries enter the kidneys, they divide into multiple segmental arteries. After splitting into multiple interlobar arteries, each segmental artery enters the renal columns, which supply the renal lobes. The renal cortex and medulla are the points where the interlobar arteries divide to form the arcuate arteries. The medullary pyramids' base is lined with arcs formed by the arcuate, or "bow-shaped," arteries. As the name implies, cortical radiate arteries extend from the arcuate arteries. The cortical radiate arteries enter the capillaries supplying the nephrons after splitting into multiple afferent arterioles. Similar in name to arteries, veins follow their course; however, segmental veins do not exist.

2.1.1. Nephron

The fundamental anatomical and functional unit of the kidney is the nephron. These are the microscopic structures made up of the renal tubule and corpuscle. The Greek word nephros, which means kidney, is where the word "nephron" originates. The nephron count in a human kidney is approximately millions.

The nephron, shown in Figure 2.3, is the functional unit of the kidney. When the kidney is sectioned sagittally, the renal cortex appears granular due to the over a million nephrons that comprise each kidney. Nephrons are classified into two types: juxtamedullary nephrons (15%), which are located in the renal cortex near the renal medulla, and cortical nephrons (85%), which are located deep in the renal cortex. Three components make up a nephron: the renal tubule, the renal corpuscle, and the network of capillaries that connects them, which comes from the cortical radiate arteries.

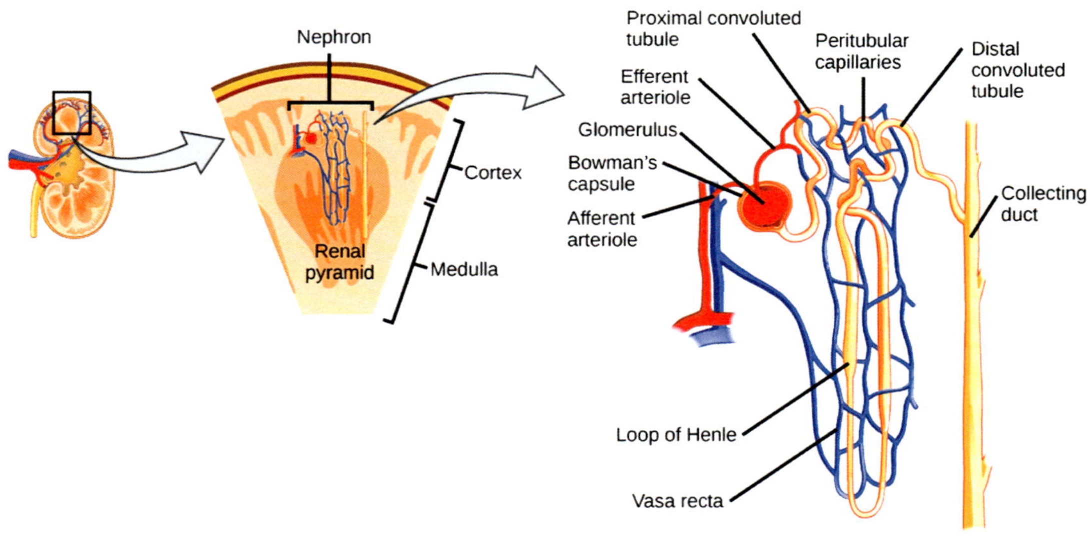

Figure 2.3. *The nephron is the functional unit of the kidney. The glomerulus and convoluted tubules are located in the kidney cortex, while collecting ducts are located in the pyramids of the medulla.*

Source: https://courses.lumenlearning.com/wm-biology2/chapter/kidneys/.

- **Renal Corpuscle:** The renal corpuscle, which is housed in the renal cortex, is composed of the glomerulus, a network of capillaries, and the glomerular or Bowman's capsule, a cup-shaped chamber that encloses the glomerulus.

- **Renal Tubule:** Based on its function, the renal tubule—a long, convoluted structure that emerges from the glomerulus—can be split into three sections. Because of its close proximity to the glomerulus, the first segment—which remains in the renal cortex—is known as the proximal convoluted tubule (PCT). Because the second section forms a loop with descending and ascending limbs that passes through the renal medulla, it is known as the loop of Henle, or nephritic loop. The distal convoluted tubule (DCT), which makes up the third segment of the renal tubule, is likewise confined to the renal cortex. The DCT, the final segment of the nephron, joins and empties into the collecting ducts that run the length of the medullary pyramids. As they approach the renal medulla's papillae, the collecting ducts combine the contents of several nephrons.
- **Capillary Network within the Nephron:** Blood that needs to be filtered enters the nephron through the capillary network that emerges from the renal arteries. The afferent arteriole is the branch that enters the glomerulus. The term "efferent arteriole" refers to the branch that leaves the glomerulus. The network of capillaries inside the glomerulus is referred to as the glomerular capillary bed. The renal tubule is surrounded by and interacts with the peritubular capillary network, which is formed when the efferent arteriole leaves the glomerulus. The PCT and DCT are surrounded by the peritubular capillary network in cortical nephrons. The peritubular capillary network, also known as the vasa recta, wraps around the loop of Henle in juxtamedullary nephrons.

2.2. Renal Anatomy

The retroperitoneum, or posterior abdominal wall, is where the kidneys are situated. They have a bean-shaped shape (Figure 2.4). A fully grown human kidney is about 12.5 cm long, 6 cm wide, and 2.5 cm deep, with a mass of about 150. Both the cortex and the medulla are clearly visible when the kidney is seen in cross-section. With a macroscopic granular appearance, the outer cortex layer has a thickness of roughly 1.4 cm. The outer cortex is the only place where the plasma filtration process occurs since there are no glomeruli anywhere else. Renal tissue with pyramidal shapes makes up the medulla, the innermost layer. Known as papillas, the apex of each pyramid is home to a papillary duct that leads into a calyx, or cavity. Two to three major calyces are formed when the roughly twelve minor calyces that make up a normal human kidney join together. Urine travels from the collecting tubules into the renal pelvis via each calyx, which functions as a funnel.

The ureter, a fibromuscular tube about 25 centimeters long, is joined by the funnel-shaped renal pelvis, which protrudes from the indented area of each kidney and narrows from there. The base of the bladder is a muscular sac with three sides that is connected to one ureter that protrudes from each kidney. The urethra begins and extends to the outside of the body at the uppermost point of this "bladder pyramid," which is downwardly oriented. As the plasma ultrafiltrate travels through the renal tubules, or nephrons, which are found in the renal cortex and medulla, urine is formed, to recapitate. Following this, the urine travels to the renal pelvis via the minor and major calyces. There, it is pushed into the bladder by the peristaltic action of smooth muscle cells in the renal pelvis. Until it is temporarily released through urination, the bladder acts as a holding tank for urine. There's a nerve reflex that starts when about 150 mL of urine builds up. If an individual does not suppress the urge to urinate (i.e., the micturition reflex), urine will pass through the urethra when the bladder muscles contract and the urinary sphincter relaxes simultaneously. About 4 cm is the length of the urethra in women and 24 cm in men, which is a canal that connects the bladder to the outside of the body.

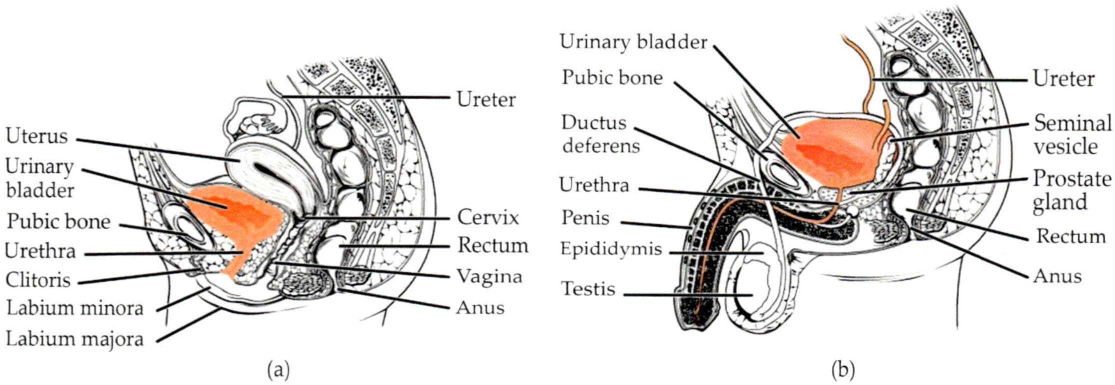

Figure 2.4. *The urethra transports urine from the bladder to the outside of the body. This image shows (a) a female urethra and (b) a male urethra.*

Source: https://courses.lumenlearning.com/suny-ap2/chapter/gross-anatomy-of-urine-transport/.

It should be noted that in a healthy individual, the urine's composition does not change significantly after entering the minor and major calyces. The main excretory product of the kidneys is urine, which is only transported by the calyces and later anatomic structures.

The functional units or tubules of the kidney, or nephrons, number about 1.3 million per kidney. Five separate regions make up a nephron, and each is crucial to the production and final makeup of urine. A nephron, its constituent parts, and their physical interactions are depicted in Figure 2.5. A capillary tuft surrounded by Bowman's capsule, a thin layer of cell epithelium, makes up the glomerulus. Bowman's space refers to the lumen of Bowman's capsule, which is actually the originating end of a renal tubule. Due to the hydrostatic pressure differential between Bowman's space and the capillary lumen, the plasma ultrafiltrate of low molecular weight solutes first gathers there.

The glomerulus is where the proximal convoluted tubule starts, and it travels a roundabout path through the cortex from there. The tubule eventually becomes the loop of Henle when it enters the medulla and straightens and turns downward. Anatomically, the loop of Henle is divided into two sections: the thick descending and ascending limbs, which are essentially straight sections of the proximal and distal tubules, and the thin descending and ascending limbs, which include a sharp hairpin turn. The distal straight tubule changes into the distal convoluted tubule upon reentry into the cortex at the macula densa, which is next to the glomerulus. Each nephron is anatomically unique up until this point in terms of both structure and function. A "shared" collecting tubule or duct, which carries the urine produced in multiple nephrons through the medulla a second time, is formed by the distal convoluted tubules after this point. The larger papillary ducts that emerge from the fusion of these collecting tubules eventually empty into the renal pelvis and the calyces of the renal pyramids. Urine travels to the bladder from the renal pelvis in preparation for excretion through the urethra.

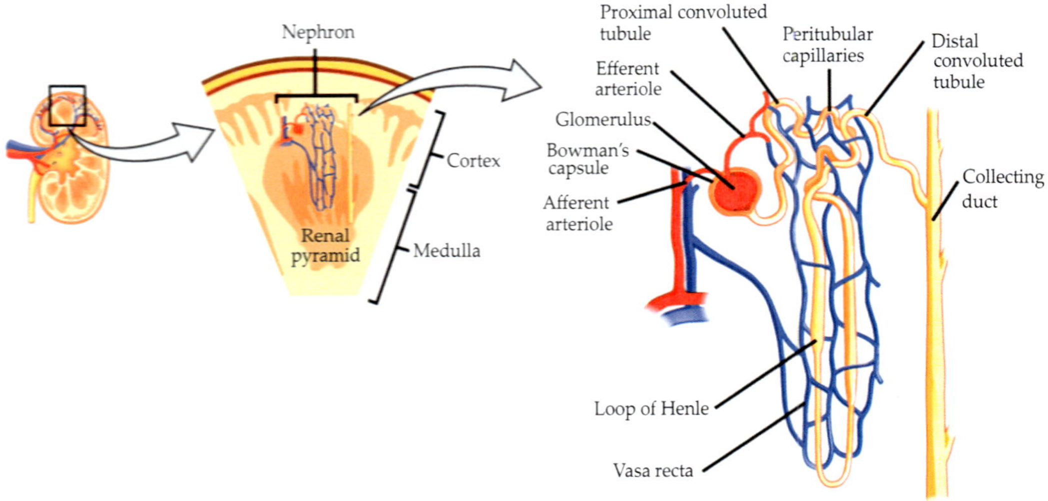

Figure 2.5. *A diagram of a nephron.*

Source: https://courses.lumenlearning.com/suny-dutchess-ap1/chapter/nephrons-structure/.

2.3. Renal Circulation

For the kidneys to carry out their main job of controlling the body's internal environment, they need a plentiful blood supply. In actuality, the kidneys receive 25% of the total cardiac output despite having a mass of only 300 g, or 0.5 percent, of the body mass. This high level of perfusion illustrates how the kidney's blood supply and functional ability are directly correlated.

A single renal artery that emerges from the aorta supplies each kidney. The renal artery creates a unique vascular configuration that is tailored to the kidney's functions as it divides in stages. The kidney is the only organ in humans that has two separate divisions of arterioles: one into a capillary bed, the other back into an arteriole, and a second division into a capillary network. Furthermore, the renal arterioles are mostly isolated end arteries that supply distinct regions of the kidney tissue.

As a result, interference with the blood supply at the glomerulus or afferent arteriole will adversely and dramatically change how the related nephron functions. Renal tissue is therefore especially vulnerable to ischemia or infarction. The lack of an arterial blood supply makes the medulla particularly vulnerable. Renal tissue damage will arise in the event of vascular stenosis or an occlusion; the degree of damage will depend on the number and location of the affected blood vessels.

Blood is supplied to each nephron's glomerulus separately by an afferent arteriole located at the vascular pole (Figure 2.6). The afferent arteriole branches into a capillary tuft upon entering the glomerulus and this structure is closely associated with the Bowman's capsule epithelial cells. As it exits the glomerulus, this branching and anastomosing capillary network joins to form the efferent arteriole. The efferent arteriole then branches into a capillary plexus a second time. The vascular configuration of this second capillary plexus is determined by the kind of nephron that the efferent arteriole services. Short Henle loops can be found on the outer cortical nephrons, and the efferent arteriole branches into the peritubular capillaries, a fine capillary plexus that completely encloses the outer cortical tubules. Henle loops are long in the mid and deep juxtamedullary nephrons. The vasa recta is a network of long, U-shaped vessels that descend deeply into the renal medulla near the loops of Henle. The efferent arterioles of these nephrons first branch into a peritubular capillary bed, which enmeshes the cortical portions of the tubules. The venous renal circulation originates from the corresponding ascending vasa recta, which emerge from deep within the medulla to form venules and drain into the renal veins. The sequential processing and exchange of solutes between the lumen fluid (ultrafiltrate) and the bloodstream throughout the nephron is made possible by the close relationship between the renal tubules and the peritubular capillaries.

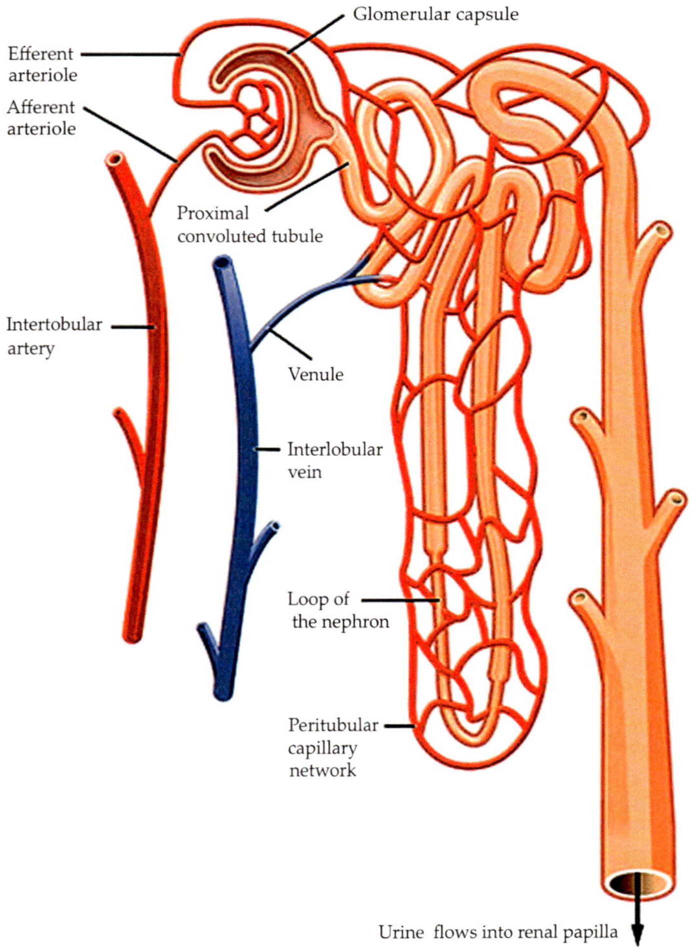

Figure 2.6. *The vascular circulation of a cortical and juxtamedullary nephron.*

Source: https://en.m.wikipedia.org/wiki/File:2611_Blood_Flow_in_the_Nephron.jpg.

The kidney can function at its best because of the special vascular configuration of the renal circulation. High hydrostatic pressure at the glomerulus is made possible by the afferent arteriole's relatively large bore.

This pressure, which drives glomerular filtration, averages 55 mm Hg, or roughly half of the mean arterial blood pressure. Because the lumen of every other capillary bed is smaller, there is more resistance to blood flow and, as a result, lower blood pressure within them. The resulting filtration force across the glomerular filtration barrier is also influenced by the ultrafiltrate itself. Bowman's space already contains plasma ultrafiltrate, which creates a hydrostatic pressure of 15 mm Hg that prevents filtration. Furthermore, in comparison to the plasma in the capillary lumen, the ultrafiltrate has a higher water content and a lower protein content. As a result, water that was able to pass through the filtration barrier unhindered tries to enter Bowman's space again. Consequently, glomerular filtration is also resisted by an oncotic pressure of 30 mm Hg brought on by the increased protein concentration in the plasma. The net filtration pressure of 10 mm Hg that results from these three pressure differentials encourages the development of a plasma ultrafiltrate in Bowman's space. It should be noted that the glomerular capillary blood pressure that powers plasma ultrafiltration is provided by the cardiac output rather than the filtration barrier, which uses no energy to create the plasma ultrafiltrate.

NFP = Glomerular blood hydrostatic pressure (GBHP) – [capsular hydrostatic pressure (CHP) + blood colloid osmotic pressure (BCOP)] = 10 mm Hg

That is: NFP = GBHP – [CHP + BCOP] = 10 mm Hg

Or: NFP = 55 – [15 + 30] = 10 mm Hg

At the vascular pole, the afferent and efferent arterioles leave Bowman's capsule close to one another. The juxtaglomerular apparatus is located in the vascular pole as well. Parts of the afferent and efferent arterioles, the extraglomerular mesangial cells (which are continuous with the supporting mesangium of the glomerulus), and the specialized region of the distal convoluted tubule (known as the macula densa) are the morphologically distinct structures that make up the juxtaglomerular apparatus. Typically, the smooth muscle cells of the afferent arteriole in the juxtaglomerular apparatus contain a significant amount of secretory granules containing the enzyme renin. The kidney's primary renin producer is the juxtaglomerular apparatus, which is essentially a tiny endocrine organ. Renin is an enzyme that eventually forms angiotensin and triggers the secretion of aldosterone when it is released into the bloodstream in response to reduced blood volume, decreased arterial pressure, sodium depletion, vascular hemorrhage, or increased potassium. The kidneys are stimulated by the secretion of aldosterone to actively retain sodium and passively retain water. Extracellular fluid volume increases, blood pressure rises, and normal potassium levels and renal perfusion are subsequently restored. On the other hand, renin secretion is inhibited and sodium excretion is enhanced by an increase in blood volume, an abrupt rise in blood pressure, or a potassium deficiency. The kidneys and the juxtaglomerular apparatus are crucial for maintaining body fluid homeostasis because of their capacity to alter fluid balance and blood pressure due to renin secretion.

2.4. Kidney Function and Physiology

Blood is filtered by kidneys in three stages. Blood that passes through the glomerulus's capillary network is first filtered by the nephrons. A procedure known as glomerular filtration is used to filter out almost all solutes—apart from proteins—into the glomerulus. Second, the renal tubules are where the filtrate is gathered. Tubular reabsorption is the process by which the majority of the solutes in the PCT are reabsorbed.

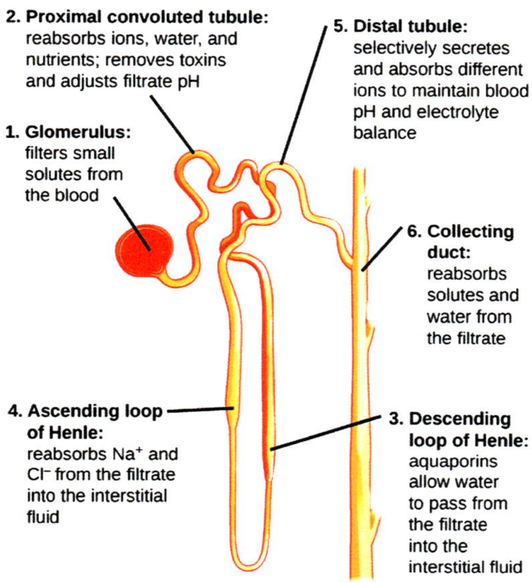

Figure 2.7. *A diagram of the nephron.*

Source: https://courses.lumenlearning.com/wm-biology2/chapter/kidney-function-and-physiology/.

The filtrate keeps exchanging water and solutes with the renal medulla and the peritubular capillary network inside the loop of Henle. In this step, water is also reabsorbed. Then, during tubular secretion—basically, the reverse of tubular reabsorption—more solutes and waste products are secreted into the kidney tubules. Filtrate from the nephrons is collected by the collecting ducts, which then merge in the medullary papillae. The filtrate, which is now known as urine, is then transported by the papillae into the minor calyces, which subsequently connect to the ureters via the renal pelvis. Figure 2.7 provides an illustration of this entire process. Each part of the nephron (Figure 2.7) performs a different function in filtering waste and maintaining homeostatic balance.

1. The glomerulus forces small solutes out of the blood by pressure.
2. The proximal convoluted tubule reabsorbs ions, water, and nutrients from the filtrate into the interstitial fluid, and actively transports toxins and drugs from the interstitial fluid into the filtrate. The proximal convoluted tubule also adjusts blood pH by selectively secreting ammonia (NH_3) into the filtrate, where it reacts with H^+ to form NH_4^+. The more acidic the filtrate, the more ammonia is secreted.
3. The descending loop of Henle is lined with cells containing aquaporins that allow water to pass from the filtrate into the interstitial fluid.
4. In the thin part of the ascending loop of Henle, Na^+ and Cl^- ions diffuse into the interstitial fluid. In the thick part, these same ions are actively transported into the interstitial fluid. Because salt but not water is lost, the filtrate becomes more dilute as it travels up the limb.
5. In the distal convoluted tubule, K^+ and H^+ ions are selectively secreted into the filtrate, while Na^+, Cl^-, and HCO_3^- ions are reabsorbed to maintain pH and electrolyte balance in the blood.
6. The collecting duct reabsorbs solutes and water from the filtrate, forming dilute urine (Alpem and Herbert, 2008; Patton and Thibodeau, 2010)

2.5. Urine Formation

The kidneys' main excretory function is the production of urine. Three steps go into making urine: the glomeruli filter plasma, the renal tubules reabsorb it, and finally, the renal tubules secrete certain components. The kidneys' functions include the elimination of waste products from metabolism, the control of water and electrolytes (e.g., sodium, and chloride), as well as upholding the acid-base balance of the body. Whatever the body has produced or consumed, the kidneys are the real regulators, choosing which chemicals to excrete and which to hold onto.

The kidneys filter about 180,000 mL (125 mL/min) of plasma every day, which ends up as 600–1800 mL of urine. Water makes up the majority of urine's contents. Urea, chloride, sodium, and potassium are the main solutes found here, followed by phosphate, sulfate, creatinine, and uric acid. The tubules essentially re-absorb other substances that were initially in the ultrafiltrate, including albumin, glucose, and bicarbonate. As a result, these solutes are not found in appreciable concentrations in the urine of healthy, normal people. eliminated as 1 percent of the filtered plasma volume, or about 1200 mL, is the average urine output, 99% of the ultrafiltrate that initially gathers in Bowman's space is reabsorbed. Furthermore, as the ultrafiltrate flows through the kidneys, the nephrons reabsorb solutes widely and selectively and secrete them.

2.6. Glomerular Filtration

The afferent arteriole's specialized membranes and high blood pressure cause glomerular filtration to remove the majority of solutes. An independent set of factors that influence systemic blood pressure maintains the blood pressure in the glomerulus. Solutes are easily able to flow through the glomerular capillary network's "leaky" connections between endothelial cells. Everything that is not a macromolecule, such as proteins, diffuses passively through the glomerular capillaries. As the filtration process reaches this point, no energy is needed. A kidney's production of glomerular filtrate per minute is measured by its glomerular filtration rate, or GFR. The global functional reserve (GFR) is a crucial measure of kidney health that is regulated by various mechanisms.

A coil of about eight capillary lobes, collectively referred to as the capillary tuft, makes up the glomerulus. It is situated inside Bowman's capsule, which marks the renal tubule's origin. Many factors affect the actual filtration process, even though the glomerulus acts as a nonselective filter for plasma substances with molecular weights less than 70,000. These include the Bowman's capsule and capillary walls' cellular structure, hydrostatic and oncotic pressures, and the feedback mechanisms of the renin-angiotensin-aldosterone system. A diagrammatic view of the glomerular areas affected by these factors is shown in Figure 2.8.

2.6.1. Cellular Structure of the Glomerulus

The visceral epithelium of Bowman's capsule, the basement membrane (basal lamina), and the capillary wall membrane are the three cellular layers that the plasma filtrate must pass through. The capillary wall's endothelial cells are known as fenestrated because they have pores, setting them apart from those in other capillaries. Although the pores make capillaries more permeable, they prevent blood cells and big molecules from passing through. As the filtrate moves through the basement membrane and the thin membranes covering the filtration slits created by the intertwining foot processes of the podocytes in the inner layer of Bowman's capsule, more restriction of large molecules takes place (Figure 2.8).

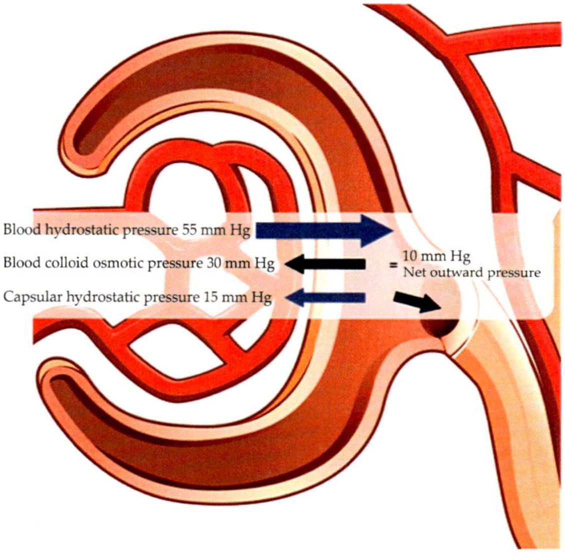

Figure 2.8. *Factors affecting the glomerular filtration in the renal corpuscle.*

Source: https://open.oregonstate.education/aandp/chapter/25-4-physiology-of-urine-formation-glomerular-filtration/.

2.6.2. Glomerular Pressure

Filtration is improved by the hydrostatic pressure created by the glomerular capillaries and the smaller size of the efferent arteriole. This pressure is required to overcome the oncotic pressure of unfiltered plasma proteins in the glomerular capillaries as well as the opposing pressures from the fluid inside Bowman's capsule. An autoregulatory mechanism in the juxtaglomerular apparatus regulates the size of the afferent arteriole to keep the glomerular blood pressure relatively constant despite variations in systemic blood pressure. When blood pressure drops, the afferent arterioles dilate and the efferent arterioles constrict, preventing a significant drop in blood flow through the kidney and an increase in the blood level of toxic waste products. Similar to this, a rise in blood pressure causes the afferent arterioles to constrict to protect the glomerulus from over filtration or injury.

2.6.3. Renin-Angiotensin-Aldosterone System

The regulation of blood flow to and within the glomerulus is carried out by the renin-angiotensin-aldosterone system (RAAS). The juxtaglomerular apparatus, comprising the distal convoluted tubule's macula densa and the afferent arteriole's juxtaglomerular cells, monitors changes in blood pressure and plasma sodium content, and the system reacts to these changes (Figure 2.9). Low plasma sodium content reduces the circulatory system's ability to retain water, which lowers total blood volume and, in turn, lowers blood pressure. A series of events take place inside the RAAS when the macula densa detects such alterations (Figure 2.10). The blood-borne substrate angiotensinogen and the enzyme renin, which is produced by the juxtaglomerular cells, combine to form the inactive hormone angiotensin I. Angiotensin converting enzyme (ACE) converts angiotensin I into the active form angiotensin II as it travels through the lungs. The following mechanisms by which angiotensin II corrects renal blood flow are: it causes constriction of the efferent arterioles and vasodilation of the afferent arterioles; it stimulates sodium reabsorption in the proximal convoluted tubules; and it causes the adrenal cortex and hypothalamus to release the hormones that retain sodium, aldosterone and antidiuretic hormone (Table 2.3). Renin secretion declines with increases in systemic blood pressure and plasma sodium content. Consequently, the nephron experiences continuous pressure due to the effects of angiotensin II.

Due to the glomerular mechanisms mentioned above, two to three million glomeruli filter about 120 mL of low-molecular-weight substances that contain water every minute. The lack of plasma protein, any protein-bound materials, and cells is the only distinction between the compositions of the filtrate and the plasma due to the nonselective nature of this filtration. It is confirmed that the filtrate is chemically an ultrafiltrate of plasma by analysis of the fluid as it exits the glomerulus, which reveals a specific gravity of 1.010. This data offers a helpful starting point for assessing the renal processes that transform the plasma ultrafiltrate into the finished urine product.

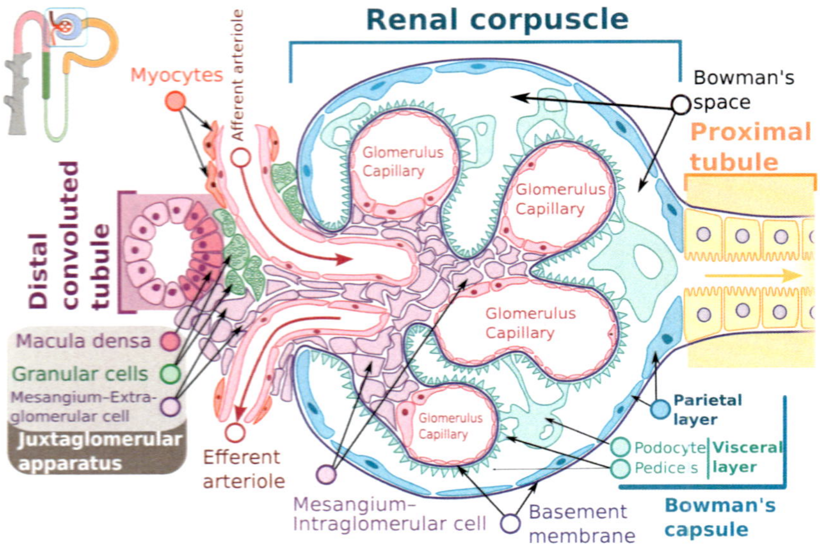

Figure 2.9. *The juxtaglomerular apparatus.*

Source: By Shypoetess - File: Renal corpuscle.svg and File: Cialko nerkowe.svg by M•Komorniczak, CC BY-SA 4.0, https://commons.wikimedia.org/w/index.php?curid=76356955.

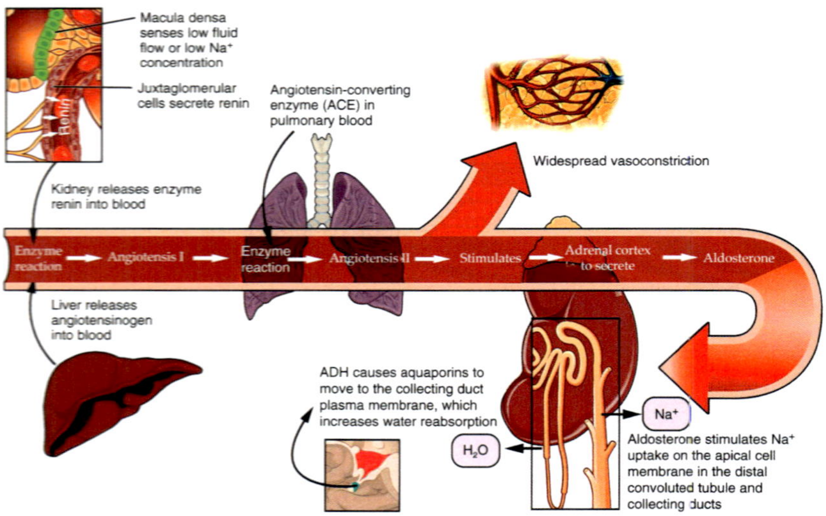

Figure 2.10. *The rennin-angiotensin-aldosterone system.*

Source: https://open.oregonstate.education/aandp/chapter/25-4-physiology-of-urine-formation-glomerular-filtration/.

2.7. Tubules

The five different regions of the nephron have different epithelium lining the renal tubules. Comprehending the different processes involved is made easier by examining the unique and specialized epithelial features of each segment.

The ultrafiltrate is only moved through the remaining tubular sections of the nephrons by hydrostatic pressure once the glomerular ultrafiltrate has formed in Bowman's space. The epithelium of each tubular segment varies distinctly, which is directly related to the distinct processes that take place there. The large convoluted part (pars convoluta) and the straight portion (pars recta) make up the first section, the proximal tubule. Proximal tubule cells are tall and heavily interdigitate with one another (Figure 2.11). Salt-transporting epithelia are characterized by intercellular interdigitations that serve to increase the total cellular surface area. Due to the large number of microvilli (typical of absorbing epithelia as in the small intestine) present, the luminal surfaces of these cells have a brush border. A maximum area for filtrate reabsorption is provided by these closely spaced microvilli, which significantly increase the luminal surface area. The proximal tubular cells also have a large number of mitochondria, indicating a high level of metabolic activity, as well as an abundance of the enzymes required for the active transport of different solutes.

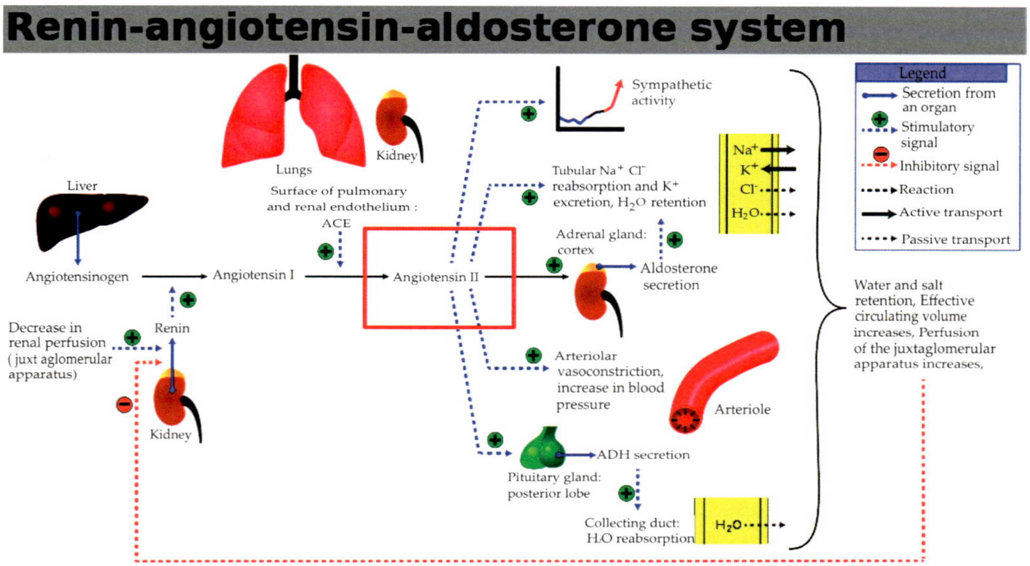

Figure 2.11. *Changes in the hormones.*

The tubular epithelium changes when the straight section of the proximal tubule enters the outer medulla to form the thin descending limb of the loop of Henle. At this stage, the epithelium is made up of simply arranged, flat, noninterdigitating cells (Figure 2.11). The cellular organization differs according to the length of the Henle loop. The cellular complexity of the longest limbs, which extend deeply into the medulla, has increased. The epithelium changes once more at the hairpin turn of the loop of Henle, regardless of the length of the limb. Despite staying flat, these epithelial cells have a lot of interdigitation. The thin ascending limb of the loop of Henle is covered in the interdigitating epithelium that is present at the hairpin turn.

The thick ascending limb of the loop of Henle, also known as the distal tubule's straight section, is primarily made up of tall, interdigitating cells (Figure 2.11). Only two to three loops of tubular convolution are required for the distal convoluted tubule to reach a collecting duct, compared to the proximal tubule's greater amount of tubular convolution.

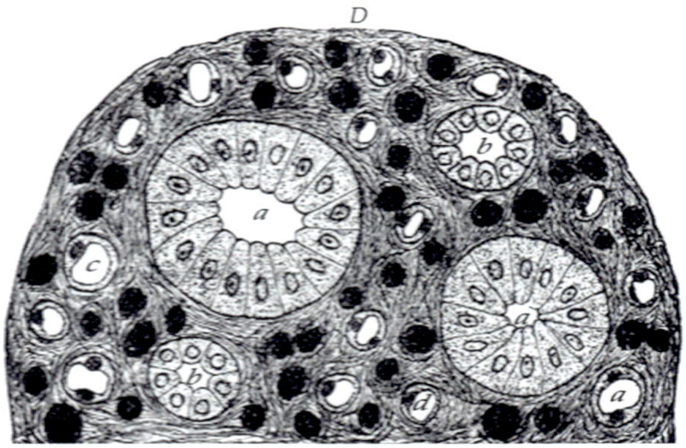

Figure 2.12. *Simple columnar epithelium and simple cuboidal epithelium in the collecting ducts of the pig kidney. The walls of the large and small connecting tubules (a and b respectively), the circular structures, are formed by simple columnar epithelium (a) and simple cuboidal epithelium (b).*

Source: By Henry Vandyke Carter - Henry Gray (1918) Anatomy of the Human Body (See "Book" section below) Bartleby.com: Gray's Anatomy, Plate 1133, Public Domain, https://commons.wikimedia.org/w/index.php?curid=567102.

The final urine concentration occurs in the collecting duct, which passes through the renal cortex and medulla. Polygonal cells with a few small, stubby microvilli and no intercellular interdigitations make up the majority of the epithelium of the collecting ducts (Figure 2.11). Intercellular junctions, or gaps, exist between these cells from their bases to their luminal surfaces. The spaces between the cells dilate when antidiuretic hormone (ADH), also referred to as arginine vasopressin, is present, making the epithelium highly permeable to water. In contrast, the spaces are joined tightly in the absence of ADH (Figure 2.12). Taller and more columnar cells reappear in the epithelium as the collecting duct gets closer to the papillary tip.

2.8. Tubular Function

The high volume of reabsorption that occurs within the renal tubules is demonstrated by the fact that only 1% (or about 1200 mL) of the initial plasma ultrafiltrate supplied to the tubules is eliminated as urine. Along with this significant volume change, the urine excreted has a drastically different solute makeup than the original ultrafiltrate, highlighting the dynamic processes that the tubules perform. The kidney's ability to regulate the excretion of water and other solutes is what makes it the most significant organ in fluid exchanges. The substances are moved either from the tubular lumen into the peritubular capillary blood and interstitium (reabsorption) or from the peritubular capillary blood and interstitium into the tubular lumen (secretion). The mechanisms causing these changes are the same: tubular reabsorption and tubular secretion.

2.8.1. Transport

The mechanisms of tubular transport (i.e., secretion, and reabsorption) are either passive or active. The passage of a material across a membrane against a gradient is known as active transport. Put another way, the chemical or electrical composition of the compartments divided by the membrane varies. Such transportation necessitates the direct or indirect use of energy. Direct active transport is the process of actively moving a substance when energy is needed, such as in the potassium-to-sodium exchange facilitated by adenosine triphosphate hydrolysis (the sodium pump). Indirect active transport, also known as cotransport, is the movement of one substance along a gradient accompanied by the movement of another substance (e.g., the proximal tubules' indirect absorption of glucose and sodium).

Certain protein-binding sites that cross the cell membrane are involved in active transport, which happens transcellularly. The steps involved in active transport are as follows: (1) the material attaches to its particular membrane-binding site; (2) it passes through the cell membrane; and (3) it is released either inside or outside the cell when the binding site changes conformation.

The movement of a substance along a gradient, or, to put it another way, from an area of higher concentration to one of lower concentration, is known as passive transport. This type of transport, like that of urea, does not require energy. Transport between cells via junctions and intercellular spaces can be either transcellular or paracellular in nature (Alpem and Herbert, 2008; Patton and Thibodeau, 2010).

Every solute has a unique transport mechanism. Cellular protein-binding sites can carry multiple solutes, frequently displaying preferential transport of one analyte over another, or they can be specific for a single solute and only carry that solute across the membrane. Furthermore, depending on the location of the tubule, the mode of transportation—passive or active—may change. For instance, chloride is passively reabsorbed in the proximal tubule but actively reabsorbed in the ascending loop of Henle (Table 2.1).

Table 2.1. Substances Secreted or Reabsorbed in the Nephron and Their Locations

Substance	PCT	Loop of Henle	DCT	Collecting Ducts
Glucose	Almost 100% reabsorbed; secondary active transport with Na^+			
Oligopeptides, proteins, amino acids	Almost 100% reabsorbed; symport with Na^+			
Vitamins	Reabsorbed			
Lactate	Reabsorbed			
Creatinine	Secreted			
Urea	50% reabsorbed by diffusion; also secreted	Secretion, diffusion in descending limb		Reabsorption in medullary collecting ducts; diffusion

Sodium	65% actively reabsorbed	25% reabsorbed in thick ascending limb; active transport	5% reabsorbed; active	5% reabsorbed, stimulated by aldosterone; active
Chloride	Reabsorbed, symport with Na^+, diffusion	Reabsorbed in thin and thick ascending limb; diffusion in ascending limb	Reabsorbed; diffusion	Reabsorbed; symport
Water	67% reabsorbed osmotically with solutes	15% reabsorbed in descending limb; osmosis	8% reabsorbed if ADH; osmosis	Variable amounts reabsorbed, controlled by ADH, osmosis
Bicarbonate	80–90% symport reabsorption with Na^+	Reabsorbed, symport with Na^+ and antiport with Cl^-; in ascending limb		Reabsorbed antiport with Cl^-
H^+	Secreted; diffusion		Secreted; active	Secreted; active
NH_4^+	Secreted; diffusion		Secreted; diffusion	Secreted; diffusion
HCO_3^-	Reabsorbed; diffusion	Reabsorbed; diffusion in ascending limb	Reabsorbed; diffusion	Reabsorbed; antiport with Na^+
Some drugs	Secreted		Secreted; active	Secreted; active
Potassium	65% reabsorbed; diffusion	20% reabsorbed in thick ascending limb; symport	Secreted; active	Secretion controlled by aldosterone; active
Calcium	Reabsorbed; diffusion	Reabsorbed in thick ascending limb; diffusion		Reabsorbed if parathyroid hormone present; active

Magnesium	Reabsorbed; diffusion	Reabsorbed in thick ascending limb; diffusion	Reabsorbed	
Phosphate	85% reabsorbed, inhibited by parathyroid hormone, diffusion		Reabsorbed; diffusion	

Source: https://courses.lumenlearning.com/suny-ap2/chapter/tubular-reabsorption-no-content/.

2.8.2. Tubular Reabsorption

Selective excretion of waste materials like creatinine and metabolic acids occurs during tubular function, while reabsorbing elements like water, salts, glucose, proteins, and amino acids that are vital for maintaining body homeostasis and function.

The body cannot lose 120 milliliters of vital substances that are contained in water per minute. Thus, through cellular transport mechanisms, the nephrons start reabsorbing these vital chemicals and water when the plasma ultrafiltrate enters the proximal convoluted tubule (Table 2.2).

Table 2.2. Tubular Reabsorption

Reabsorption of Major Solutes by the PCT	
Basal Membrane	Apical Membrane
Active transport	Symport with Na^+
Na^+ (exchange for K^+)	K^+
Facilitated diffusion	Cl^-
K^+	Ca^{++}
Cl^-	Mg^{++}
Ca^{++}	HCO_3^-
HCO_3^-	PO_4^{3-}-PO_4^{3-}
PO_4^{3-}-PO_4^{3-}	Amino acids
Amino acids	Glucose
Glucose	Fructose
Fructose	Galactose
Galactose	Lactate
Lactate	Succinate
Succinate	Citrate
Citrate	Diffusion between nephron cells
	K^+
	Ca^{++}
	Mg^{++}

Source: https://courses.lumenlearning.com/suny-ap2/chapter/tubular-reabsorption-no-content/.

2.8.2.1. Reabsorption Mechanisms

The substance is transferred across cell membranes and back into the bloodstream by the electrochemical energy produced by this interaction. Reabsorbing glucose, amino acids, and salts in the proximal convoluted tubule, chloride in the ascending loop of Henle, and sodium in the distal convoluted tubule is all due to active transport.

All areas of the nephron experience passive reabsorption of water, with the exception of the ascending loop of Henle, whose walls are impermeable to water. The proximal convoluted tubule and the ascending loop of Henle both passively reabsorb urea, and the ascending loop passively reabsorbs sodium in tandem with the active transport of chloride.

The concentration of the material being transported can have an impact on both active and passive transport. A substance that is normally fully reabsorbed becomes visible in urine when its plasma concentration rises to an abnormally high level and the filtrate concentration surpasses the tubules' maximal reabsorptive capacity (T_m). The renal threshold is the plasma concentration at which active transport ends. When the plasma concentration of glucose hits the renal threshold of 160 to 180 mg/dL, glucose starts to show up in the urine. Renal tubular damage and excess solute filtration can be distinguished from one another using knowledge of the renal threshold and plasma concentration. For instance, tubular damage, not diabetes mellitus, is the cause of glucose showing up in the urine of a person with a normal blood glucose level. (Figure 2.13).

Water is passively reabsorption occurs in tandem with the active transport of over two-thirds of the filtered sodium out of the proximal convoluted tubule. Thus, the fluid exiting the proximal convoluted tubule retains the same concentration as the ultrafiltrate.

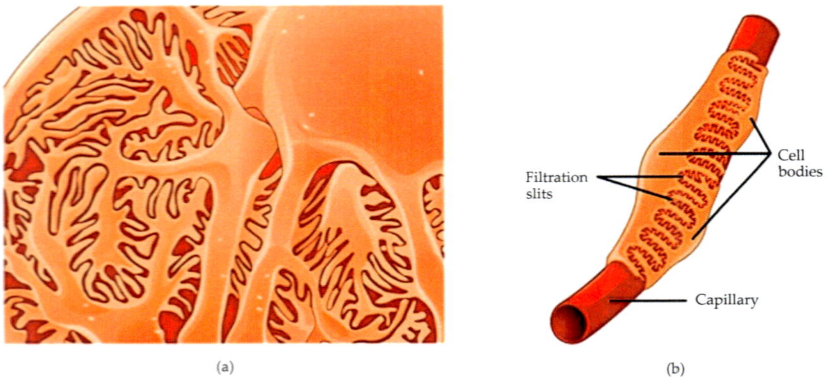

Figure 2.13. *Podocytes interdigitate with structures called pedicels and filter substances into the glomerular capsule. In (a), the large cell body can be seen at the top right corner, with branches extending from the cell body. The smallest finger-like extensions are the pedicels.*

Source: https://open.oregonstate.education/aandp/chapter/25-2-microscopic-anatomy-of-the-kidney-anatomy-of-the-nephron/.

2.8.2.2. Tubular Concentration

The high osmotic gradient of the renal medulla is exposed to the filtrate in the descending and ascending loops of Henle, where renal concentration starts. In the descending loop of Henle, water is eliminated through osmosis, while in the ascending loop, sodium and chloride are reabsorbed. Water-impermeable walls of the ascending loop prevent excessive reabsorption of water as the filtrate passes through the highly concentrated medulla. This process of selective reabsorption, known as the countercurrent mechanism, keeps the medulla's osmotic gradient intact. The water reabsorbed from the descending loop does not dilute the medullary interstitium because the sodium and chloride leave the filtrate in the ascending loop. When the filtrate reaches the collecting duct, its final concentration depends on the maintenance of this osmotic gradient. The reabsorption of salt rather than water in that section of the tubule is the reason for the relatively low actual concentration of filtrate exiting the ascending loop. The hormone aldosterone now regulates sodium reabsorption in the distal convoluted tubule, which is still occurring in response to the body's need for sodium.

2.8.2.3. Collecting Duct Concentration

The late distal convoluted tubule is where the filtrate's final concentration from water reabsorption starts, and it continues in the collecting duct. The osmotic gradient in the medulla and the hormone vasopressin (antidiuretic hormone [ADH]) are necessary for reabsorption. Passive reabsorption of water is expected to occur as the diluted filtrate in the collecting duct comes into contact with the medullary interstitium's higher osmotic concentration. The distal convoluted tubule and collecting duct walls' water permeability or impermeability, on the other hand, is determined by the presence or lack of ADH. A high ADH level increases permeability, which enhances water absorption and produces concentrated urine with a low volume. Similar to how the walls become impermeable to water when ADH is absent, this causes a significant amount of diluted urine. The body's level of hydration affects the synthesis of ADH in the same way that sodium concentration affects aldosterone production. Urine volume and concentration are therefore ultimately determined by the body's chemical balance. ADH function is summarized as follows:

$\uparrow$Body Hydration = $\downarrow$ADH = $\uparrow$Urine Volume

$\downarrow$Body Hydration = $\uparrow$ADH = $\downarrow$Urine Volume

2.8.3. Tubular Secretion

Tubular secretion is the process by which substances leave the blood in the peritubular capillaries and enter the tubular filtrate, as opposed to tubular reabsorption, which involves removing substances from the glomerular filtrate and returning them to the blood (Figure 2.14). Two primary purposes of tubular secretion are the removal of waste materials that the glomerulus is unable to filter and the secretion of hydrogen ions, which helps to maintain the body's acid-base equilibrium. Since many foreign substances are attached to plasma proteins, the glomerulus is unable to filter them. Examples of these substances include medications. Nevertheless, these protein-bound materials gain a greater affinity for tubular cells and separate from their carrier proteins upon entering the peritubular capillaries. This allows the tubular cells to transport the materials into the filtrate. The proximal convoluted tubule is the main location where these unfiltered substances are removed.

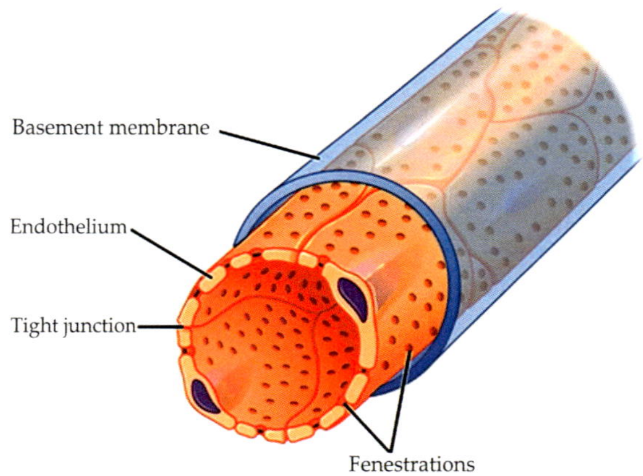

Figure 2.14. *Fenestrated capillaries in the nephron.*

Source: https://open.oregonstate.education/aandp/chapter/25-2-microscopic-anatomy-of-the-kidney-anatomy-of-the-nephron/.

Tubular secretion occurs throughout the nephron, just like tubular reabsorption. The primary functions of the renal secretory process are to: (1) remove waste products from metabolism and substances that aren't typically found in plasma; and (2) modify the body's acid-base balance. These two roles overlap because the body's acid-base balance is directly impacted by the weak acids and bases found in many foreign substances and metabolic byproducts. Some of the significant secreted ultrafiltrate solutes and the tubular secretion locations are compiled in Table 2.3.

Table 2.3. Substances Filtered and Reabsorbed by the Kidney Per 24h

Substance	Amount Filtered (grams)	Amount Reabsorbed (grams)	Amount in Urine (grams)
Water	180 L	179 L	1 L
Proteins	10–20	10–20	0
Chlorine	630	625	5
Sodium	540	537	3
Bicarbonate	300	299.7	0.3
Glucose	180	180	0
Urea	53	28	25
Potassium	28	24	4
Uric acid	8.5	7.7	0.8
Creatinine	1.4	0	1.4

Source: https://open.oregonstate.education/aandp/chapter/25-5-physiology-of-urine-formation-tubular-reabsorption-and-secretion/.

Apart from hydrogen ions, ammonia, and potassium, the majority of substances secreted are weak acids or bases. These weak bases and acids come from external or metabolic sources. They are (1) substances that the body has not fully metabolized (e.g., thiamine), (2) substances secreted unaltered and not metabolized at all (e.g., as mannitol and radiopaque contrast media), or (3) materials that aren't typically found in plasma (e.g., salicylate, penicillin). Certain substances are bound to plasma proteins, mainly albumin, which prevents them from excreting through the glomerular filtration barrier (e.g., drugs, unconjugated bilirubin). They consequently have a significant increase in size overall and may lose some of their initial molecular charge. However, tubular secretion offers a way to get rid of them. These comparatively big, protein-bound materials are carried into renal tubular cells, where they interact with endothelium-binding sites before being secreted into the tubular lumen as they pass through the peritubular capillaries.

2.8.4. Regulation of Acid-Base Equilibrium

A basic understanding of the body's endogenous production of bases and acids is necessary to comprehend the function of tubular secretion in maintaining acid-base equilibrium. Normal blood pH in healthy individuals ranges from 7.35 to 7.45, which is alkaline. Nonetheless, the pH can be as high as 7.80 or as low as 7.00 in pathologic disease states. Blood has an alkaline pH, and the endogenous production of acids from regular food metabolism continuously jeopardizes this pH. These endogenous acids are produced in three ways: (1) by the oxidative metabolism of food, which produces carbonic acid, (2) by the breakdown of dietary proteins and phospholipids, or (3) by the production of acids under specific pathologic or physiological conditions, such as lactic acid with exercise or acetoacetic acid in uncontrolled diabetes mellitus.

Three bodily systems—the pulmonary system, the renal system, and the blood buffer system, which includes hemoglobin, bicarbonate, proteins, and inorganic phosphates—are involved in keeping the blood pH at a level that is conducive to life. While the three systems collaborate to sustain homeostasis, the pulmonary and blood-buffer systems can react promptly to pH variations, albeit to a limited extent. However, the renal system can fully correct deviations in blood pH, even with its relatively slow response.

The kidneys excrete acid or alkali in urine according to blood pH variations. Excess alkali is removed by excreting sodium salts like sodium bicarbonate and disodium phosphate, while excess acids are removed by excreting titratable acids like monosodium phosphate and ammonium salts like NH_4Cl,$[NH_4]_2SO_4$, etc.

The tubular secretion of H^+ ions is a prerequisite for each of the three secretory mechanisms that regulate blood pH, either directly or indirectly. Renal tubular cells secrete H^+ ions (acids) in exchange for sodium and bicarbonate ions (alkali) in acidotic conditions. Tubular H^+ ion secretion is reduced in alkalotic conditions, aiding in the body's removal of excess alkali.

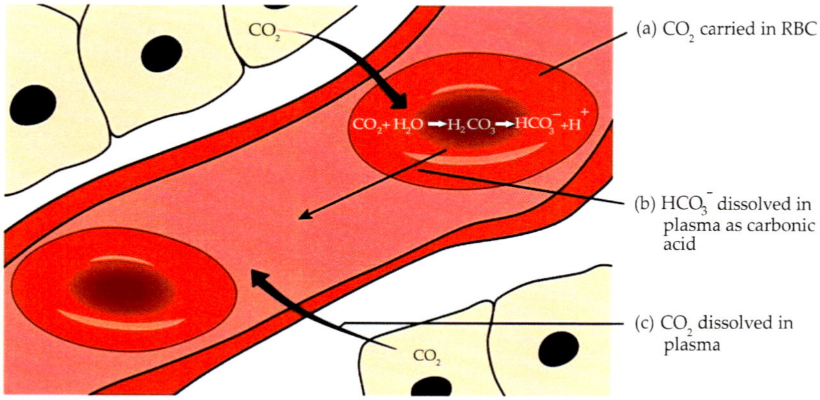

Figure 2.15. *The blood buffer.*

Source: By OpenStax College - Anatomy & Physiology, Connexions Web site. http://cnx.org/content/col11496/1.6/, Jun 19, 2013., CC BY 3.0, https://commons.wikimedia.org/w/index.php?curid=30148398.

In the first secretory mechanism, the loss of bicarbonate, an essential part of the blood-buffer system, is directly prevented by the secretion of H^+ ions into the proximal tubular lumen. In Figure 2.15, carbonic acid (H_2CO_3) is formed in the tubular lumen as a result of a reaction between bicarbonate ions (HCO_3^-), which easily cross the glomerular filtration barrier, and the released H^+. However, due to the high concentration of the enzyme carbonic anhydrase found in the brush border of the proximal tubular cells, this carbonic acid is quickly catalyzed to carbon dioxide and water. As the carbon dioxide permeates into the proximal cell, intracellular carbonic anhydrase again converts it to HCO_3^- and H^+. Thus, H^+ ions are once again available for tubular secretion and for the reabsorption of HCO_3^- ions from the lumen of the tubule. Reabsorbed bicarbonate replenishes the blood-buffer system by diffusing into the interstitial fluid and peritubular capillaries (Lumen Learning; Alpem and Herbert, 2008; Patton and Thibodeau, 2010).

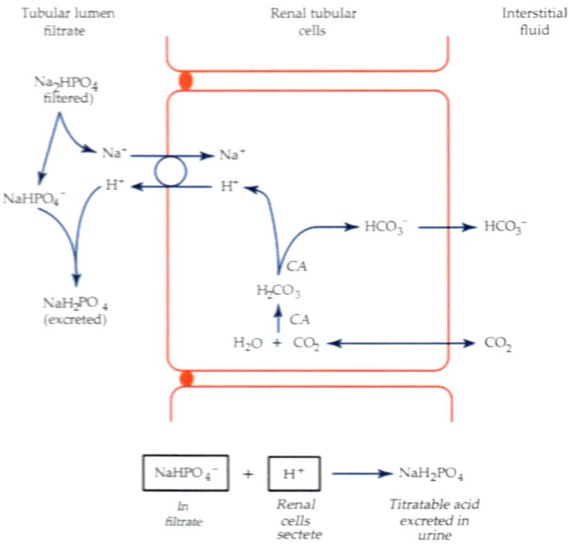

Figure 2.16. *Hydrogen ion secretion and the formation of titratable acids. This is a mechanism of urine acidification in the collecting ducts. CA, Carbonic anhydrase..*

Source: By OpenStax College - Anatomy & Physiology, Connexions Web site. http://cnx.org/content/col11496/1.6/, Jun 19, 2013., CC BY 3.0, https://commons.wikimedia.org/w/index.php?curid=30148398.

The second secretory mechanism, as seen in Figure 2.16, is contingent upon the ultrafiltrate's phosphate content. The blood quickly transforms phosphoric acids, which are created during food metabolism, into neutral salts (e.g., Na_2HPO_4) and are carried to the renal system. Disodium phosphate (Na_2HPO_4) is converted to monosodium phosphate (NaH_2PO_4) in the tubular lumen of the nephrons by the exchange of secreted hydrogen ions with sodium ions (Equation 2.1). Titratable acids are those monobasic phosphates that are specifically mixed with hydrogen ions and eliminated in the urine. The name derives from the ability to titrate urine to a pHof7.4(pH of normal plasma) using a standard base (e.g., NaOH), to determine the amount of acid present as a result of the se monobasic phosphates. Note that hydrogen ions combined with other solutes are not measured by this titration.

These phosphates in the ultrafiltrate cause the body to release acid and acidify the urine; additionally, they restore sodium and bicarbonate ions to the blood in the peritubular capillaries.

As seen in Figure 2.17, the third secretory mechanism for acid removal is dependent on the secretion of ammonia and the subsequent exchange of sodium ions for ammonium ions. The renal tubular cells produce ammonia (NH_3) when the enzyme glutaminase reacts with glutamine, which is derived from the blood in the peritubular capillaries. NH_3 is lipid soluble and easily diffuses through tubular cell membranes and into the tubular lumen because it is not ionized. Ammonium ions (NH_4^+) are created when NH_3 quickly combines with H^+ ions inside the lumen. Due to their charge, these ions are essentially nondiffusible; as a result, they stay in the tubular lumen where they may mix with neutral salts like sodium sulfate, a metabolic byproduct, or sodium chloride. Equations 2.2 and 2.3 depict the chemical reactions that take place in the tubular lumen.

$$\begin{array}{ll} \text{In blood} & H_3PO_4 + 6Na^+ \rightarrow 3Na_2HPO_4 \\ \text{In ultrafiltrate} & Na_2HPO_4 + H^+ \rightarrow NaH_2PO_4 + Na^+ \\ & Na^+ + HCO_3^- \rightarrow NaHCO_3 \text{ (reabsorbed)} \end{array} \quad (2.1)$$

$$\begin{array}{c} NH_3 + H^+ \rightarrow NH_4^+ \\ NH_4^+ + NaCl + HCO_3^- \rightarrow NH_4Cl \text{ (excreted)} + NaHCO_3 \text{ (reabsorbed)} \end{array} \quad (2.2)$$

$$NH_3 + H^+ \rightarrow NH_4^+$$

$$2NH_4^+ + Na_2SO_4 + 2HCO_3^- \rightarrow (NH_4)_2SO_4 \text{ (excreted)} + 2NaHCO_3 \text{ (reabsorbed)} \quad (2.3)$$

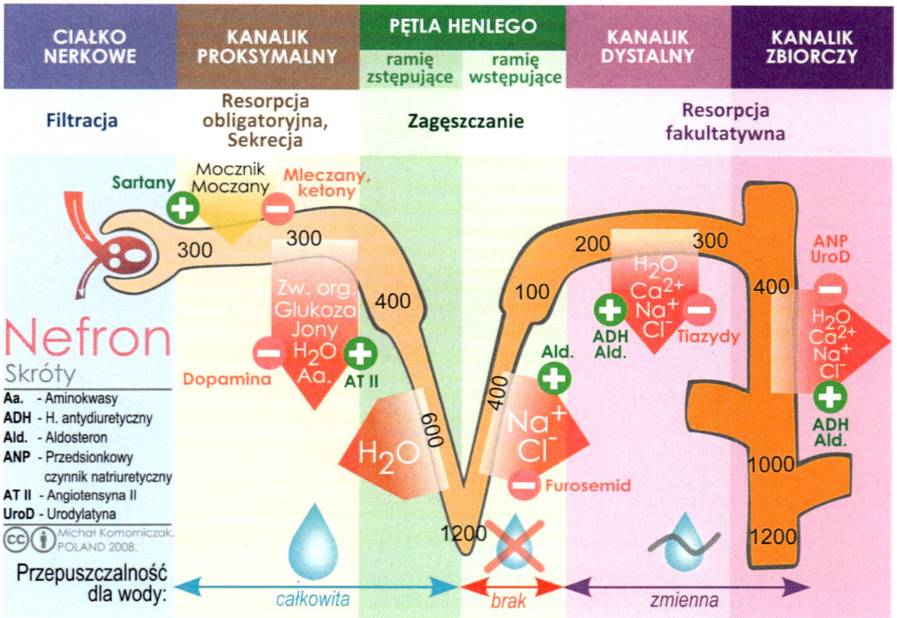

Figure 2.17. *Ion movement in the nephron.*

Source: By Nephron-urine.svg: M.Komorniczak, polish wikipedist.Kidney nephron molar transport diagram.png: *Nephron-urine.svg: M.Komorniczak, polish wikipedist.derivative work: Juvo415derivative work: Mcstrother - Nephron-urine.svgKidney nephron molar transport diagram.png, CC BY-SA 3.0, https://commons.wikimedia.org/w/index.php?curid=12880243.

It should be noted that sodium and bicarbonate are restored and made available for tubular reabsorption in both reactions. The renal tubules are the main source of ammonia excreted in urine. Ammonia is produced by both the proximal and collecting duct cells, and the collecting ducts are primarily where final urine acidification takes place. However, the body's acid-base status directly affects how quickly ammonia is synthesized. For instance, in acidotic conditions, there is an increase in ammonia production.

In conclusion, the kidney uses three renal secretory mechanisms to control the body's acid-base equilibrium: (1) H^+ ion secretion to recover bicarbonate; (2) H^+ ion secretion to produce urine titratable acids (e.g., monosodium phosphate); and (3) H^+ ion and NH_3 secretion to yield ammonium salts (e.g., ammonium chloride, ammonium sulfate). Through all of these methods, the secretion of hydrogen ions (i.e., the acid loss) causes the reabsorption of sodium or bicarbonate (i.e., the alkali's gain). As a result, the kidney adjusts the amount of hydrogen ions and ammonia it secretes based on the body's changing acid-base requirements.

2.8.5. Tubular Transport Capacity

The substance involved determines the renal tubules' capacity for both secretion and reabsorption. For some substances, the rate of tubular reabsorption increases along with the amount of solute presented to the renal tubules, reaching a maximal rate of reabsorption. Even if the solute's concentration rises further, this maximal reabsorptive rate won't change. Urine then contains extra solute that has not been reabsorbed. The maximal tubular reabsorptive capacity refers to this reabsorptive property of the renal epithelium. The amount of solute (milligrams) reabsorbed per minute is indicated by the symbol T_m. The particular solute and additional variables, like the glomerular filtration rate, affect the T_m. Among the solutes with a T_m-limited tubular reabsorptive capacity are glucose, proteins, amino acids, phosphate, sulfate, and uric acid. Additionally, the blood concentration of these solutes has a Tm-specific value known as the renal threshold level. For instance, the glucose T_m is roughly 350 mg/min (corrected to 1.73 m^2 body surface area), meaning that a glucose plasma renal threshold level of 160–180 mg/dL is associated with this value. Put another way, a maximum of 350 mg of glucose can be reabsorbed per minute, independent of the amount of glucose present in the renal tubular lumen. Urine contains glucose excreted when the plasma glucose level surpasses 160 to 180 mg/dL, meaning that the ultrafiltrate glucose concentration surpasses the capacity of tubules to reabsorb (T_m). Maximal tubular secretory capacity or T_m is seen for a weak organic acid like Hippurate.

Conversely, the amount of some solutes that can be reabsorbed is unrestricted (e.g., sodium) or released (e.g., potassium). Several factors, including the tubular flow rate, the duration of the solute's contact with the renal epithelium, the concentrations of other solutes in the filtrate, the presence of transport inhibitors, and variations in hormone levels, all affect the rate of transport for these substances (e.g., ADH).

2.8.6. Proximal Tubular Reabsorption

The proximal tubule reabsorbs over 66% of the filtered sodium, chloride, and water. Furthermore, a cotransport mechanism coupled to sodium essentially reabsorbs all of the proteins, amino acids, and glucose. The proximal tubule is also where other solutes like bicarbonate, phosphate, sulfate, magnesium, calcium, and uric acid are reabsorbed. The proximal tubule fluid exits osmotically unaltered despite these reabsorptive processes drastically reducing the volume and concentrations of particular solutes. To put it another way, even though there is a significant amount of water and solute reabsorption in the proximal tubule, the total number of solute particles (osmoles) in a kilogram of water is still the same as in the original ultrafiltrate, which is the same as the plasma in the peritubular capillaries (assuming it is made protein-free). The solute particles in the filtrate also vary greatly (e.g., more chloride and less sodium) compared to those in the initial ultrafiltrate.

In conclusion, the fluid volume has decreased by more than two-thirds as the filtrate exits the proximal tubule; important solutes such as proteins, glucose, and salts have been significantly reabsorbed either actively or passively; and the fluid's osmolality has not changed.

2.8.7. Water Reabsorption

All throughout the nephron, water is reabsorbed, except the thick and thin ascending limbs of the renal medulla's loops of Henle (Figure 2.18). Despite a significant osmotic gradient between the tubular lumen fluid and the medullary interstitium, the tubular epithelium in the ascending limbs is selectively impermeable to water. Water reabsorption in the remaining regions of the nephron is accomplished by osmosis working in concert with the tubular epithelium. The membrane or barrier that prevents water from diffusing into the interstitium (paracellular diffusion) or into the cells themselves (transcellular diffusion) is provided by the epithelium. Throughout the nephron, changes occur in the tubular epithelium's anatomic structure, particularly in the features of its intercellular spaces. The amount of water that is eventually reabsorbed by the nephron, as well as the location and timing of this absorption, are determined by these epithelial properties, which are governed by physiological demands and hormonal regulation.

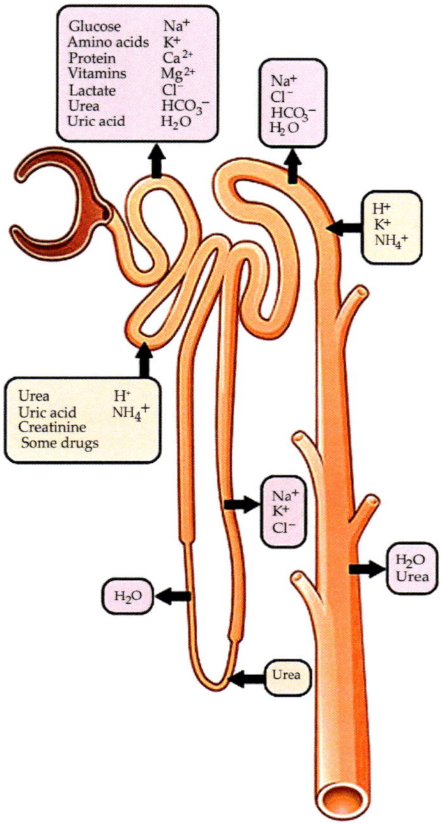

Figure 2.18. *Tubular reabsorption.*

Source: By OpenStax College – Anatomy & Physiology, Connexions Web site. http://cnx.org/content/col11496/1.6/, Jun 19, 2013., CC BY 3.0, https://commons.wikimedia.org/w/index.php?curid=30148548.

The transfer of water across a membrane from a solution with a low osmolality to one with a higher osmolality is known as osmosis. Because the cell membrane is semipermeable, some solutes can pass through it while others cannot. A gradient of osmolality (i.e., two regions with different concentrations of solute particles per volume of solvent) causes water to diffuse across the membrane to achieve an osmotic equilibrium. The massive reabsorption of water by the renal tubules is exclusively the result of this passive mechanism. The renal medulla's high solute concentration, or hypertonicity, is essential to this process because it creates the required osmotic gradient.

2.8.8. Renal Concentrating Mechanism

The renal medulla is body's only tissue that is hypertonic in comparison to normal plasma. The renal medulla (its osmolality is greater than 290 mOsm/kg). Hypertonicity gradually rises in medullary tissue; it is lowest near the border with the isosmotic cortex and highest in the renal pyramid papillary tips. All the constituents in the medullary interstitium—tissue cells, interstitial fluid, blood vessels, and blood—share this growing hypertonicity.

Two countercurrent mechanisms: (1) an "active" countercurrent multiplier mechanism occurring in the loops of Henle, and (2) a "passive" countercurrent exchange mechanism involving the vasa recta, are responsible for establishing and maintaining the gradient hypertonicity of the medullary interstitium. The name "countercurrent mechanism" refers to the perfectly symmetric parallel structures of the vasa recta and the Henle loops, which lie near one another and contain fluid flowing in opposing directions in their ascending and descending segments. The ascending limb of the loop of Henle is practically impermeable to water, actively reabsorbing sodium and chloride into the medullary interstitium (Figure 2.18). The tonicity of the interstitium rises during this active process, i.e., the lumen fluid's tonicity drops as the solute concentration rises. Water easily enters the interstitium in the descending limb at the same time that solutes—aside from urea—are not reabsorbed. As a result, the osmolality of the fluid in the descending limb and the interstitium equalize and rise above that of the fluid in the ascending limb (Figure 2.19, A). A gradient of hypertonicity forms as a result of this process, with the interstitium and the descending limb fluid getting increasingly more concentrated. Observe that the lumen fluid's intratubular osmolality difference from cortex to medulla is noticeably larger than the difference observed laterally (i.e., in ascending and descending tubules, at the same level). Countercurrent processes, in which sodium and chloride are actively reabsorbed in the ascending limb while water is passively reabsorbed in the descending limb, have essentially "multiplied" the osmotic gradient within the tubule from the cortex to the medulla.

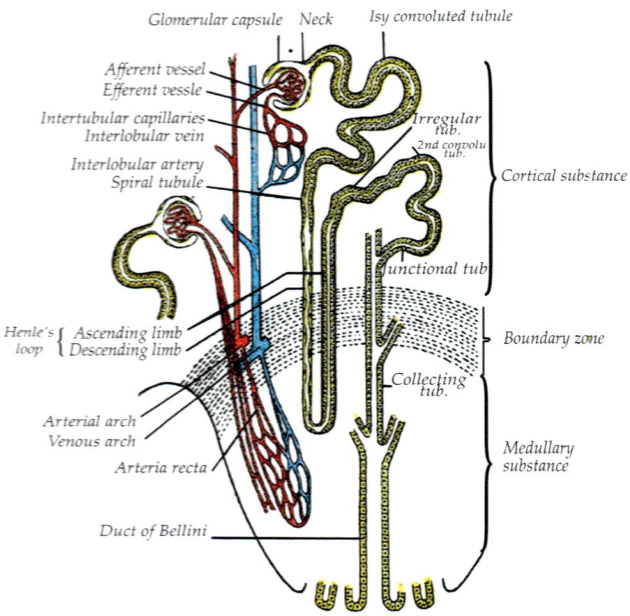

Figure 2.19. *The countercurrent mechanism.*

Source: By Henry Vandyke Carter - Henry Gray (1918) Anatomy of the Human Body (See "Book" section below) Bartleby.com: Gray's Anatomy, Plate 1128, Public Domain, https://commons.wikimedia.org/w/index.php?curid=567094.

When the lumen fluid in the loop of Henle becomes concentrated in the descending limb and then becomes diluted (by solute removal) in the ascending limb, it seems that the countercurrent multiplier mechanism has not done much at first. Overall, the fluid inside the tubular lumen is somewhat hypotonic compared to what was initially supplied to the Henle loop. However, the main function of the countercurrent multiplier mechanism is to create and preserve the gradient hypertonicity in the medullary interstitium rather than to concentrate the lumen fluid. The lumen fluid then condenses or dilutes to form the final urine when it reaches the collecting tubules, which pass through every part of the renal cortex and the medulla. The second countercurrent mechanism, on the other hand, is a "passive" exchange process that takes place in the renal medulla's deep vascular bed. Here, water and reabsorbed solutes in the medullary interstitium diffuse into the vasa recta passively. The blood's osmolality increases as it moves toward the papillary tips but gradually decreases as it ascends to the renal cortex, much like the countercurrent mechanism in the tubular lumens. Both the removal of reabsorbed water for distribution throughout the body and the supply of nutrients to medullary tissue are made possible by this vascular countercurrent mechanism. As a result, these activities also keep the renal medulla hypertonic.

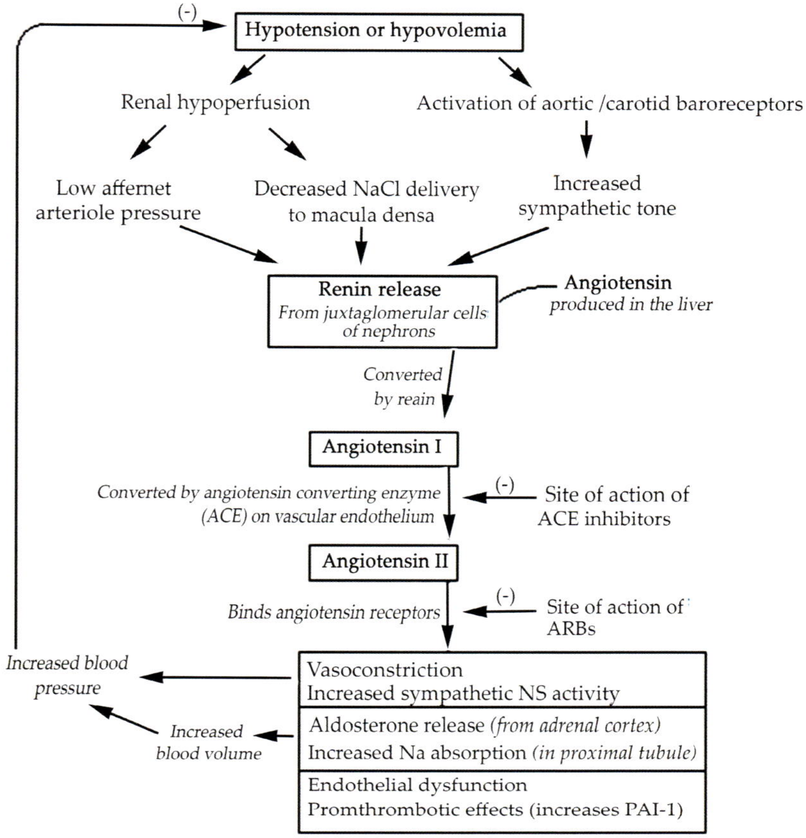

Figure 2.20. *Renin-angiotensin system-scheme.*

Source: By Npatchett - Own work, CC BY-SA 4.0, https://commons.wikimedia.org/w/index.php?curid=39235263.

The lumen fluid exiting the distal tubules is isosmotic, despite the significant solute and water exchanges occurring in the tubules until this point. The last osmolality change takes place in the collecting tubules (or ducts), the final tubular segment of the nephron; the final urine is either concentrated, diluted, or stays unchanged. It is significant to remember that the tubules selectively avoid reabsorption of water rather than secreting it.

Hormonal control governs the simultaneous processes of solute exchange and water reabsorption in the collecting tubules. Two separate and independent hormonal processes regulate the absorption of water and sodium as the isosmotic lumen fluid enters the cortical collecting tubules. For sodium reabsorption, the renin-angiotensin aldosterone system is in charge. Reduced sodium, blood volume, or blood pressure causes the juxtaglomerular apparatus to release renin into the bloodstream, as is briefly discussed in the renal circulation section and illustrated in Figure 2.20. The fast formation of angiotensin II causes the adrenal cortex to release more aldosterone. Aldosterone then causes the distal and cortical collecting tubules to begin reabsorbing sodium (Goldman and Bennet, 2000; Pincus et al., 2001; Alpem and Herbert, 2008).

ADH (arginine vasopressin) must be present for the collecting tubules to reabsorb water. The hormone ADH is produced in the hypothalamus and travels to the posterior pituitary (neurohypophysis) via the neuronal stalk, where it is released into the bloodstream. The heart's vascular baroreceptors track arterial blood pressure. The hypothalamus receives a signal when arterial blood pressure rises, which inhibits the release of ADH into the bloodstream. A negative feedback mechanism is the term for this interactive process, which is depicted in Figure 2.21. The epithelium of collecting tubules changes as the plasma level of ADH drops, which results in a decrease in the amount of water moving from the lumen fluid into the medullary tissue. As a result, water is held in the lumen fluid, which causes the urine to become diluted (hypotonic or hypo-osmotic). On the other hand, ADH release is elevated when baroreceptors detect a drop in blood pressure. ADH stimulation results in changes to the collecting tubule epithelium, increased medullary osmolality that causes increased water reabsorption, and concentrated urine that is either hyperosmotic or hypotonic. Keep in mind that reabsorption of sodium and chloride is unaffected by ADH secretion.

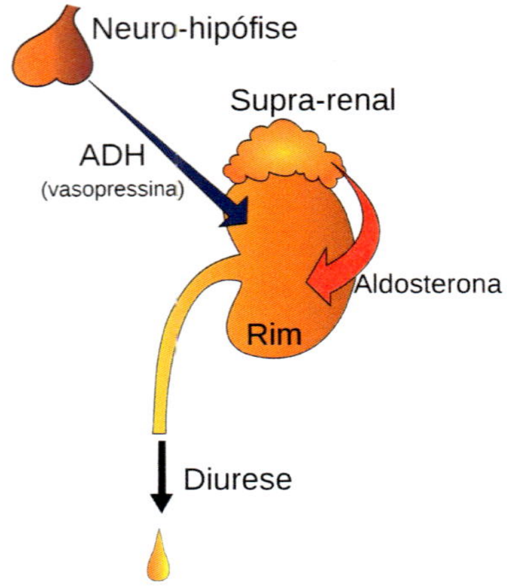

Figure 2.21. *The role of ADH.*

Source: By Rodrigo H. Castilhos – Own work, Public Domain, https://commons.wikimedia.org/w/index.php?curid=1577278.

As the lumen fluid moves deeper into the medulla toward the papillary tips, the osmolality difference between the fluid in the tubules and the medullary interstitium increases. An initial ultrafiltrate osmolality of 290 mOsm/kg in Bowman's space can be concentrated in the final urine to as high as 900 to 1400 mOsm/kg due to this enormous gradient. Urine osmolality can never be higher than that of the medullary interstitium because the final urine excreted is formed in equilibrium with the renal interstitium.

Urea cycle, which keeps the medullary concentration of urea high, is responsible for half of the solutes present. As a consequence of protein breakdown, urea readily crosses the glomerular filtration barrier and enters the tubules as ultrafiltrate. 40 to 70% of urea is passively reabsorbed into the medullary interstitium, even though it is a metabolic waste product that the body does not need. Subsequently, urea diffuses into the lumen fluid in the Henle loops along its concentration gradient. In the presence of ADH, water is reabsorbed when the lumen fluid enters the cortical collecting tubules, but urea is not. Any additional reabsorption of water helps to concentrate the amount of urea in the lumen fluid. Within the medullary collecting tubules, urea and water (influenced by ADH) easily diffuse into the interstitium when the lumen fluid reaches them. Stated differently, the collecting tubule's cortical epithelium is impervious to urea, while the medullary epithelium is easily permeable. As a result, urea diffuses into the interstitium from the concentrated lumen fluid in the medullary collecting tubules along its concentration gradient until the urea concentration in both of these regions is equal. This urea equilibrium leads to two things happening: (1) the final urine's nonurea solutes are osmotically balanced by the sodium salts in the hypertonic medulla; and (2) urea itself determines the final urine's urea concentration. Urine flow rate is another factor that influences the final urine's urea concentration. More urea is reabsorbed when urine flows slower than 2 mL/min, but urea can still be reabsorbed at constant, minimal flow rates when urine flows faster than 2 mL/min.

In conclusion, the urea cycle and the countercurrent multiplier mechanism cause the medullary interstitium to become hypertonic. The presence of ADH controls the hypertonic medulla, which is created by these two processes and offers a strong osmotic force for water reabsorption from the collecting tubules in response to physiological demands. The concentration of the final urine excreted is ultimately determined by the collecting tubules' regulation of water content, even though solutes like sodium (under aldosterone control) can be selectively reabsorbed or excreted in the distal and collecting tubules. Therefore, whether a concentrated (hypertonic) or diluted (hypotonic) final urine is produced depends on the reabsorption of water by the collecting tubules under ADH control (Goldman and Bennet, 2000; Pincus et al., 2001; Alpem and Herbert, 2008).

A Closer Look

Acid-Base Balance

To maintain the normal blood pH of 7.4, the blood must buffer and eliminate the excess acid formed by dietary intake and body metabolism. The buffering capacity of the blood depends on bicarbonate (HCO_3^-) ions, which are readily filtered by the glomerulus and must be expediently returned to the blood to maintain the proper pH. As shown in Figure 2.22, the secretion of hydrogen ions (H^+) by the renal tubular cells into the filtrate prevents the filtered bicarbonate from being excreted in the urine and causes the return of a bicarbonate ion to the plasma. This process provides for almost 100% reabsorption of filtered bicarbonate and occurs primarily in the proximal convoluted tubule.

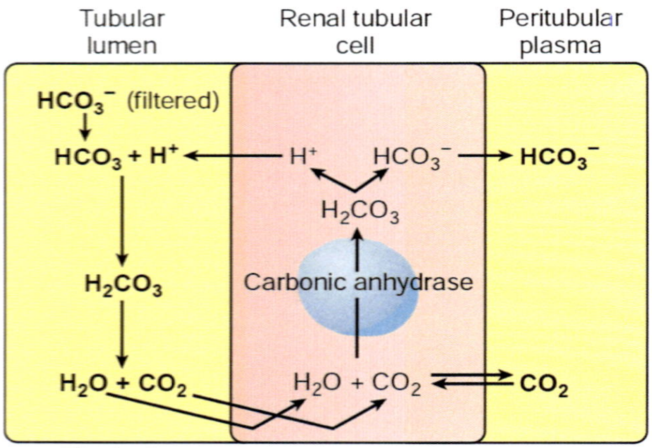

Figure 2.22. *Reabsorption of filtered bicarbonate.*

Source: Susan King Strasinger and Marjorie Schaub Di Lorenzo. Urinalysis and Body Fluids. Fifth Edition. Copyright © 2008 by F. A. Davis Company.

As a result of their small molecular size, hydrogen ions are readily filtered and reabsorbed. Therefore, the actual excretion of excess hydrogen ions also depends on tubular secretion. Figures 2.23 and 2.24 are diagrams of the two primary methods for hydrogen ion excretion in the urine. In Figure 2.23 the secreted hydrogen ion combines with a filtered phosphate ion instead of a bicarbonate ion and is excreted rather than reabsorbed. Additional excretion of hydrogen ions is accomplished through their reaction with ammonia produced and secreted by the cells of the distal convoluted tubule. In the proximal convoluted tubule, ammonia is produced from the breakdown of the amino acid glutamine. The ammonia reacts with the H^+ to form the ammonium ion (NH_4^+) (Figure 2.24). The resulting ammonium ion is excreted in the urine.

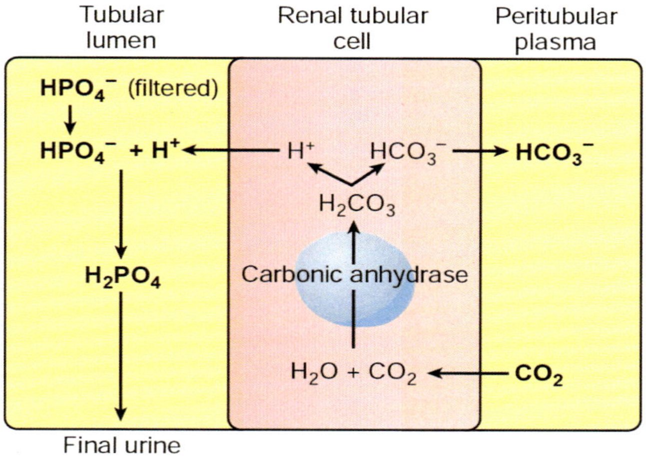

Figure 2.23. *Excretion of secreted hydrogen ions combined with phosphate.*

Source: *Susan King Strasinger and Marjorie Schaub Di Lorenzo. Urinalysis and Body Fluids. Fifth Edition. Copyright © 2008 by F. A. Davis Company.*

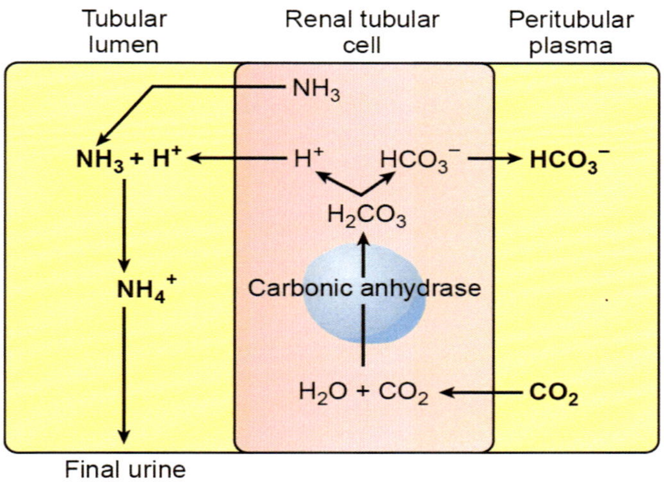

Figure 2.24. *Excretion of secreted hydrogen ions combined with ammonia produced by the tubules.*

Source: Susan King Strasinger and Marjorie Schaub Di Lorenzo. Urinalysis and Body Fluids. Fifth Edition. Copyright © 2008 by F. A. Davis Company.

All three of these processes occur simultaneously at rates determined by the acid-base balance in the body. A disruption in these secretory functions can result in metabolic acidosis or renal tubular acidosis, the inability to produce an acid urine.

Summary

- The structure of the human kidney can be seen as two reddish bean-shaped organs that are located below the rib cage on each side of the spine. They are almost a fistful in size, measuring around 10-12cm. Kidneys are the main organs in the human excretory system, which take part in the filtration of the blood before the urine is formed.
- A nephron is the basic structural and functional unit of the kidney. They are microscopic structures composed of a renal corpuscle and a renal tubule. The word nephron is derived from the Greek word – nephros, meaning kidney. There are millions of nephrons in each human kidney.
- The renal corpuscle, located in the renal cortex, is made up of a network of capillaries known as the glomerulus and the capsule, a cup-shaped chamber that surrounds it, called the glomerular or Bowman's capsule.
- The kidneys require a rich blood supply to execute their primary function of regulating the internal environment of the body. In fact, despite their mass of only 300 g, or 0.5% of the total body mass, the kidneys receive 25% of the total cardiac output. This high degree of perfusion reflects the direct relationship of the kidney's functional ability to its blood supply.
- Urine formation is the primary excretory function of the kidneys. Urine formation consists of three processes: plasma filtration at the glomeruli followed by reabsorption and secretion of selective components by the renal tubules.
- Glomerular filtration filters out most of the solutes due to high blood pressure and specialized membranes in the afferent arteriole. The blood pressure in the glomerulus is maintained independent of factors that affect systemic blood pressure.
- The tubular function is selective, reabsorbing the substances necessary for the maintenance of body homeostasis and function, such as water, salts, glucose, amino acids, and proteins, while excreting waste products such as creatinine and metabolic acids.
- Passive transport is the movement of molecules across a membrane as a result of differences in their concentration or electrical potential on opposite sides of the membrane. These physical differences are called gradients.
- Active transport, like passive transport, can be influenced by the concentration of the substance being transported. When the plasma concentration of a substance that is normally completely reabsorbed reaches an abnormally high level, the filtrate concentration exceeds the maximal reabsorptive capacity (T_m) of the tubules, and the substance begins appearing in the urine.

References

1. Alpern, R. J., & Hebert, S. C. (Eds.). (2008). *Seldin and Giebisch's the Kidney: Physiology and Pathophysiology* (4th ed.). Amsterdam: Academic Press/Elsevier.
2. Anderson, S. C., & Cockayne, S. (2003). *Clinical Chemistry: Concepts and Applications*. New York: McGraw-Hill.

3. Goldman, L., & Bennett, J. C. (Eds.). (2000). *Cecil Textbook of Medicine* (21st ed.). Philadelphia: W.B. Saunders.

4. Longmire, M., Choyke, P. L., & Kobayashi, H. (2008). Clearance properties of nano-sized particles and molecules as imaging agents: Considerations and caveats. *Nanoscience, 3*, 703–717.

5. Patton, K. T., & Thibodeau, G. A. (2010). Urinary system. In *Anatomy and Physiology* (7th ed.). St. Louis: Mosby/Elsevier.

6. Pincus, M. R., Preuss, H. G., & Henry, J. B. (2001). Evaluation of renal function, water, electrolytes, acid-base balance, and blood gases. In J. B. Henry (Ed.), *Clinical Diagnosis and Management by Laboratory Methods* (20th ed.). Philadelphia: W.B. Saunders.

7. Schrier, R. W., & Gottschalk, C. W. (2001). *Diseases of the Kidney and Urinary Tract* (7th ed.). Philadelphia: Lippincott Williams & Wilkins.

Chapter

3

RENAL FUNCTION

Contents

Introduction

The term "renal function" describes the essential role the kidneys play in preserving the body's homeostasis through the regulation of fluid balance, electrolyte levels, acid-base equilibrium, and the removal of metabolic waste products from the bloodstream.

Urine, the end result of renal function, is made up of various solutes, water, electrolytes, and metabolic waste products like urea, creatinine, and uric acid. The bladder, urethra, and ureters are the routes by which urine is eliminated from the body.

Renal function plays a crucial role in maintaining homeostasis. Renal dysfunction can result in several illnesses and imbalances, underscoring the vital role renal function plays in general health and wellbeing.

Orientation and Directional Terms

Term	Definition	Illustration
Osmolality	Osmolality indicates the concentration of all the particles dissolved in body fluid.	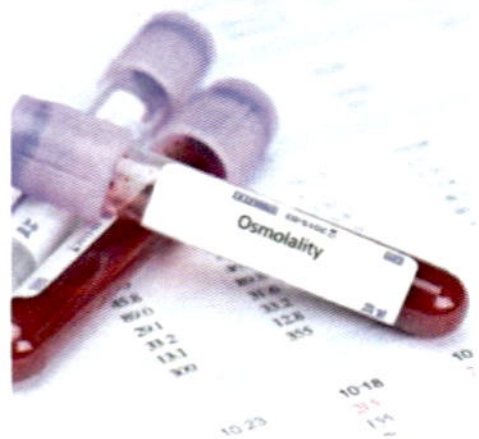
Medullary interstitium	The medullary interstitium is a tissue that surrounds the loop of Henle in the medulla of the kidney.	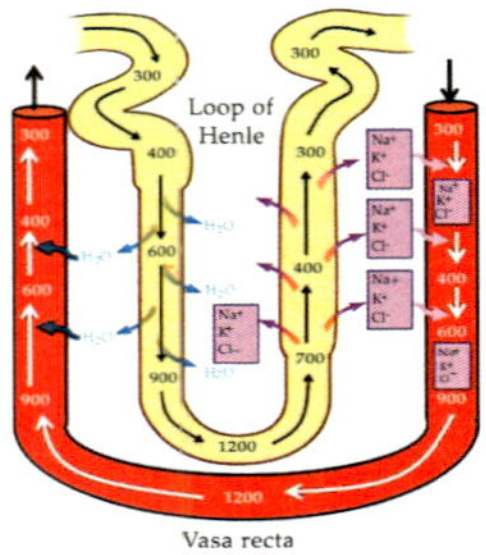
Tubules	Tubule pertains to a small tube-like structure that is lined with glandular epithelium.	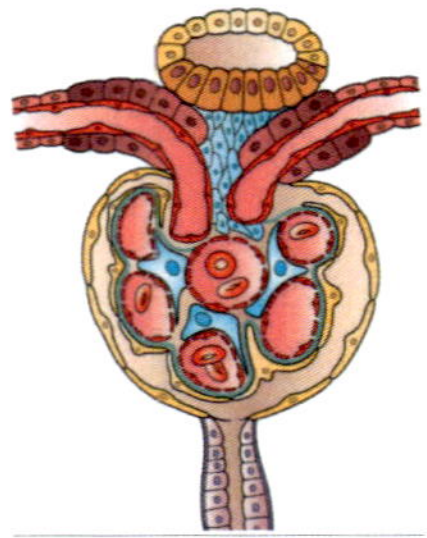
Water diuresis	Water diuresis is a condition where the kidneys filter too much bodily fluid, resulting in increased urine flow.	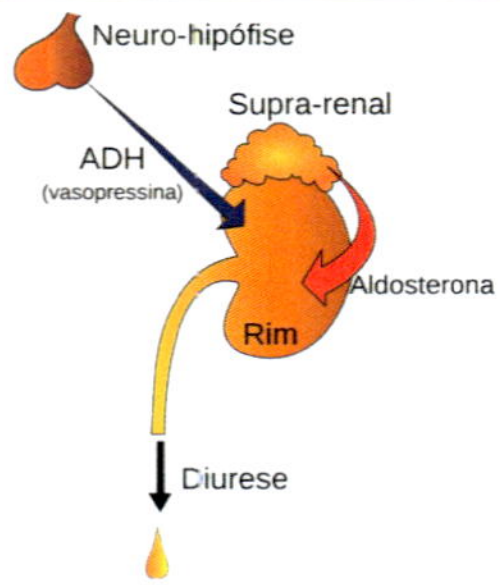
Diabetes insipidus	Diabetes insipidus (DI), also known as water diabetes, is a rare condition that causes excessive thirst and urination.	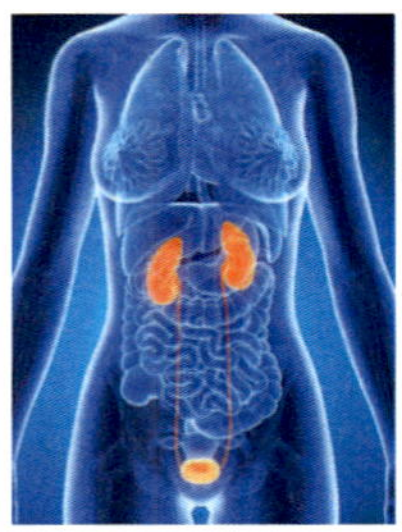

3.1. Urine Composition

The amount and type of substances found in urine can vary greatly based on factors such as diet, activity level, and overall health. Due to these variables, determining the standard values for each component in urine is challenging. Urine is a filtered form of plasma with some substances being reabsorbed and others being secreted, while the volume of water is dependent on the body's hydration level. In a healthy individual, urine will contain the unnecessary solutes and excess water from the body. Typically, urine is made up of 94% water and 6% solutes. The kidneys play a crucial role in regulating the body's fluid balance and composition by adjusting the excretion of water and solutes (Guyton and Hall textbook of medical physiology; Seldin and Giebisch's the kidney: physiology and pathophysiology; Anderson and Cockayne, 2003; Patton, 2010; Hall, 2011; Goldman-Cecil medicine, 2015).

3.2. Solute Elimination

Renal excretion is the main mechanism through which soluble metabolic wastes (e.g., salt) are eliminated, in addition to its function in selectively preserving electrolyte (e.g., organic bases and acids) and external materials (e.g., medications, radiographic contrast media). Renal excretion is not necessary for carbon dioxide and water, which are typical byproducts of the metabolism of triglycerides and carbohydrates. On the other hand, the body can only excrete soluble substances like urea, creatinine, uric acid, and other inorganic solutes through urine as a result of the metabolism of proteins and nucleic acids. Urea and creatinine, two of these compounds that are only eliminated by the kidneys, are particularly useful for tracking and assessing renal function, more especially glomerular filtration. Additionally, urine contains high concentrations of creatinine and urea, which make them useful markers for differentiating urine from other bodily fluids.

The amounts and masses of the main components of urine are compared in Table 3.1. Keep in mind that mass indicates the "weight" of a component, while amount, measured in millimoles, corresponds to the number of particles present. For instance, there are fewer inorganic phosphate molecules than there are potassium molecules, but there are actually more inorganic phosphate molecules overall. This distinction between the mass and number of solute particles is crucial because it directly affects the measurements of specific gravity and osmolality, respectively. The amount of solutes in urine is measured using osmolality and specific gravity, which indicates how well the kidneys can produce concentrated urine.

Table 3.1. Typical Design Values for the Concentrations of Constituents in Fresh Urine, Based on Data in Sweden and Switzerland

Parameter	Value
pH	6.2
Total nitrogen	8830 mg/L
Ammonium/ammonia-N	460 mg/L
Nitrate and nitrite	0.06 mg/L
Chemical oxygen demand	6000 mg/L
Total phosphorus	800 – 2000 mg/L
Potassium	2740 mg/L
Sulphate	1500 mg/L
Sodium	3450 mg/L
Magnesium	120 mg/L
Chloride	4970 mg/L
Calcium	230 mg/L

However, it is important to note that lesser amounts

* Average 24-hour urine volume with a glomerular filtration rate of 125 mL/min.

Source: https://en.wikipedia.org/wiki/Urine.

3.3. Measurements of Solute Concentration

3.3.1. Osmolality

The concentration of a solution, measured in osmoles of solute particles per kilogram of solvent, is known as osmolality. A substance's dissociation amount in a solution that yields one mole of particles (6.023×10^{23} particles, Avogadro's number) is known as an osmole (Osm). The unit of measurement most commonly used to describe solute concentrations in bodily fluids is milliosmole (mOsm). One millimole (mmol) of particles "in solution" is known as a mOsm. Since urea in solution, for instance, does not dissociate, 1 mmol of urea (60 mg) is equal to 1 mOsm. On the other hand, one mmol of NaCl (58 mg) is equal to two mOsm because NaCl in solution dissociates into two particles, Na^+ ions and Cl^- ions. Put differently, because of dissociation, the osmolality of a 1 mmol/L NaCl solution is roughly twice that of a 1 mmol/L urea solution. Water serves as the solvent in urine, while additional solutes secreted by the renal tubules and particles that cross the filtration barrier and are not reabsorbed make up the solute particles.

Although albumin and other high-molecular-weight solutes found in the bloodstream are absent from the ultrafiltrate in Bowman's space, it contains the same solute composition as the plasma. As a result, this initial filtrate's osmolality is equal to that of the plasma, which is why it is referred to as isosmotic. The filtrate's solute composition (type and concentration) varies continuously as it passes through the nephron's tubules. On the other hand, until the filtrate reaches the thin descending limb of the loop of Henle, the osmolality stays constant (isosmotic at $\approx$300 mOsm). The filtrate in the Henle loops gradually becomes hyperosmotic in the descending limb and hypoosmotic in the ascending limb due to the countercurrent multiplier mechanism. Upon entering the distal tubules, the filtrate exhibits a slight hypoosmotic condition ($\approx$100 mOsm).

The distal tubules and collecting ducts are where urine's ultimate osmolality is measured. When antidiuretic hormone (ADH) is present, the hypertonic concentration gradient in the surrounding medullary interstitium facilitates the reabsorption of water. The filtrate once more becomes isosmotic ($\approx$300 mOsm) in the distal tubules when ADH is present, matching the hypertonicity of the cortical interstitium. If ADH is present, the filtrate's osmolality can rise further as it moves through the collecting tubules (as water is absorbed) until it reaches the same level as the surrounding hypertonic medullary interstitium. Keep in mind that the medullary interstitium's osmolality determines the maximum urine osmolality that can be achieved, which is 1200 to 1400 mOsm/kg. Until an osmotic equilibrium is reached, the collecting tubules can only passively reabsorb water without exchanging solutes (Figure 3.1).

A random urine specimen's osmolality can range from 50 mOsm/kg to 1400 mOsm/kg. Its osmolality typically ranges from one to three times (275 to 900 mOsm/kg) that of serum (275 to 300 mOsm/kg) in normal conditions. U/S, or urine-to-serum osmolality ratio, is a useful measure of the kidneys' capacity to concentrate urine. Normal people have an average fluid intake, and their U/S ratio falls between 1 and 3.

The kidneys modify the amount of water in which solutes are eliminated, which alters the osmolality of urine. An individual must excrete 100–1200 mOsm of solutes daily on a typical American diet. However, a higher volume of urine is needed to excrete the increased solute load from diets high in protein and salt. Certain illnesses (e.g., diabetes mellitus) can generate up to

5000 mOsm of solutes per day for excretion. As a result, it takes a lot of water to eliminate them in the urine. Enough fluid intake is required because the kidneys cannot directly replace excessive water loss. As a result, these people have extreme thirst, or polydipsia, to keep the water balance and eliminate the required solutes.

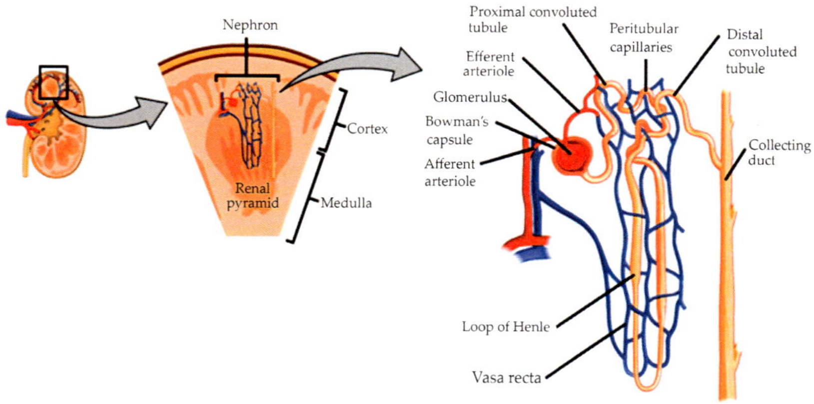

Figure. 3.1. *The nephron is the functional unit of the kidney. The glomerulus and convoluted tubules are located in the kidney cortex, while collecting ducts are located in the pyramids of the medulla.*

Source: https://courses.lumenlearning.com/suny-dutchess-ap1/chapter/nephrons-structure/.

3.3.2. Specific Gravity

Another way to express the concentration of a solute is its specific gravity (SG), which compares the density of urine to that of an equivalent volume of pure water. Urine specific gravity measurements are always greater than 1 point000 because specific gravity is a ratio that compares the mass of the solutes present in urine to pure water. Similar to osmolality, the initial ultrafiltrate in Bowman's space has a specific gravity of 1.010, which is the same as protein-free plasma. The specific gravity of the filtrate varies as it moves through the tubules and solute exchange takes place. The normal range of urine specific gravity values is between 1.002 and 1.035. The filtrate's final concentration (SG >1.010) or dilution (SG <1.010) during the nephrons' passage is indicated by the SG value. Similar to osmolality, urine specific gravity is based on the quantity of water and solutes eliminated; this is influenced by a person's fluid intake and level of hydration.

Specific gravity and osmolality have a close but nonlinear relationship because density is dependent on the quantity and relative mass of solute particles present. In healthy individuals, this relationship is largely stable; however, in certain conditions, the excretion of high-molecular-weight solutes, like glucose, urea, or proteins, causes this relationship to disappear. The specific gravity values of water with added NaCl, urea, and glucose are displayed in Table 3.2. Every solute addition corresponds to nearly the same quantity of particles—roughly 5.2 x 10^{23} particles—added to the solution. Observe that even when the same number of particles are present, the specific gravity value varies. This happens as a result of the impact that solute mass has on various specific gravity calculation techniques. Refractive index and reagent strip measurements measure density indirectly, while the urinometer—a method dating back centuries—is a direct indicator of density (Figure 3.2).

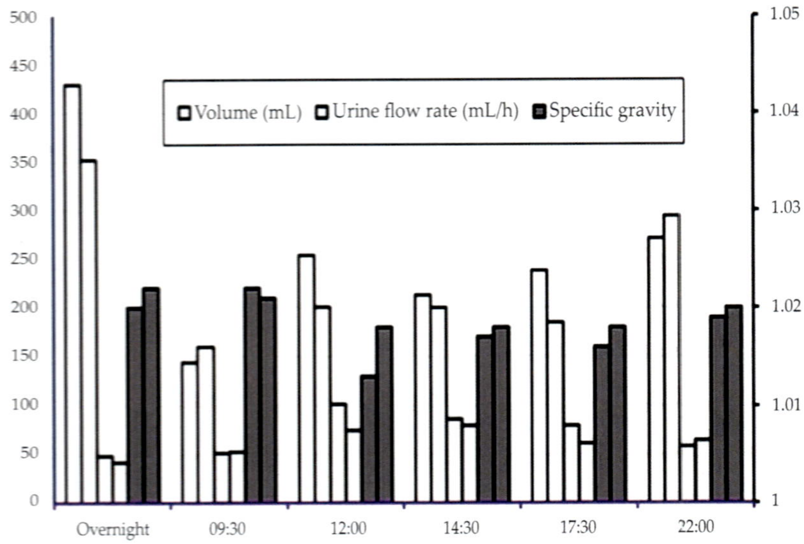

Figure 3.2. *A comparison of urine specific gravity and urine osmolality.*

Source: Sallsten G, Barregard L. Variability of Urinary Creatinine in Healthy Individuals. International Journal of Environmental Research and Public Health. 2021; 18(6):3166. https://doi.org/10.3390/ijerph18063166.

Table 3.2. Urine Characters

Characteristic	Normal values
Color	Pale yellow to deep amber
Odor	Odorless
Volume	750–2000 mL/24 hour
pH	4.5–8.0
Specific gravity	1.003–1.032
Osmolarity	40–1350 mOsmol/kg
Urobilinogen	0.2–1.0 mg/100 mL
White blood cells	0–2 HPF (per high-power field of microscope)
Leukocyte esterase	None
Protein	None or trace
Bilirubin	<0.3 mg/100 mL
Ketones	None
Nitrites	None
Blood	None
Glucose	None

Source: https://open.oregonstate.education/aandp/chapter/25-8-urine-transport-and-elimination/.

The "actual" specific gravity of urine will rise significantly when large-molecular-weight solutes like protein, urea, or glucose are present, irrespective of the technique employed, in contrast to small solutes like sodium or chloride ions.

Urine specimens may occasionally have a specific gravity value of $\geq$1.050, which is much higher than what is physiologically feasible ($\approx$1.040). In these specimens, there should be a suspicion of the excretion of a high molecular weight substance, such as mannitol or radiopaque contrast media (x-ray dye). Patients receive these exogenous substances intravenously, and they are eliminated through urine. They do not signify a disorder or disease process; rather, they are thought of as a urine contaminant. It should be noted that these urine specimens have normal osmolality values despite having specific gravity results that are physiologically impossible. This is because the "number" of solutes present is the only factor that affects osmolality values, and there are not enough of these high-molecular-weight solutes in relation to all the other solutes in the urine (e.g., urea, sodium). Put another way, the mass of solutes present is important and influences the specific gravity of urine, but their quantity is insufficient to have a noticeable impact on the osmolality of urine. These urine samples are deemed unfit for analysis because they are contaminated. When the prescribed amount of time has elapsed and the exogenous substance is no longer being eliminated, a fresh specimen ought to be obtained.

Urine concentration is measured using physical attributes such as specific gravity and osmolality. Urine osmolality measures only the total number of solutes present, independent of solute type, while specific gravity measures the mass and number of solutes combined in the urine (Guyton and Hall textbook of medical physiology; Seldin and Giebisch's the kidney: physiology and pathophysiology; Anderson and Cockayne, 2003; Patton, 2010; Hall, 2011; Goldman-Cecil medicine, 2015).

3.4. Urine Volume

To maintain balance, the kidneys must produce a daily urine volume of at least 500mL to eliminate 600 to 700 mOsm of solutes. The kidneys adjust their urine volume based on the body's water intake and metabolic processes to achieve water homeostasis. When the body lacks water or is dehydrated, the kidneys excrete solutes in a minimal urine volume. Conversely, when the body has excess water, the kidneys excrete solutes in a larger volume of urine, up to 25 L/day.

The excretion of more than three liters of urine per day is known as polyuria. If urine osmolality is less than >200 mOsm/kg, the causes of polyuria can be classified into two categories based on diagnostic criteria: (1) conditions with water diuresis and (2) conditions with solute diuresis (urine osmolality greater than $\geq$300 mOsm/kg). An assessment flowchart for polyuria is offered by Figure 3.3. There is one common factor among conditions that cause water diuresis: ADH. ADH secretion is insufficient or ADH's effect on the renal receptors is ineffective in these disorders. Solute diuresis, on the other hand, is associated with conditions that typically involve glucose, urea, or sodium but lack a common feature.

The Greek word diabainein, which means "to pass through or siphon," is where the terms diabetes mellitus and diabetes insipidus originate. The term refers to the excessive amounts of urine that people with these conditions produce. Both conditions share intense thirst (polydipsia) and large volumes of urine excretion (polyuria), despite being completely different. Diabetes mellitus is a disorder of the metabolism of carbohydrates that is caused by insufficient insulin secretion or utilization, which leads to the excretion of glucose in the urine. Diabetes insipidus is a condition marked by decreased ADH function or production, which makes it difficult to regulate the excretion of water in the urine.

Urine production can also be reduced by other conditions like renal tubular dysfunction, urinary obstruction, or additional fluid loss. The word "oliguria," which is defined as a daily urine volume of less than 400 mL/day, is frequently used to characterize these conditions. A typical daily solute load cannot be eliminated with this volume of urine, and if it is left untreated, death will result. The condition is known as anuria, and if treatment is not received, death is likely to occur. Anuria typically appears gradually following an initial presentation of oliguria in progressive renal disease. A sharp drop in renal perfusion can result in anuria very quickly (e.g., hemorrhage, shock) or as a result of abrupt, severe kidney damage.

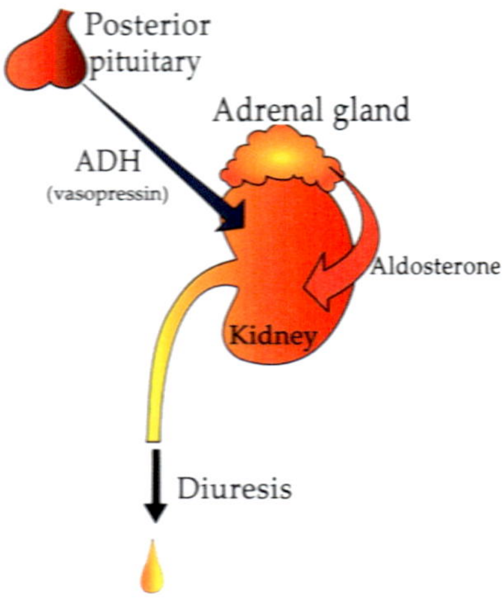

Figure 3.3. *Polyuria.*

Source: By Rodrigo H. Castilhos - Own work, Public Domain, https://commons.wikimedia.org/w/index.php?curid=1577278.

The amount of urine eliminated in a 24-hour period can range from roughly 500 to 1800 mL. The amount of solutes consumed, the amount of fluid consumed, and the activity of ADH are all reflected in this total daily volume. Urine volume, however, can increase to up to 15 times normal when renal and metabolic diseases are present, or it can decrease to zero output (anuria) (Guyton and Hall textbook of medical physiology; Seldin and Giebisch's the kidney: physiology and pathophysiology; Anderson and Cockayne, 2003; Patton, 2010; Hall, 2011; Goldman-Cecil medicine, 2015).

3.5. Assessment of Renal Concentrating Ability/Tubular Reabsorptive Function

3.5.1. Osmolality Versus Specific Gravity

Osmolality and specific gravity are ways to measure the amount of solutes in a liquid. These values can change in urine based on how much water and solutes are being excreted. Therefore, a simple test to check kidney function and water conservation ability is to see if the tubules can produce concentrated urine, indicated by an osmolality greater than 800 mOsm/kg or a specific gravity higher than 1.025.

For the assessment of renal concentrating ability, osmolality determinations are preferred even though they are simpler and take less time to complete. Since every solute particle contributes equally to the osmolality value, as was previously mentioned, osmolality measurements are thought to be a more accurate assessment. Specific gravity measurements, on the other hand, compare densities and are more influenced by some solutes than by others. Remember from Table 3.1 that sodium, chloride, and urea are the three most common solutes found in urine. Both active and passive tubular transport mechanisms selectively reabsorb sodium and chloride throughout the nephrons.

Consequently, keeping an eye on the sodium and chloride concentrations in urine provides insight into the kidney's capacity to concentrate and process ultrafiltrate. On the other hand, because urea is only passively processed in the nephrons, it is not a reliable measure of the kidney's capacity to concentrate urine (i.e., urea cycle), and the amount of this exchange fluctuates depending on many variables (e.g., flow rate in tubes).

Osmolality measurements are superior to specific gravity measurements in evaluating the kidneys' capacity to concentrate because small amounts of high-molecular-weight solutes, such as e. g., protein, and glucose) will influence specific gravity readings but not osmolality readings. In the proximal tubules, solutes like protein and glucose are practically totally reabsorbed. Rather than a shift in the kidney's capacity to concentrate urine, their presence in urine is indicative of a disease process. Urine containing glucose and protein has a relatively constant osmolality, in contrast to specific gravity measurements. Due to the high molecular weight of the protein and glucose in such urine, the density is greatly increased; however, the increase in particle numbers is negligible in comparison to the total solutes present. It should be noted that a change in specific gravity signifies a shift in solute density, not always a sign of a change in the kidney's capacity to concentrate urine. Furthermore, because osmolality increases in direct proportion to an increase in solute number, regardless of the type of solute, it is preferred over specific gravity measurements.

The tubular concentrating ability gradually decreases in certain chronic renal diseases until the urine's specific gravity and osmolality become fixed or unchanging. The ultrafiltrate's solute concentration doesn't change because the tubules can no longer actively reabsorb and secrete particular solutes from it as it passes through the nephron. Urine therefore has the same osmolality and specific gravity as the original ultrafiltrate in Bowman's space, with an osmolality of roughly 300 mOsm/kg (i.e., 1.010) and a specific gravity of 1.010. i.e., the same as plasma devoid of proteins). A common characteristic of chronic renal diseases is the fixation of the urine solute composition, which results in polyuria and nocturia, or excessive nighttime urination.

While nocturia is typically associated with renal disease, it can also occur in conditions where the bladder's capacity is reduced (e.g., pregnancy, kidney stones, prostate enlargement), or just drinking a lot of fluids at night.

Urine concentration is measured using nonspecific tests such as specific gravity and osmolality. All they can do is point to or corroborate a possible decline in renal function. These tests are unable to identify the underlying issue, which could be renal disease, diabetes insipidus, or the side effects of diuretic therapy.

3.5.2. Fluid Deprivation Tests

As shown in Figure 3.3, polyuria caused by water diuresis may occur due to either excessive water consumption or conditions affecting ADH (vasopressin). In cases where ADH production or secretion is deficient, it is known as neurogenic diabetes insipidus. On the other hand, when there is a lack of response in the kidneys to ADH, it is referred to as nephrogenic diabetes insipidus. To determine the underlying cause of water diuresis, a fluid deprivation test can be conducted.

The capacity of renal tubular cells to selectively absorb and secrete solutes is assessed using a fluid deprivation test. Put another way, it evaluates the renal capacity for renal concentration. The patient is not allowed to drink any more water during this test, and the urine's concentration is measured on a timed basis. According to standard protocol, the patient has a regular evening meal and then abstains from all liquids from 6 PM until 8 AM the following day. Urine is taken at eight in the morning, and its osmolality is measured. The test is over if the urine osmolality is more than 800 mOsm/kg, which indicates that the kidneys' capacity for renal concentrating is normal.

If the osmolality level is lower than 800 mOsm/kg, fluid deprivation will continue. At 10 AM, both serum and urine samples will be collected for osmolality tests. If the urine osmolality is higher than 800 mOsm/kg or the U/S ratio is greater than 3.0, it shows normal renal concentrating ability and the test will stop. If neither condition is met, ADH will be given subcutaneously and at 2 PM and 6 PM, more samples will be collected for osmolality testing. The test will end at 6 PM regardless of the patient's response. A positive response to ADH means the urine osmolality is higher than 800 mOsm/kg or the U/S ratio is 3.0 or more, indicating the kidneys can respond to ADH but there is inadequate production of ADH by the patient (a neurogenic issue). A negative response to ADH indicates a nephrogenic issue, where the renal receptors for ADH are not functioning properly.

Urine specific gravity measurements are used in other tests that evaluate renal concentrating ability. The patient in the Fishberg concentration test follows the previously mentioned fluid deprivation protocol. Urine samples are taken and their specific gravities are ascertained at predetermined intervals. The test is over if the urine specific gravity reaches 1.025 or higher, indicating normal renal concentrating ability.

In contrast to the tests that have already been covered, Mosenthal's test calls for a unique 24-hour urine collection while allowing patients to continue with their regular dietary and hydration regimen. The 12-hour day portion and the 12-hour night portion of the 24-hour urine collection are two distinct 12-hour urine collections, which makes it unique. It is determined the specific gravity and volume of each 12-hour urine collection. A daytime urine volume that is greater than the nighttime volume and a nighttime urine specific gravity of 1.020 or higher are indicators of a normal Mosenthal test.

3.5.3. Osmolar and Free-Water Clearance

Measuring the clearance of water and solutes not reabsorbed by the kidneys by comparing renal clearance of solutes with solute-free water clearance can provide valuable diagnostic information to clinicians. This requires measuring osmolality in timed urine and serum samples, and calculating the osmolar clearance (C_{Osm}) by multiplying the ratio of urine osmolality to serum osmolality by the timed urine volume. This information can help differentiate between diseases like neurogenic diabetes insipidus and nephrogenic diabetes insipidus.

$$C_{Osm}\ (\text{mL plasma per minute}) = \frac{U_{Osm}\ (\text{mOsm/kg})}{S_{Osm}\ (\text{mOsm/kg})} \times V\ (\text{mL/min}) \quad (1)$$

where V is the amount of urine excreted per minute, S_{Osm} is the serum osmolality, and U is the urine osmolality. The amount of plasma water (in milliliters) removed by the kidneys in a minute is known as the osmolar clearance, or C_{Osm}. The normal range for fasting osmolar clearance values is 2 to 3 mL/min, and it is independent of urine flow.

The two distinct volumes that make up the total volume (V) of urine eliminated by the kidneys are solute-free water (CH_2O) and osmolar clearance water (C_{Osm}).

$$V\ (\text{mL/min}) = C_{Osm}\ (\text{mL/min}) + C_{H_2O}\ (\text{mL/min}) \quad (2)$$

The amount of water needed to remove the solutes from plasma is known as the osmolar clearance water (C_{Osm}), while extra water that is consumed more than what the body requires is known as solute-free water (CH_2O), which is then excreted in urine through the tubules.

It is clear from Equation 1 that the total urine volume (V) must equal the osmolar clearance volume ($V=C_{Osm}$) for the urine and plasma to be isosmotic ($U_{Osm} = S_{Osm}$). The solute-free water clearance (CH_2O) is zero at this point. By rearrangement, the solute-free or free-water clearance (CH_2O) can be found.

$$C_{H_2O}\ (mL/min) = V\ (mL/min) - C_{Osm}\ (mL/min) \quad (3)$$

The U_{Osm} is lower than the S_{Osm} and the total volume of urine cleared (V) is higher than the osmolar clearance water (C_{Osm}) when urine is diluted due to water diuresis. The urine is hypoosmotic or hypotonic as a result, and the solute-free water clearance (CH_2O), which measures excess water elimination, is positive. The total urine volume (V) cleared is less than the osmolar clearance water when the U_{Osm} is greater than the S_{Osm}, which happens with dehydration. Consequently, the solute-free water clearance is negative. The kidneys are reabsorbing water and producing hyperosmotic or hypertonic urine when there is a negative free-water clearance.

It is crucial to remember that urea is the main solute in urine that contributes to its osmolality, while sodium and chloride ions are the main cause in serum. Because of this, the only uses for osmolar and free-water clearances are to determine the volume and concentration of urine solutes. When figuring out the cause of polyuria or diuresis, these clearances are useless.

Water excretion is controlled by the kidneys to preserve the body's overall fluid homeostasis. Unwanted solutes must be removed with a certain amount of water, and any extra water can be removed or reabsorbed. The kidneys' primary function is to maintain normal plasma osmolality, which is accomplished by the selective removal and reabsorption of water and solutes.

3.6. Assessment of Glomerular Filtration

3.6.1. Renal Clearance

Adequate renal plasm flow (RPF) through the glomeruli is necessary for the kidneys to eliminate metabolic wastes and selectively reabsorb water and solutes. The amount of plasma ultrafiltrate processed by the kidney's nephrons is determined by the RPF. The urine excretion volume and composition are directly influenced by the amount of renal plasma that the glomeruli filter. The renal tubules actively and selectively remove some plasma solutes for excretion from the peritubular capillaries where the portion of the plasma that does not pass the glomerular filtration barriers flows. A solute's concentration in urine can be linked to the renal processing of a volume of plasma when it is filtered but not secreted or absorbed by the nephrons. This volume of plasma, measured in milliliters, that is totally cleared of a material per unit of time is known as renal clearance.

Renal clearance tests offer a quick and reasonably simple approach to evaluate a patient's renal status because renal disease is frequently a slow process and large amounts of renal tissue can become nonfunctional before the disease is discovered. The ability of the kidneys to remove a substance from the blood can be ascertained by measuring the concentration of the substance in the plasma and in a timed urine specimen. Renal clearance (C), which is this capacity, is calculated as follows:

$$C\ (mL/min) = \frac{U\ (mg/dL) \times V\ (mL/min)}{P\ (mg/dL)} \quad (4)$$

V represents the amount of urine eliminated during the scheduled collection (mL/min), U denotes the substance concentration in the urine (e.g., mg/dL) in the scheduled collection, P is the drug's concentration in plasma (or serum) (e.g., mg/dL) that were gathered throughout the timed interval, and C represents the drug's renal clearance (mL/min). Keep in mind that in order for the renal clearance equation to work, the units for the plasma and urine concentrations must match. For the majority of substances, a 24-hour timed collection is recommended; however, it is required for analytes or physiological functions that exhibit diurnal variations.

3.6.2. Clearance Tests

A clearance test can help assess renal blood flow as well as tubular reabsorption, tubular secretion, and glomerular filtration. It is necessary to use drugs with well-established and strictly restricted renal excretion modes to assess each of these renal functions. For instance, compounds that are only eliminated through glomerular filtration (e.g., GFR) can be calculated using glomerular filtration rate (GFR) as an example. However, materials eliminated exclusively through renal tubular secretion (e.g., p-aminohippurate, and phenolsulfonphthalein) are used to evaluate the nephrons' solute-processing capacity.

The majority of clearance tests are carried out in a clinical laboratory to assess GFR. Theoretically, GFR can be ascertained by any substance that: (1) keeps the plasma level constant; (2) is eliminated only by glomerular filtration; and (3) is not secreted or reabsorbed by the tubules. Finding the perfect material for measuring GFR is still a challenge, though.

It is possible to run clearance tests using endogenous (e.g., urea, and creatinine) or external materials. Many exogenous agents have been tested to find a straightforward, accurate, and safe way to measure GFR. These exogenous materials can be separated into two groups: those that have a radioisotope label (inulin, iohexol, and iothalamate) and those that do not (^{51}CrEDTA [chromium ethylenediaminetetraacetic acid], ^{125}I-iothalamate, and ^{125}I-diatrizoate). A single (bolus) intravenous injection or a subcutaneous injection have taken the place of the ongoing intravenous infusion due to more recent methods utilizing exogenous agents. Exogenous substances offer a more precise way to measure GFR, but these clearance tests are more costly, time-consuming, and uncomfortable for the patient. The GFR that is obtained through a clearance test is commonly known as the measured GFR, or mGFR. In contrast, when one or more biomarkers and an equation are used to "estimate" the GFR (e.g., eGFR, an acronym for creatinine, cystatin C, is utilized.

3.6.2.1. Inulin Clearance

Even though it's not often used in clinical settings, the inulin clearance test is still the gold standard for determining GFR. Since the gastrointestinal tract is unable to absorb inulin, an exogenous nontoxic fructopolysaccharide with a molecular weight of 5200, it must be injected intravenously both prior to and during the test. Since inulin is not altered by the body, it easily gets past the glomerular filtration barriers without being secreted or reabsorbed by the renal tubules. Even though inulin is the best substance to measure GFR, routine or periodic GFR measurements cannot be achieved by conducting an inulin clearance test.

3.6.2.2. Creatinine Clearance

The goal has been to find an endogenous substance with a renal clearance similar to inulin to eliminate the drawbacks associated with exogenous agents. Due to their high urinary concentrations and simplicity of measurement, urea and creatinine have been thoroughly studied. On the other hand, urea is reabsorbed by the tubules, and the urine flow rate directly influences the concentration of urea. Furthermore, diet has an impact on plasma urea levels. Urea clearances are therefore rarely done and are imprecise and inaccurate. On the other hand, creatinine is not impacted by urine flow rate, is not reabsorbed by the renal tubules, and is not changed by a typical diet when it comes to plasma levels. As a result, the most popular clearance test for regular GFR evaluation is the creatinine clearance test. Patients find this test to be inconvenient because the most accurate creatinine clearance can only be obtained through a 24-hour urine collection. Studies conducted recently have shown the importance and practical utility of estimating GFR (eGFR) to identify and track kidney disease.

It has been known since 1938 that the clearance of creatinine and inulin are nearly identical. Creatinine is a byproduct of phosphocreatine and creatine metabolism in muscles. It is produced steadily, which maintains both the plasma concentration and the rate of excretion of urine. Because creatinine production is directly correlated with muscle mass, it is affected by the patient's age, gender, and level of physical activity. Specifically, males and muscular female athletes produce higher levels of creatinine than non-athletic females, children, or the elderly. The normalization of creatinine clearance values to the external body surface area of an average individual is necessary due to the dependence of these values on individual muscle mass. This is achieved by dividing the calculated body surface area of the patient by the average individual's body surface area, or 1.73 m^2 /SA, in the computation of the normalized creatinine clearance (C) (Equations 4 and 5).

$$C\,(mL/min) = \frac{U \times V}{P} \times \frac{1.73\,m^2}{SA} \quad (5)$$

where SA is the patient's body surface area, P is the creatinine concentration in plasma, V is the amount of urine excreted in milliliters per minute, and U is the creatinine concentration in urine.

The patient's height and weight are used to calculate their body surface area. It can be computed using the following equation or obtained from a nomogram.

$$\log SA = (0.425 \times \log W) + (0.725 \times \log H) - 2.144 \quad (6)$$

where W represents the patient's weight (mass) in kilograms, H is the patient's height in centimeters, and SA is the body surface area in square meters.

The creatinine clearance test's normalization allows comparison of clearance outcomes (i.e., GFR) in comparison to those of other people, irrespective of the patient's body surface area. Based on age and gender, Table 3.3 provides typical reference intervals for creatinine clearance and serum creatinine levels.

3.6.2.3. Advantages and Disadvantages

It is quick and simple to measure creatinine in urine and serum (or plasma), and each measurement method's accuracy and dependability are well-established and verified.

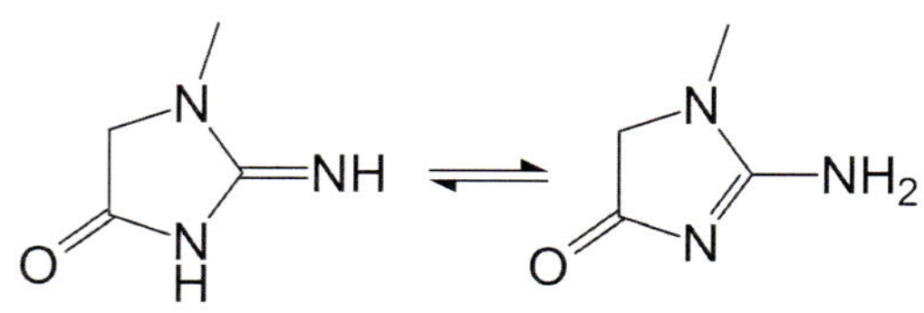

Figure 3.4 *Creatinine.*

Source: By Original: Ben Mills (Benjah-bmm27) Vector: gesamtszenario - Own work based on: Creatinine-tautomerism-2D-skeletal.png by Ben Mills (Benjah-bmm27), Public Domain, https://commons.wikimedia.org/w/index.php?curid=126318673.

The creatinine clearance test has a few drawbacks despite its benefits that need to be fixed to guarantee accurate results interpretation. Actually, the renal tubules(≈7% to 10%) secrete a tiny quantity of creatinine. (Figure 3.4).

Table 3.3 Creatinine Levels

Groups		Number of individuals	Mean ± SD	P2.5	P97.5
Age	**Sex**				
Infant (1–12 months)	M	2,227	0.26 ± 0.07	0.12	0.39
	F	1,527	0.25 ± 0.07	0.11	0.39
1–2 years	M	1,653	0.29 ± 0.07	0.15	0.42
	F	1,367	0.29 ± 0.07	0.15	0.42
2–3 years	M	1,230	0.33 ± 0.07	0.19	0.46
	F	1,012	0.31 ± 0.07	0.17	0.45
3–4 years	M	1,011	0.35 ± 0.07	0.21	0.49
	F	824	0.34 ± 0.07	0.20	0.48
4–5 years	M	946	0.37 ± 0.07	0.23	0.51
	F	708	0.37 ± 0.07	0.23	0.50
5–6 years	M	842	0.39 ± 0.07	0.25	0.53
	F	662	0.38 ± 0.07	0.24	0.52
6–7 years	M	723	0.42 ± 0.08	0.26	0.57
	F	565	0.41 ± 0.08	0.25	0.56
7–8 years	M	602	0.44 ± 0.08	0.28	0.59
	F	495	0.44 ± 0.08	0.28	0.60
8–9 years	M	559	0.46 ± 0.08	0.30	0.61
	F	454	0.46 ± 0.08	0.30	0.61
9–10 years	M	519	0.49 ± 0.08	0.33	0.63
	F	452	0.47 ± 0.08	0.31	0.62
10–11 years	M	491	0.52 ± 0.08	0.36	0.68
	F	371	0.49 ± 0.07	0.35	0.63
11–12 years	M	496	0.54 ± 0.09	0.36	0.71
	F	381	0.51 ± 0.09	0.33	0.70
12–13 years	M	517	0.58 ± 0.10	0.38	0.78
	F	399	0.54 ± 0.09	0.36	0.73
13–14 years	M	487	0.64 ± 0.11	0.42	0.85
	F	397	0.58 ± 0.08	0.42	0.74
14–15 years	M	465	0.72 ± 0.11	0.50	0.94

	F	419	0.61 ± 0.09	0.43	0.79
15–16 years	M	619	0.79 ± 0.12	0.55	1.02
	F	550	0.62 ± 0.10	0.42	0.81
16–17 years	M	726	0.82 ± 0.12	0.58	1.05
	F	708	0.63 ± 0.09	0.45	0.82
17–18 years	M	1,278	0.84 ± 0.11	0.62	1.05
	F	1,229	0.64 ± 0.09	0.46	0.82

Source: Chuang G-T, Tsai I-J and Tsau Y-K (2021) Serum Creatinine Reference Limits in Pediatric Population—A Single Center Electronic Health Record-Based Database in Taiwan. Front. Pediatr. 9:793446. doi: 10.3389/fped.2021.793446

Because of this secretion, the urine excretion concentration (U in Equation 4) is elevated, leading to an overestimation of the GFR. However, this increase is negated when creatinine is measured using the widely used, nonspecific alkaline picrate method (Jaffe reaction). The plasma creatinine result (P in Equation 4) is likewise overestimated due to the reaction of plasma noncreatinine chromogens by this method. Thankfully, these two effects cancel each other out, and there is a strong correlation between the inulin and creatinine clearances. When more specific creatinine methods (e.g., enzymatic) are employed, these elements don't cancel one another out. In the latter instance, tubular secretion causes the urine creatinine to be overestimated but not the measured plasma creatinine. Consequently, the clearance results do not compare as well to the inulin clearance, and the creatinine clearance (C in Equation 4) is overestimated.

Individuals whose renal function is compromised (i.e., it can be challenging to assess using the creatinine clearance, given their elevated plasma creatinine concentration. Because of the elevated plasma concentration in these patients, the renal tubular secretion of creatinine (a process restricted by maximal tubular secretory capacity) increases; this leads to an increased concentration in the urine (U in Equation 4), and once more an incorrect GFR is determined. Exogenous agents like salicylate, trimethoprim, and cimetidine are known to cause disruptions in the renal secretion of creatinine. These medications prevent creatinine from being secreted through the tubules, which lowers urine creatinine concentration and results in an artificially low creatinine clearance or GFR.

In conclusion, a number of variables influence creatinine tubular secretion, and the technique employed for measuring creatinine can have a direct impact on the measured creatinine clearance. Notwithstanding these drawbacks, the creatinine clearance remains a valuable tool for medical professionals to assess GFR. The periodic performance of a creatinine clearance offers important diagnostic and prognostic information about a patient's ongoing renal status because creatinine methods have been thoroughly studied and shown to be reliable.

3.6.2.3. Importance of Time Interval

It is necessary to collect a timed urine specimen to do a creatinine clearance test. The specimen must be supplied with the period during which the urine is collected. A 24-hour urine collection is thought to be the best specimen to use when determining creatinine clearance due to the diurnal variation in the GFR. Throughout the 24-hour period, the plasma specimen needed for the clearance determination can be obtained at any time. Reduced collection times (e.g., 12-hour or 2-hour intervals) may be employed, particularly in patients who need recurrent GFR assessments to track their kidney health. In these situations, the urine sample should be collected at the same time of day for comparison, the patient needs to be kept well hydrated throughout the test, and the plasma sample is typically taken halfway through the collection. 24-hour collections are preferred because creatinine clearance results within a single individual can vary by as much as 15–20%. Collections made over a shorter period of time may exhibit even greater variability.

It is impossible to overstate the significance of the urine collection and its timing. Urine excretion in milliliters per minute is calculated for the clearance equation using the time interval and the total volume of urine collected. It is clear from Equation 5 that the creatinine concentration (U) and urine volume (V) have a direct impact on the magnitude of clearance results.

Examining a few elements that may have an impact on the clearance equation's parameters is crucial. Because of pH fluctuations, improper storage of the urine specimen can lead to bacterial proliferation, which in turn can cause creatinine breakdown to creatine or degradation of creatinine by bacterial creatinases. Under either scenario, the urine creatinine value (U) is artificially lowered. However, the clearance results are also void if the urine volume (V) that was utilized to calculate the clearance is off. Evaluating the acceptability of data (urine volume, collection interval) submitted with a specimen for creatinine clearance is practically impossible. The laboratory technician can be made aware of discrepancies in the data by analyzing individual plasma and urine creatinine results and deriving conclusions about their meaning regarding renal function and the clearance equation.

The creatinine clearance test is still a crucial diagnostic tool for assessing renal function, particularly glomerular filtration, in spite of its drawbacks. The GFR will be affected by pathologic conditions that alter the glomerular filtration barrier or the renal blood flow to glomeruli. For instance, if the glomeruli receive less blood plasma for processing, the glomerular function falls. It should be noted that the afferent and efferent arterioles alter blood flow to the glomeruli in response to variations in renal hemodynamics, not the kidney, which regulates the GFR. Consequently, a steady blood flow keeps the GFR steady. Given the strong correlation between renal blood flow and GFR, the creatinine clearance test offers important insights into renal function. (Myers et al., 2006)

3.6.3. Alternate Approaches to Assessing Glomerular Filtration Rate

3.6.3.1. Estimated GFR (eGFR)

Every time a patient who is 18 years of age or older has a serum creatinine test, laboratories should compute the eGFR. When it comes to high-risk patients, such as those with diabetes, hypertension, cardiovascular disease, or a family history of kidney disease, the eGFR is a straightforward and useful tool that can help medical professionals identify chronic kidney disease. A formula based on the patient's age, gender, and ethnicity as well as their serum creatinine level can be used to estimate their GFR. The Modification of Diet in Renal Disease (MDRD) Study developed and validated the suggested formula. Depending on how serum creatinine is measured, the equation changes. When the creatinine method is not calibrated to an isotope dilution mass spectrometry (IDMS) reference method, Equation 7 displays the original MDRD equation.

$$GFR\,(mL/min/1.73\,m^2) = 186 \times (S_{cr})^{-1.154} \times (\text{Age in years})^{-0.203} \times (0.742\ \textit{if female}) \times (1.212\ \textit{if African American}) \quad (7)$$

Equation 8 is the equation used when the creatinine method is calibrated to an IDMS reference method.

$$GFR\,(mL/min/1.73\,m^2) = 175 \times (S_{cr})^{-1.154} \times (\text{Age in years})^{-0.203} \times (0.742\ \textit{if female}) \times (1.212\ \textit{if African American}) \quad (8)$$

Research contrasting the MDRD equation with other formulas, like the Cockcroft-Gault, and with results from 24-hour creatinine clearance have shown the MDRD equation's applicability and validity.

Additionally, it has received the greatest validation in populations of African Americans and Caucasians. Still, efforts are being made to develop an even more precise and accurate equation that works over a larger range of GFR.

When the eGFR is less than or equal to 60 mL/min/1.73 m^2 body surface area, the MDRD equation yields the most accurate values. According to the guidelines of the National Kidney Disease Education Program (NKDEP), only eGFR values of 60 or less should be reported numerically. Values for eGFR that fall outside of this range ought to be stated as "greater than 60." A clinical chemistry text should be consulted for more information on the clinical utility of eGFR measurements.

3.6.3.2. Cystatin C and β_2-Microglobulin

Renal disease causes the kidneys' remaining functional nephrons to increase in functional capacity to make up for their declining number. Therefore, before creatinine results show a significant decline in GFR and reduced renal function, 50–60% of the nephrons must be lost. This phase of "creatinine blindness" has prompted efforts to find more accurate biomarkers of renal function and to assess low-molecular-weight proteins like cystatin C and β2-microglobulin. Both of these proteins are not the best indicators of renal function in all patient populations, but research has shown that they can be more sensitive and specific biomarkers of renal function in some clinical settings (i.e., GFR) as opposed to creatinine.

A low-molecular-weight protein with 13,000 Daltons, cystatin C, may be used as a biomarker for long-term renal function monitoring. It is a cysteine proteinase inhibitor that is continuously produced by all nucleated cells. Cystatin C, akin to β_2-microglobulin, is easily absorbed by the proximal tubular cells, undergoes catabolization, and subsequently leaves the bloodstream. Cystatin C levels in the serum are essentially constant and unaffected by age, gender, or muscle mass. Blood levels of cystatin C rise in tandem with a decline in GFR. When compared to a serum creatinine or creatinine clearance test, several studies have indicated that cystatin C analysis offers comparable and, in certain patient populations, enhanced detection of adverse early changes in GFR. Cystatin C's drawbacks, however, may include increased intraindividual variation and higher analysis costs.

A single polypeptide chain with a molecular weight of 11,800 Daltons is known as β_2-microglobulin. All nucleated cells have the β_2-microglobulin (also known as the β-chain of human leukocyte antigens) on their surface. As a result, its concentration in all bodily fluids, including plasma, is practically constant. In a healthy state, β_2-microglobulin easily crosses the glomeruli and is fully reabsorbed (99.9%) by the proximal tubular cells, where it undergoes catabolization. Therefore, in the case of normal renal function, the excretion of β_2-microglobulin in urine is low and its concentration in plasma stays constant (i.e., 0.03 to 0.37 milligrams daily). A more accurate indicator of decreased renal tubular function than glomerular function is β_2-microglobulin (i.e., GFR). The concentration of β_2-microglobulin in urine increases significantly, while its concentration in serum remains essentially normal when tubular reabsorptive function is reduced or lost. To accurately identify this change in renal processing, simultaneous measurements of serum and urine β_2-microglobulin levels are helpful in two clinical settings: (1) identifying allograft rejection in kidney transplant recipients; and (2) differentiating renal diseases that are tubular and glomerular in nature.

A decrease in GFR is accompanied by elevated levels of β_2-microglobulin in plasma. Regretfully, β_2-microglobulin is also elevated in several diseases linked to higher cell turnover, including multiple myeloma, autoimmune diseases, viral infections, and inflammatory disorders. Furthermore, treatments like corticosteroid drugs and hemodialysis raise the level of β_2-microglobulin in the blood.

The sensitivity of β_2-microglobulin to degradation in acidic environments is a technical drawback. Degradation is a concern when collecting urine specimens, but it is not a problem with serum specimens. When obtaining and handling urine samples for β_2-microglobulin analysis, care must be taken to guarantee that the urine is alkalinized during collection or that patients are medicated in a way that causes their excreted urine to be alkaline. In conclusion, β_2-microglobulin has limited utility as a GFR marker but can be a useful indicator of renal tubular function.

For many patient populations, long-term renal function monitoring is essential. These include people with renal disease that is currently recognized, as well as people who may develop renal disease in the future, such as those with diabetes, hypertension, or autoimmune diseases, as well as people who are taking nephrotoxic medications (e.g., chemotherapeutics, antirejection medications for transplants, and specific antibiotics). The search for a more accurate biomarker than creatinine continues because prompt detection of detrimental changes in renal function allows for prompt intervention. It is yet to be determined what exactly the levels of cystatin C and β2-microglobulin will contribute to the long-term surveillance of renal function.

3.6.4. Screening for Albuminuria

Early on in the development of diabetic nephropathy, proteinuria of glomerular origin manifests. Consequently, tracking urine albumin excretion in diabetics helps identify and treat early nephropathy earlier. In diabetics, albuminuria is also indicative of elevated cardiovascular morbidity and mortality. Microalbuminuria, or low levels of increased urine albumin excretion, is an early indicator of cardiovascular risk factor reduction and the need for further screening for potential vascular disease.

Changes in the glomerular filtration barrier lead to increased glomerular permeability, even though the precise mechanism causing this proteinuria is unclear. Hyperglycemia is the single most significant factor linked to the glomerular proteinuria's development. Glucose appears to interact with proteins of the glomerular filtration barrier through nonenzymatic binding, resulting in alterations in glomerular permeability and promoting the formation of the mesangial matrix.

Urine albumin excretion greater than 30 mg/day (20 μg/min) indicates glomerular changes. Urine collected for 24 hours yields accurate results and permits the simultaneous determination of creatinine clearance; however, collecting this specimen is not the simplest. On the other hand, precise information regarding albumin excretion can be obtained from a readily available random urine specimen. The albumin-to creatinine ratio is calculated by normalizing the amount of albumin present against the creatinine concentration using a random urine specimen. Before a person is diagnosed with microalbuminuria, at least two of the three urine collections examined over three to six months should show elevated albumin concentrations.

This is because daily excretion of albumin can vary greatly. Excretion of more than 30 mg of albumin per gram of creatinine (>30 mg albumin/g creatinine) is the definition of microalbuminuria based on a random urine specimen (Guyton and Hall textbook of medical physiology; Seldin and Giebisch's the kidney: physiology and pathophysiology; Anderson and Cockayne, 2003; Patton, 2010; Hall, 2011; Goldman-Cecil medicine, 2015)

3.7. Assessment of Renal Blood Flow and Tubular Secretory Function

3.7.1. Determination of Renal Plasma Flow and Renal Blood Flow

Sufficient renal blood flow is necessary for normal renal function (RBF). The capacity of nephrons to reabsorb and secrete water and solutes, as well as glomerular filtration, are all affected by changes in blood flow to the kidneys. The glomeruli use the plasma component of the circulating blood to create an ultrafiltrate. It should be noted that the unfiltered portion of blood plasma enters the peritubular capillaries where the tubules process it.

Not every blood clot that enters the kidney is cleared. Actually, only about 8% of the RBF is in direct contact with healthy renal tissue. RBF and renal plasma flow (RPF) are not the same. Equation 9, where Hct represents the hematocrit, explains the relationship between RPF and RBF.

$$RBF = \frac{RPF}{1 - Hct} \tag{9}$$

The optimal clearance material for measuring RPF and then RBF needs to: (1) only be found in the blood's plasma fraction; (2) be extracted from the plasma mainly by renal tubular secretion; and (3) be eliminated entirely from the plasma during the kidney's initial passage through it, leaving practically no concentration in the venous renal blood. The conventional clearance equation (see Equation 4) can be used to calculate the actual plasma flow in milliliters per minute when a substance has been fully extracted from the plasma after passing through the glomeruli and the peritubular capillaries. Keep in mind that a normal RPF is required to assess the renal tubules' secretory function. On the other hand, normal tubular secretory function is required for the evaluation of RPF.

The renal tubular secretory function is evaluated by clearance tests employing phenolsulfonphthalein and p-aminohippurate. The renal tubules actively secrete both substances; however, phenolsulfonphthalein is not entirely eliminated as it passes through the kidney and is therefore inadequate for determining the RPF. While the p-aminohippurate clearance test is a useful method for determining the RPF, other methods that involve radioactive substances (e.g., ^{131}I-orthoiodohippuran) have been employed. Since secretory function and RPF measurements necessitate the intravenous infusion of an external substance, they are not routinely carried out.

The p-aminohippurate clearance test is the most widely used test to determine RPF. The proximal tubules secrete p-aminohippurate, an exogenous, weak, nontoxic organic acid (a small amount is filtered through the glomerulus). When normal secretory function is known, the p-aminohippurate clearance test not only provides an excellent indicator of renal tubular secretory function, but it also provides a way to determine the RPF and the RBF because at certain plasma levels, p-aminohippurate is secreted completely during its first pass through the kidneys. The current techniques for analyzing p-aminohippurate in urine and plasma are challenging and time-consuming, although the p-aminohippurate clearance test is the reference method for measuring the RPF. Another disadvantage of p-aminohippurate's regular clinical use is that it needs to be infused because it is an exogenous substance.

According to the results of the p-aminohippurate clearance test, a normal RPF is between 600 and 700 mL/min. By applying Equation 7 and assuming an average normal hematocrit of 0.42 (42%), normal values for the RBF range from roughly 1000 to 1200 mL/min. With this data and a typical resting cardiac output of about 6 L/min, it is possible to determine that the kidneys receive 16–20% of the cardiac output. The 8% of the RBF that never makes contact with functional renal tissue is not taken into consideration in this measurement. The kidneys receive about 25% of the total cardiac output when the 8% is added.

3.7.2. Assessment of Tubular Secretory Function for Acid Removal

In reaction to variations in the body's acid-base balance, the renal tubules actively secrete acids. Phosphoric and sulfuric acids are produced as a consequence of the metabolism of proteins and phospholipids. Bicarbonate quickly neutralizes these acids, forming CO_2 and the neutral salts Na_2SO_4 and Na_2HPO_4. Although the kidneys pass the neutral salts into the ultrafiltrate, the lungs expel CO_2. The neutral salts undergo additional modification to become ammonium salt (e.g.) as the renal tubules secrete hydrogen ions and ammonia. e.g., $[NH_4]_2SO_4$) or acid that can be titrated (i.e., NaH_2PO_4) for excretion; as a result, measuring ammonium salts and titratable acids is necessary to assess the renal tubular ability to generate an acid urine. An average person's daily urine excretion of acid is between 50 and 100 mmol.

3.7.2.1. Measurement of Titratable Acid Versus Urinary Ammonia

Acid (H^+) plus ammonia are typically excreted in urine at a ratio of twice that of titratable acid. The amount of phosphate ions present in the ultrafiltrate determines how much titratable acid can form. The ultrafiltrate concentration is typically low because the plasma concentration of phosphate ions is normally low. On the other hand, the renal tubules directly produce and secrete ammonia in response to the body's need to expel acid. The production of ammonia is not restricted, and in healthy renal tubules, the production is increased to eliminate extra amounts of metabolic acids. For instance, titratable acid excretion only rises to 100 to 200 mmol/day in patients with diabetic ketoacidosis, while ammonium salt excretion can reach 400 mmol/day. On the other hand, sick tubules are unable to generate and release ammonia in addition to losing the capacity to release hydrogen ions. Under these circumstances, the daily excretion of total acids may drop to 3 to 35 mmol. Simultaneously, the ratio of excreted ammonium salts to titratable acids may diminish to the extent that a greater amount of acid is eliminated as free titratable acid than is mixed with ammonia.

Because the kidneys are essential for preserving a healthy acid-base equilibrium, a disruption in tubular secretory function results in systemic acidosis. Retinal failure is actually typically linked to acidosis. Titratable acid and ammonium salts provide useful information about the total hydrogen ion excretion in urine, which in turn provides valuable insights into tubular secretory function.

3.7.2.2. Oral Ammonium Chloride Test

Ammonium chloride, which metabolizes to urea and HCl, is administered orally as part of the oral ammonium chloride test. The kidneys excrete more titratable acid and ammonium salts to make up for the increased acid, which makes the urine more acidic. Measurements of plasma bicarbonate are taken both before and during the test to track the body's loss of bicarbonate reserves. The test shouldn't be run if the initial plasma bicarbonate level is low (less than 20 mmol/L). Before the test, a 2-hour urine specimen is collected in the morning. Acid excretion is normal if the specimen's pH is less than 5.3, so there's no need to run the test. Urine is taken for the test eight to ten hours every two hours. The pH, titratable acid, and ammonium excretion are measured after every two-hour collection.

The urine pH can be lowered to less than 5 points by normal individuals with a total hydrogen ion excretion of more than 60 mmol/min (titratable acid plus ammonium salts). Both the excretion of ammonium salt and titratable acid should be greater than 25 mmol/min. The plasma bicarbonate level should decrease to less than 26 mmol/L at the same time. A diagnosis of renal tubular acidosis is supported if, following this challenge test, there is no acidic urine excretion. Defective tubular ammonia production, defective tubular hydrogen ion secretion, or defective bicarbonate reabsorption in the proximal tubules are the hallmarks of renal tubular acidosis. Patients with renal tubular acidosis excrete alkaline urine despite having systemic acidotic urine, regardless of the specific defect involved.

To measure titratable acids, a sample of well-mixed urine is titrated with 0.1 N NaOH using a pH meter until it reaches a pH of 7.4. This matches the pH levels of blood and urine. The amount of ammonium in the urine is then determined by subtracting the total acidity from the titratable acids present in the sample.

While it is possible to measure the nephron's localized functions, clinical settings do not often employ this technique. Rather, the most popular and useful urine tests for routinely assessing renal function are the urine protein electrophoresis to assess glomerular permeability to plasma proteins, the urine osmolality determination to assess tubular concentrating ability, and the creatinine clearance test to assess GFR. Furthermore, eGFR computations and plasma creatinine levels offer continuous signs of impaired or altered renal function (Coresh and Stevens, 2006; Levey et al., 2009).

3.8. Functional Aspects

3.8.1. Effects of Abnormal Renal Function on Body Fluid

Numerous types of renal disease can result in excesses or deficiencies in the body's supply of water, sodium, potassium, and magnesium as well as protein shortages brought on by significant protein losses in the urine. The inability of the kidney to function normally can result in the retention of other nitrogenous compounds, such as creatinine, and waste products of protein metabolism, such as urea and uric acid, in the blood. There might be unusually high blood phosphate levels, which can cause low blood calcium levels (for reasons that remain somewhat unclear). In the process of bringing the blood and tissue fluid's calcium levels back to normal, calcium may be lost from the bones. Tetany, a condition characterized by painful and spastic muscles, can result from a calcium deficiency. Although these disturbances can and frequently do coexist, changes in volume, changes in composition, and protein depletion of renal origin will be discussed separately for descriptive purposes.

The main cation in intracellular fluids, which make up 33% of body weight, is potassium. These distinct bodily fluid "compartments" are in osmotic equilibrium, meaning that if a solute (e.g., the concentration of the extracellular solution is increased by adding sodium chloride, which is then followed by the addition of water to lower the concentration and increase the extracellular compartment. If there is a significant increase in extracellular fluid, it may manifest clinically as edema, which is a swelling of the tissues caused by fluid and usually relieved by applying firm pressure. Edema can occur in three different conditions: acute kidney inflammation (nephritis), protein deficiency of renal origin, and chronic kidney inflammation complicated by heart failure linked to abnormally high blood pressure. All of these conditions are characterized by the kidneys' inability to adequately excrete sodium and water.

The kidneys don't need to be diseased for them to be in such edematous states; for instance, normal kidneys in a patient with heart failure may retain sodium when their ability to function is impaired by inadequate circulation and abnormally high levels of hormones that retain sodium, like aldosterone. The only volume change associated with renal disease that is both common and easily noticeable is an increase in extracellular fluids. Conversely, the opposite condition, sodium depletion or clinical dehydration, is more frequently brought on by vomiting and diarrhea when these are side effects of terminal renal disease. Sodium and water depletion can be identified by signs of poor circulation, such as a drop in blood pressure and an increase in pulse rate, as well as by a lack of elasticity in the superficial tissues and poor blood vessel filling. Although certain diseases cause changes in intracellular fluid volume, particularly when the body's potassium content is compromised, it is difficult to identify these changes.

3.8.2. Properties of Body Fluids

Osmolality, or the total osmotic concentration of a bodily fluid, is a crucial characteristic because osmotic forces play a significant role in regulating fluid distribution within the body. This is contingent upon the solute concentration. All solutes have an impact on osmolality, but small particles like sodium or chloride ions have a much greater impact than their weight and actually account for more than 90% of plasma's osmolality. Changes in osmolality in the context of renal disease are primarily dependent on the kidney's water handling capacity. A state of water depletion, marked by an increase in the osmolality of bodily fluid, occurs when the kidneys are either unable to conserve water or are not stimulated to do so by the pituitary's ADH. Other times, the kidneys may retain too much water, particularly in the presence of too much hormone; in this scenario, the excess water leads to a clinical state known as water intoxication, which is characterized by a decrease in the osmolality of bodily fluids.

The degree of acidity or alkalinity in bodily fluids is another significant general characteristic. Impaired kidney function results in the retention of hydrogen ions, a condition known as renal acidosis. The kidneys are involved in the excretion of hydrogen ions. Renal acidosis can arise from a specific disease of the renal tubules, which is responsible for converting the slightly alkaline glomerular filtrate into the typically acidic urine, or from general renal failure.

In addition to these general alterations in bodily fluid, renal illness can cause distortions in the pattern of specific constituents. The issue with many substances is that they are not excreted, which leads to an increase in concentration in bodily fluids. The increase in concentration may aid excretion if filtration is used to attain it, allowing for longer periods of equilibrium at the expense of higher but usually manageable concentration levels. For instance, a person suffering from renal failure needs to excrete the same amount of urea as a healthy person following the same diet, but they can only do so at a blood-urea concentration of 100 mg/100 mL, as opposed to the normal blood-urea concentration of 25 mg/100 mL. Urea, creatinine, uric acid, phosphate, sulfate, urochrome, and all other typical urine constituents—aside from those that are "regulated" as opposed to merely "excreted"—are among the substances whose concentration rises in this manner. Potassium should be discussed due to the unique risk of its retention, which can result in lethal irregularities in heart function. This is a known risk of acute renal failure, which is currently typically avoided by using an artificial kidney with semipermeable membranes and occasionally by using resins that will absorb potassium from the alimentary tract.

Traces of protein are present in normal urine, and increased excretion of protein in the urine is seen in many forms of renal disease. This is typically indicative of increased permeability of the tuft of capillaries that forms the glomerulus. This elevated proteinuria, which is more accurately termed albuminuria but is often called proteinuria, usually amounts to 0–5 grams per day or more. When it reaches five grams per day and stays there, the amount of protein lost in the urine surpasses the liver's ability to reprocess the materials into new protein; the blood's concentration of protein falls, which causes the bloodstream to release more fluid into the tissues. This is because the physical pressure in capillaries, which tends to push fluid out, and the osmotic pressure of plasma proteins, which has the effect of holding fluid in, are normally in equilibrium. A deficiency of plasma proteins upsets this balance of forces. Massive edema results from a general loss of fluid in the tissues, to which the kidneys additionally contribute by retaining salt and water. Nephrotic syndrome is the term for the confluence of high protein levels in the urine, low blood protein levels, and ensuing edema. This is an excellent illustration of a syndrome, which is characterized as a discernible pattern of manifestations with multiple potential causes. Acute and chronic renal failure are two more instances of syndromes in renal disease.

3.8.3. Disorders of Urine Flow

If there is little to no urine production, it could indicate either oliguria (little urine production) or anuria (no urine production). It could also indicate a blockage in the urethra or bladder that is preventing both kidneys from excreting urine. One kidney is present at birth in about one in every 500 people, and kidney loss due to illness or trauma is not uncommon. As long as the remaining kidney continues to function normally, the loss of one kidney does not significantly impair a person's capacity to eliminate waste. Patients will experience symptoms comparable to lower urinary tract obstruction if the remaining ureter becomes completely blocked. The section on acute renal failure treats partial or total inability to form urine, and the section on diseases of the urinary tract treats obstructive conditions.

Certain common clinical scenarios that correspond to distinct modes of disordered urinary flow can be distinguished in cases of damage to nervous control: (1) Lack of conscious inhibition of micturition due to cerebral cortex damage or, more frequently, psychological causes results in an involuntary need to micturitate, even in cases where the bladder volume may be relatively small; micturition is precipitate and continues until the bladder is empty. (2) Transverse lesions or other damage to the spinal cord above the sacral reflex centers, which results in lower limb paralysis, initially resulting in an atonic (physiologically tone-deficient) bladder. The detrusor relaxes, causing the bladder to swell significantly and eliminating reflex micturition. Urine is finally released in small amounts when the pressure finally increases enough to overcome the sphincters' spasm. Additional build-up and partial overflow voiding reoccur (overflow incontinence). These circumstances make it easy for the bladder to inflame, which increases the risk of a chronic ascending urinary infection that could be fatal.

To prevent overdistension and eventually create an "automatic" bladder, intermittent catheter drainage of the bladder may be required, as well as firm abdominal wall pressure. This organ has a limited capacity (about 150 milliliters) and needs to be emptied frequently. The sacral segments of the spinal cord mediate reflex control, the higher centers do not inhibit the detrusor, and the internal sphincter relaxes more easily. If the abdominal muscles aren't also paralyzed, they can provide voluntary assistance in this case. Nonetheless, there's always a chance of infection and some leftover pee from an incomplete emptying. Sometimes the kidneys can become infected due to pressure buildup in the bladder; in these situations, the kidneys will suffer harm if medication or more frequent bladder emptying isn't taken to relieve the pressure. Alternatively, damage to the nerves supplying the bladder and urethra or to the central nervous system below the sacral cord reflex centers can result in an isolated, or "autonomous," bladder. The bladder tenses up but contracts very weakly, leaving behind 200–300 milliliters of residual urine despite only small amounts being void. Unlike automatic bladder overflow incontinence, this condition is referred to as active incontinence. Once more, better bladder emptying through catheter drainage might be beneficial in this situation.

3.8.4. Diseases and Disorders of the Kidney

This section covers the syndromes of acute and chronic renal failure, which have various causes, in addition to particular kidney diseases. Kidney infections are treated later, as they are a subset of urinary tract infections in general.

3.8.4.1. Acute Renal Failure

When renal function abruptly drops to extremely low levels, the body retains the materials—including water—that the kidneys would normally eliminate, resulting in little to no urine production. This condition is known as acute renal failure. Acute renal failure can result from two main mechanisms. The renal circulation is further suppressed when the cardiac output, or the volume of blood the heart pumps into the general circulation, is reduced due to bleeding or medical or surgical shock. More significantly, however, the kidney tissue cannot tolerate a protracted disruption of its blood supply and experiences either patchy or massive necrosis, which results in tissue death. This directly causes inefficient excretion. Treatment for acute renal failure is based on the hope that kidney tissue may regenerate given enough time. The most common and significant causes of acute renal failure caused by low blood supply (ischemia) are multiple injuries, sepsis (bloodstream infections), abnormal or excessive bleeding during abortions, internal or external hemorrhage, loss of bodily fluid from burns or severe diarrhea, transfusion reactions, and severe heart attacks. Transplanted kidneys are an exception, as they frequently experience an acute renal failure phase that is separate from potential rejection.

Toxicology is the second common mechanism of acute renal failure. Many poisons are eliminated by the kidney; during this process, they concentrate and, like other urine constituents, reach levels in the tubular fluid that cause damage to the tubule lining cells. If the patient can be kept alive during the period of reduced renal function and is not killed by other effects of the poison, regeneration can occur even though the tubular cells die and are shed in the urine. Many poisons can harm the kidney in this way, but the primary categories include organic solvents (carbon tetrachloride, propylene glycol, methanol), heavy metals (mercury, arsenic, uranium), other organic substances (aniline, phenindione, insecticides), antibacterial agents (sulfonamides, aminoglycosides, amphotericin), and certain fungi (e.g., Ammonita phalloides. Apart from the ischemic and toxic origins of acute renal failure, fulminating forms of acute renal diseases, which are typically mild, should also be mentioned e.g., the acute form of immunologic rejection that can irreversibly damage a kidney within minutes of transplantation, as well as acute glomerulonephritis (see below). Acute obstruction of the urine flow from the kidneys is another mechanism of acute renal failure. This condition is easily treated by restoring adequate urinary drainage from at least one kidney.

Three phases are helpfully distinguished in the course of acute renal failure: the onset phase, the phase of established acute renal failure, and the recovery phase. The second of these phases is typically, though not always, marked by a low urine output (oliguria), and the third by an increasing urine output (polyuria). Acute renal failure episodes begin during the onset phase, which is characterized by general illness. During this phase, symptoms such as blood in the urine or pain in the loins may indicate that renal damage is imminent. If circulatory failure is treated quickly, renal damage may be reversible at this early stage (e.g., by maintaining appropriate blood oxygen levels and by transfusion sufficient amounts of plasma, whole blood, or electrolyte replacement fluids. Treatment for any infection or underlying condition needs to happen right away.

Small amounts of urine, frequently containing hemoglobin or red blood cells, are passed in the second phase; total absence of urine is uncommon and indicates that something is blocking the passage of urine. Quantitatively speaking, significant oliguria is defined as a urine volume of less than 500 milliliters per day; this is the lowest amount at which the excretory demand imposed by a typical diet can be satisfied. Since many of the causes of acute renal failure are also causes of increased tissue breakdown generally, the excretory demands in the actual situation of acute renal failure may actually be much higher. The amount of tissue breakdown and the severity of renal failure both influence how quickly blood urea levels rise. The kidney can no longer adequately excrete potassium, sodium, or water in addition to nitrogen.

These different deficiencies indicate how acute renal failure should be managed, which involves avoiding the ingestion of any hazardous substances that the kidneys are no longer able to process. To reduce tissue breakdown, the diet needs to be either low in high-quality protein or completely absent from protein. It must also be devoid of potassium and sodium. Acute toxic effects on the heart caused by elevated blood potassium levels have killed some renal failure patients, while pulmonary edema, a correlation between sodium retention and renal failure, has killed many others. Water cannot be completely eliminated from the diet, but it must be consumed in amounts that are estimated to be equivalent to the water lost through breathing and skin perspiration. The patient's weight and the blood sodium level are reliable indicators of how much water restriction is appropriate. A progressive decline in serum sodium suggests that too much water is being consumed when there are no ongoing sodium losses from the body, such as those caused by vomiting or diarrhea. Renal function can return, usually within seven to ten days. Renal recovery is accelerated by the use of dialysis, which removes waste products from the blood by filtering it through semipermeable membranes. Resins can extract potassium from the body, but if dialysis is available, this is less frequently necessary.

The convalescent kidney takes time to regain its full regulatory function, and electrolytes and water may be lost at an unusual rate during this stage, necessitating replacement. Despite this, the recovery phase presents fewer challenges than the oliguric phase. The majority of people who survive acute renal failure recover fully, but some people continue to have residual renal damage. Some experience this to such an extent that it effectively places them in the category of chronic renal failure. One of the medical miracles of the past few decades is the artificial kidney, which, along with advancements in the use of stronger antibiotics to control infection, has changed the prognosis for many patients suffering from acute renal failure.

3.8.4.2. Chronic Renal Failure

Although the term "uremia" is sometimes used synonymously with "chronic renal failure," it actually refers to an increase in the blood's urea concentration. This can occur in a variety of acute illnesses where the kidney is not the primary organ as well as the previously mentioned acute renal failure. Although uremia should be understood as a purely chemical statement, it is occasionally used to indicate a severe renal insufficiency clinical picture.

Chronic renal failure can be caused by a variety of factors, just like acute renal failure. The two most frequent causes are glomerulonephritis, or inflammation of the kidney involving the glomeruli, and pyelonephritis. Other common causes include renal damage resulting from obstructive conditions of the lower urinary tract and renal damage caused by the effects of high blood pressure. These are the main disorders that are explained below. They are all characterized by a progressive loss of nephrons, which can occur down to less than 20% of normal. Most of the changes seen in chronic renal failure can be directly attributed to the quantitative loss of nephrons; glomerular filter loss is the cause of excretion failure, and other characteristics like the large amounts of diluted urine indicate a change in tubular function that may be explained by the increased load that each remaining nephron must support. Beyond the four prevalent causes, there exist numerous other reasons for chronic renal failure. These include connective tissue diseases, tuberculosis, congenital anomalies, other hereditary disorders, the consequences of diabetes and other metabolic disorders, and several primary disorders of the kidney tubules. A few of the numerous causes are more significant than others due to their reversibility. These include uric acid buildup in gout, renal amyloidosis (abnormal deposits of the complex protein substance amyloid in the kidney), which may have treatable causes, damage to the kidney from excessive calcium or potassium deficiency, and the effects of analgesic agents (substances used to relieve pain) and other toxic substances, including drugs.

The patient with renal failure, particularly in the early stages, may be completely asymptomatic or may be experiencing intermittent convulsions and frequent urination—a tendency that many healthy individuals share—or he may be in a coma. The patient may have a sallow overall appearance as a result of both anemia and urine pigment retention. The affected individual may exhibit withdrawn behavior, twitching of the muscles, and more widespread convulsions, even if they are not in a true coma. It is believed that poisoning is the cause of the coma, and convulsions are frequently linked to the intensity of hypertension, which frequently exacerbates advanced renal failure. High blood pressure is also linked to symptoms like blurred vision. Hemorrhages and bruises could be apparent. Even though the toxin (or toxins) causing uremia are still unknown, the quick recovery that occurs after dialysis strongly suggests that there is a toxic component. By itself, urea is not particularly toxic. Not every chemical change associated with uremia is a straightforward retention. Deep breathing is a clinical sign of a condition called ketoacidosis, which is characterized by a decrease in the alkalinity of blood and tissue fluids as the lungs attempt to expel carbon dioxide. Electrolyte abnormalities are frequent because the kidney's ability to adapt to changes in salt, potassium, and water intake gradually deteriorates. Patients with uremia frequently experience poor appetite, nausea, vomiting, and diarrhea, all of which contribute to chemical disturbance. Because phosphate is retained in the blood and is linked to low blood calcium levels, renal failure is associated with overactive parathyroid glands and lower-than-normal levels of vitamin D, as the kidneys produce less of the vitamin's active form (1,25-dihydroxycholecalciferol). Calcium is released from the bones by parathyroid hormone and calcium absorption from the intestines is facilitated by vitamin D. Because bone calcium is lost and calcium stores are not sufficiently replenished, these alterations can cause severe bone disease in people with renal failure.

Excessive renin production by the kidney in chronic renal failure can cause severe hypertension, which may even take center stage in the clinical picture. Hypertension may cause direct heart failure in addition to damage to the brain and retina. Due to its effects on the renal blood vessels themselves, hypertension can also hasten the progression of renal damage, creating a vicious cycle that can be challenging to break. The inability to produce enough erythropoietin can also contribute to severe anemia.

Advanced renal failure patients require special care because they are more susceptible to infection and other complications like vomiting or diarrhea. A strict low-protein diet that includes 18–20 grams of high-quality protein per day can halt the progression of advanced renal failure symptoms before they manifest. Only a type of dialysis can save a person with terminal renal failure, after which dialysis or a transplant can be used to sustain them.

3.8.4.3. Glomerulonephritis

The condition often referred to as nephritis or Bright's disease, is glomerulonephritis. The glomerular tuft's vessels are the main target of the illness. Glomerulonephritis is linked to infection in the restricted sense that it may start soon after a streptococcal infection and may be made worse by other infections later on. The suffix "-itis" denotes an inflammatory lesion. It appears, however, to be an immunologic disorder in the sense of the formation of antibodies in response to the presence of a foreign protein (antigen) elsewhere in the body; these form antigen–antibody complexes that lodge in the glomerular tuft or, in a small number of cases, themselves become deposited on the capillary glomerular walls. This is despite compelling evidence that glomerulonephritis does not represent a direct attack on the kidney by an infectious agent. The process is commonly known as circulating complex disease, and in each instance, the antibody or antigen–antibody complex enters the kidney through the circulation. Damage to the glomeruli results from the subsequent response within the glomeruli. These foreign protein deposits and complexes react with other blood proteins (refer to the article complement) and draw circulating platelets and white blood cells to the area. These cells then release protease enzymes and other chemical mediators of tissue damage (Walmsley and White; Schrier and Gottschalk, 2000; Levey et al., 2003).

This theory of glomerulonephritis is based in part on comparisons to the renal damage that allergies can cause in animals, as well as the observation that an allergic reaction's protein component gets lodged in the sick glomerulus. A wide range of initial stimuli and subsequent immunologic disease-causing mechanisms can both be included in the broad definition of an immunologic disorder. These include the potential for primary glomerular damage, which could lead to the glomerulus becoming antigenic and triggering a secondary antibody response, as well as the involvement—or lack thereof—of T lymphocytes. Such diversity is strongly suggested by the different ways the disease manifests in the affected individual as well as by the differences in the glomerular tissues seen under both an ordinary and an electron microscope.

Glomerulonephritis usually manifests as a sudden illness within one to two weeks of a sore throat, or occasionally after a prolonged streptococcal infection of the skin. Although other infectious agents such as viruses and protozoans can also be to blame, a few drugs acting as foreign macromolecules may have similar effects.

The afflicted individual has noticeable bloodstains in their urine and facial and ankle puffiness. Examining the patient reveals loose tissues with edema; the fluid is easily removed with light pressure, and there is a slight to moderate increase in blood pressure and urea levels. Although the condition is concerning, there is actually no special treatment required for an acute episode of glomerulonephritis other than eliminating the infection or stopping the offending medication, along with some protein and fluid restriction. Nine times out of ten affected individuals fully recover. Occasionally, exceptional outbreaks with a higher fatality rate have been reported. Only a small percentage of patients, though, may pass away during the acute attack or within a few months if the disease's effects are exceptionally severe. An alternative scenario is that the afflicted individual might seem to have fully recovered, showing no signs of illness; however, the disease process is still ongoing, resulting in a gradual loss of nephrons and eventually chronic renal failure. The patient may experience no overt symptoms of latent nephritis during the many years that this process takes, other than the presence of protein and a low concentration of red blood cells in the urine. However, it should not be assumed that the presence of protein in the urine (proteinuria) in the absence of symptoms indicates that the patient has kidney disease; in fact, young individuals without any subsequent signs of renal disease may have symptomless proteinuria for a variety of reasons.

In conclusion, glomerulonephritis can result in renal failure in a matter of weeks or months, following years of proteinuria without symptoms, or following a phase of severe proteinuria that gives rise to the nephrotic syndrome. Sometimes people who have never experienced an acute attack or who cannot recall ever having one will exhibit all of these symptoms. Numerous patients with glomerulonephritis exhibit a variety of glomerular reactions on renal biopsies, including increased cellularity, thickening and damage to the basement membrane, and varying degrees of progressive glomeruli destruction. Complete resolution of the glomerular disease happens in those who make a full recovery.

A peculiar type of glomerulonephritis that is particularly prevalent in children is linked to minimal structural damage to the glomerulus, at least when viewed under a standard light microscope. By using electron microscopy, characteristic abnormalities affecting podocytes can be identified. Nephrotic syndrome and excessive proteinuria are typically present with the condition. Contrary to other forms of glomerulonephritis, this one lacks evidence of an immunologic cause, and the triggering antigen is unknown. However, when the patient receives treatment with corticosteroids or other immunosuppressive medications, the disorder typically resolves quickly, and renal failure never happens (Walmsley and White; Levey et al., 2003).

3.8.4.4. Vascular Disease

During the discussion of chronic renal failure, the cycle wherein high blood pressure resulting from renal disease can exacerbate kidney damage was brought up. It is obvious that a primary vascular disease, or illness affecting the blood vessels, could just as easily be the reason for kidney damage.

Malignant hypertension, also referred to as accelerated hypertension, is the most dramatic example of this. It is a condition in which the blood pressure reaches abnormally high levels, with the diastolic Figure (the blood pressure in between heartbeats) being 140 millimeters of mercury or higher (the normal being approximately 80). The smallest arteries, the arterioles, suffer severe damage from prolonged exposure to this degree. The damage is widespread and results in the rapid destruction of renal substance, leaving the kidneys scarred. Malignant hypertension is a medical emergency because it can be fatal in a matter of months if left untreated. Early treatment is particularly effective in treating this condition. The affected individual usually experiences a severe headache and may initially notice blurring or loss of vision because the retinas are damaged at a faster rate than the kidneys. Treatment must be started right away to prevent damage to other organs and stroke. Even slightly higher blood pressure can lead to progressive kidney damage in the elderly or those who age prematurely due to widespread arteriosclerosis, also known as "hardening of the arteries." This illness causes scarring that progresses gradually and damages the larger arteries rather than the arterioles. Numerous conditions that hinder the healthy operation of the blood vessels, including diabetes mellitus, disorders of the collagen, bacterial inflammation of the heart lining, and many more, can also cause renal damage through a variety of mechanisms.

Though rare, a particular renovascular cause of hypertension that is significant for blood pressure regulation in healthy individuals involves the juxtaglomerular apparatus (JGA) and renin secretion. Renal artery stenosis, or constriction of one of the main renal arteries, can occur occasionally as a result of vascular disease or after trauma. When blood pressure drops below the constriction point, the JGA secretes more renin, which causes the vasoactive angiotensin II to form. The blood pressure increases as a result. Normal blood pressure and blood renin levels are typically restored by removing the damaged kidney, surgically repairing the constriction, or performing percutaneous transluminal angioplasty, which involves inserting a balloon catheter through the skin and inflating it inside the artery to flatten plaque buildup (Walmsley and White; Schrier and Gottschalk, 2000; Levey et al., 2003)

3.8.4.5. Tumors

General tumors are covered in the Cancer article. This section provides a brief discussion of the local effects of excretory system-specific tumors. When a tumor is benign, its effects include pressure on nearby structures and obstruction of hollow organs; when a tumor is malignant, additional effects include the potential for local invasion and organ-to-organ bloodstream or lymphatic-mediated dissemination (metastasis).

3.8.4.6. Carcinoma

Renal cell cancer, also known as a hyperendocrine tumor, is the most common type of tumor affecting the kidneys. It is a malignant tumor that originates from epithelial cells, which are the cells that line and cover the body. It was previously believed to originate from cortical cells of the adrenal gland located inside the kidney substance. It has since been shown to be false. Renal carcinomas make up one to two percent of all tumors, and the majority of those affected are between the ages of 40 and 60. The tumor may not cause any symptoms at all or it may become noticeable when it spreads to the lungs, resulting in blood in the breath, or to the bones, causing pathological fractures.

Much more frequently, blood in the urine serves as the initial sign of a tumor. This may be painless or, if clots are being passed, may result in ureteric obstruction. Additionally, a dull pain in the loins could be experienced due to the kidney capsule stretching. The tumor may be palpable or detectable through ultrasonography or X-rays. A rounded swelling on the kidney may distort its outline or an injection of contrast medium may cause the renal pelvis to become visible and may cause it to shift or distort. An obscure fever or polycythemia (an excess of red blood cells in the blood) as a result of excessive erythropoietin production are less common initial signs of renal carcinoma. Using a device known as a cystoscope, a direct visual examination of the urinary tract can reveal the side that is afflicted, with blood coming from a single ureteric opening. A renal pelvis tumor is a possible cause of this bleeding, so a renal pelvis examination is usually necessary. Sometimes an exploratory procedure is required, and the kidney has to be removed if carcinoma is discovered. There is some evidence to suggest that radiation therapy may somewhat enhance surgical outcomes. With a five-year survival rate of less than 50%, the prognosis is dire overall. Nonetheless, there have been reports of arrest or even regression in this type of malignant tumor.

3.8.4.7. Nephroblastoma (Wilms' Tumor)

While other types of cancer are less common in childhood, nephroblastoma is a less common but still significant tumor. The tumor may be present from birth, but about half of the cases happen between the ages of two and four. Chemotherapy, prompt surgery, and early diagnosis are the best chances for recovery (Walmsley and White; Levey et al., 2003).

3.8.4.8. Other Tumors

Apart from tumors of the renal substance, fern-like growths of the epithelium, called papillomas, can also affect the renal pelvis. Benign kidney substance tumors are rare, but cysts—abnormal kidney sacs filled with liquid or semisolid substance—are more common. Despite this, kidney cysts are not strictly speaking tumors; rather, they are malformations caused by the embryonic tubules' inability to reach a proper outlet. Nephrotic syndrome manifests in infancy in a number of forms, the majority of which are fatal. There are several types of solitary cysts, and if they produce symptoms, they might require local surgical intervention. The type of polycystic (multiple-cyst) renal disease that permits survival into adulthood is inherited; multiple family members experience minimal symptoms until middle age before developing progressive kidney dysfunction. Urinary tract infections and episodes of blood in the urine are frequent, and the kidneys are big and irregular. other organ cysts—e.g., the liver—might be there. Because of the pressure from the cysts, X-rays reveal irregularities in the renal pelvis.

Although puncturing the cysts is a possibility, the prognosis is not promising. The standard of care for chronic renal failure now includes kidney transplantation and removal.

3.8.5. Obstruction to the Flow of Urine

Urinary obstruction causes problems in the lower urinary tract, which will be discussed later. In the meantime, it is appropriate to think about the impact of urinary obstruction on the kidney (obstructive nephropathy). It should be noted, however, that obstructions can develop at the junction of the ureter and the renal pelvis due to pressure from an abnormal blood vessel crossing the pelvis or from improper smooth muscle action. In these cases, a plastic operation on the renal pelvis or division of the abnormal vessel can be beneficial. Whether the blockage starts this way or somewhere else, it can cause kidney pain, cause irregular urine flow when the obstruction is intermittent, and eventually result in a kidney mass if it continues. The disease known as hydronephrosis, in which a severely enlarged sac is surrounded by a mere rind of atrophied renal tissue, is caused by the renal pelvis swelling and the renal tissue shrinking. A severe case of hydronephrosis with very little renal substance left could indicate kidney removal.

The kidney can sustain a closed injury, where it ruptures, be bruised, or suffer damage, usually in conjunction with other viscera. Due to the kidney receiving only about 5% of the blood pumped by the heart, bleeding into the urine, tissues, and kidneys can occur frequently. This can result in hematomas, which are large masses of blood that can cause surgical shock. Renal biopsy procedures (which involve removing a sample of kidney tissue for analysis) may cause some bleeding, but this is not dangerous if done carefully. Radiation nephritis, or chronic renal damage, was once the result of massive radiation exposure to the kidney region. However, with proper precautions, this is no longer the case.

Blood in the urine and the appearance of a tender mass in the loin are typical indicators of traumatic kidney injury, along with progressive signs of shock (pallor, perspiration, drop in blood pressure). Such symptoms necessitate both surgical exploration and resuscitation if the bleeding persists. By sealing the tear, the surgical procedure can be used to stop the bleeding. If the kidney is not salvageable, surgery to remove it is required. It is not unknown for abnormal solitary kidneys to exist, and because of their size or location, these kidneys are more vulnerable to damage. If such a kidney cannot be transplanted, removal of the organ can only result in death (Schrier and Gottschalk, 2001; Levey et al., 2003; Robbins and Cotran pathological basis of disease).

3.9. Substituting for Renal Function

In the case of the kidneys, there are two ways to replace renal function: dialysis and transplantation. Normally, the loss of a vital function results in death.

3.9.1. Transplantation

The easier of these two could theoretically be accomplished by transplanting a kidney from a donor—ideally, an identical twin. The article transplant discusses the immunologic and surgical aspects of transplantation. Only the role that renal transplantation plays in the overall management of renal disease is taken into account here. In most cases of acute renal failure, when function loss is mostly reversible, the issue of a transplant is not raised; in cases of chronic renal failure, it is only brought up when the remaining renal function is hardly sufficient to sustain life.

3.9.2. Dialysis

Dialysis and transplantation are complementary, not competing, procedures. Dialysis is administered to patients in the waiting period for a transplant as well as during periods of oliguria or threatened rejection; however, patients who find dialysis to be a psychological burden may be considered for transplant consideration. Dialysis can be used independently to maintain patients with chronic renal failure in addition to its complementary role in a transplant program. It can also be used to preserve life in cases of acute renal failure and acute poisoning, allowing patients more time to recover (Figure 3.5).

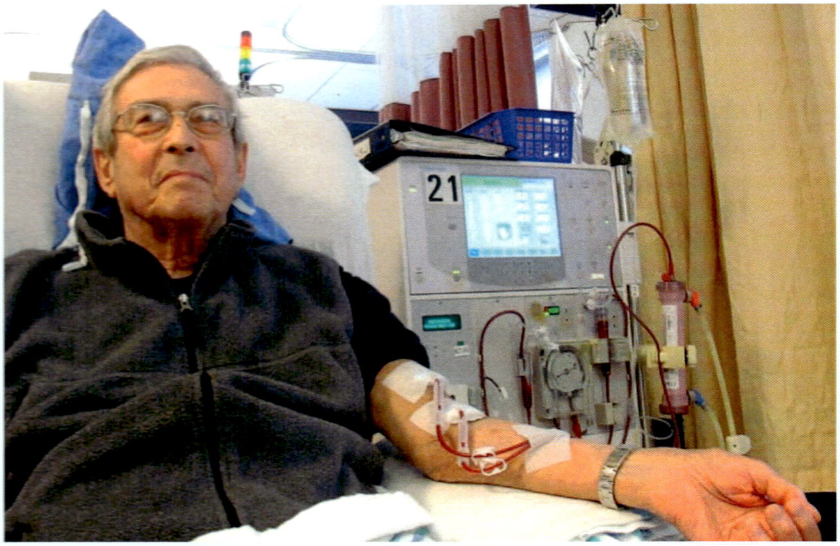

Figure 3.5. *Patient undergoing dialysis treatment.*

Source: By Anna Frodesiak – Own work, CC0, https://commons.wikimedia.org/w/index.php?curid=19317170.

There are currently two primary dialysis methods in use. The fluid used in peritoneal dialysis is run into the patient's own abdominal cavity, where it reaches equilibrium before being removed, carrying wastes and urea with it. The procedure has proven effective in treating acute renal failure in the short term, particularly in infants, and it can also be used to treat people with chronic, irreversible renal failure. Many patients can now perform peritoneal dialysis on their own for brief periods of time thanks to new techniques.

Since the invention of the artificial kidney in the 1940s, hemodialysis—the filtration of blood through semipermeable membranes—has also been used to treat acute renal failure. The issue with chronic use, however, has been recurrent access to the arterial bloodstream. This was largely resolved by the installation of an arteriovenous fistula, a permanent shunt that connects an adjacent artery to a suitable vein, typically found in the arm. The vein enlarges, making it possible to puncture it repeatedly and obtain blood, which can then be redirected through the "artificial kidney" as needed. In some later models, streams of dialyzing fluid and blood are made to flow in opposite directions and are separated by plastic sheets. In the original artificial kidney, the patient's blood was pumped through cellophane tubing submerged in a large bath of physiological fluid, which is a solution with the same osmotic pressure as blood. Disposable versions of both patterns are now available, and the apparatus can now be smaller thanks to the introduction of the "countercurrent" principle. Some hemodialysis patients have been kept alive for almost 20 years with intermittent treatment. The majority of continuous hemodialysis is still performed in hospitals or specialized facilities, but some patients have been effectively trained to perform the treatment at home with automated equipment.

3.9.3. Diseases and Disorders of the Urinary Tract

3.9.3.1. Obstruction

The urethra and ureters are much more susceptible to blockage than the urinary tract, even though a large mass (tumor, stone, or foreign body) resting in the bladder may obstruct the tract. A congenital valve or diaphragm (membranous malformation), stones (calculi) developed in the bladder or kidneys, or fibrous contraction of the urethral wall (urethral stricture) can all obstruct the urethra. The prostate, which is located near the bladder neck but is not a part of the excretory tract, is a major cause of obstruction in older men. Fibrous diseases of the bladder neck can also result in obstruction. The ureters can also become blocked by tumors, though the latter is more likely to result in blood in the urine (hematuria); strictures and calculi; and fibrosis, or scarring, of the surrounding tissue (retroperitoneal fibrosis).

The size of urinary calculi varies widely. They typically contain cystine, calcium oxalate, uric acid, or calcium phosphate. A high rate of calcium excretion, a low rate of urine formation, infections, and a number of metabolic disorders, most notably gout, are predisposing factors. Due to their size or ability to enter the ureter or urethra, they may cause problems. These include hematuria, colic, and, in the case of impaction, obstructive kidney disease. Although surgery is the primary method of treating calculi, a lithotriptor may occasionally be used to fragment the stone in place. The patient requires a thorough examination to rule out any underlying causes (e.g., a parathyroid tumor in operation that results in excessive calcium excretion).

At least historically, gonorrhea—a condition in which the urethra becomes inflamed and then scars and becomes strictured—was a common cause of urethral stricture. It is also possible for treatment-related instrument-induced urethral bruises. The affected person's bladder enlarges and they have increasing difficulty passing pee. Surgery or repeated stricture dilatation are the two possible forms of treatment.

3.9.3.2. Trauma

Except the urethra, the urinary tract is only likely to sustain damage from severe general trauma or from inadvertent ureter ligation during pelvic surgery. However, a blow to the perineum (crotch) or a fall can rupture the urethra. The inability to pass pee, bleeding from the urethra, and the appearance of a swelling containing blood and urine are signs of damage if there isn't an external wound. After experiencing a shock, the patient requires immediate surgical repair of the urethra and drainage of the possibly infected swelling.

3.9.3.3. Infection of Urinary Tract

Urinary tract infections are a frequent and significant cause of both minor and serious illnesses. At one extreme, a bladder infection, or cystitis, may only cause minor discomfort; on the other hand, once an infection is established, it can cause discomfort for the rest of one's life, be largely untreated, and even significantly shorten one's lifespan. Although a wide range of organisms can cause infection, the most prevalent ones are those that typically live in the bowel, where they are generally benign and only cause illness when they infiltrate susceptible tissue. Urinary tract infections are more common in women than in men due to the shorter urethra in women. This is especially true during pregnancy, when pressure on the urinary tract may cause partial urine stagnation. Urinary tract infections become more of an issue for men as they age and prostatic disease becomes more prevalent. Infancy is another vulnerable time, as using diapers likely makes it easier for organisms to enter the urethra. To relieve urethral obstruction, it might be necessary to insert a catheter into the bladder; however, this procedure is not taken lightly because there is always a chance of infection.

Urine may be murky and contain higher than normal levels of ammonia in all types of urinary infections. When the urethra is inflamed, urinating is typically painful; when the bladder is involved, urination is both painful and frequent. A bladder infection can also result in vomiting, a fever, and a dull pain in the lower abdomen. If the infection spreads to the kidneys, the symptoms worsen and one or both sides of the loins may hurt, along with occasionally having a high temperature.

A urine test and the patient's symptoms can usually be used to diagnose a urinary infection. Usually, the course of treatment involves giving out broad-spectrum antibiotics or sulfonamides. However, research has shown that interstitial nephritis, or chronic inflammation within and between the renal tubules, has existed for many years. This includes direct histological examination of the kidneys. A few of these patients acknowledge using nonsteroidal pain relievers like phenacetin excessively and for an extended period of time. Others may have had renal damage and urinary tract infections since childhood, which may have been exacerbated by urine refluxing into the pelvis and ureter due to an ineffective ureterovesical valve (vesicoureteric reflux). This process not only causes direct kidney damage at a young age, but it also promotes the growth of infections and results in kidneys that are later deformed by scar tissue and fibrosis. Regardless, the two most common causes of chronic renal failure severe enough to require dialysis or a kidney transplant are pyelonephritis and glomerulonephritis.

The excretory system is susceptible to tuberculous infection, just like other tissues. These days, this is rather rare, and when it does happen, general chemotherapy tailored to the specifics of the tuberculous infection can often treat it. Seldom does advanced renal tuberculosis necessitate kidney removal.

3.9.4. Renal Disorders in Pregnancy

Preeclampsia and acute urinary tract infection are two renal disorders that pregnant women are particularly susceptible to. As previously mentioned, the most frequent pregnancy complication is acute urinary tract infection, which causes significant discomfort and distress but has no effect on the mother's or the fetus's mortality.

Blood pressure elevation may occur at the beginning of pregnancy, but rising blood pressure in the final three months of pregnancy is especially concerning as it signals the beginning of preeclampsia, a condition that is more likely to occur in first-time mothers. Rapid weight gain, fluid retention, and proteinuria are present along with elevated blood pressure. Since the condition's etiology is still unknown, it has been called a "disease of theories." However, the placenta and fetus's existence inside the uterus (womb) undoubtedly affects its development. It appears likely that inadequate blood flow to the uterus is the initial event that causes placental ischemia; i.e., portions of the placental tissue deteriorate or perish. This consequently causes the blood to release chemicals into the bloodstream that heighten the risk of blood clotting in renal capillaries and other small blood vessels throughout the body. Subsequently, there is an increase in hypertension and subsequent organ damage, including renal failure. Untreated illness results in convulsions and widespread seizures (eclampsia). A dangerous illness, eclampsia has a high rate of maternal and fetal mortality. When preeclampsia is treated appropriately early on, it does not develop. Drug therapy is required to control hypertension, and the baby should be delivered a few weeks ahead of full term (Walmsley and White; Schrier and Gottschalk, 2000; Levey et al., 2003).

A Closer Look

Glomerular Filtration

One essential physiological function of the kidneys is glomerular filtration, which takes place in the renal corpuscles inside the nephrons. It is vital to the production of urine because it filters blood and separates waste and surplus substances from those that the body needs to hold on to.

The filtration site is the glomerulus, a network of capillaries surround by the Bowman's capsule. The afferent arteriole, which is wider than the efferent arteriole, allows blood to enter the glomerulus and creates pressure inside the structure. This pressure, also referred to as glomerular hydrostatic pressure, is necessary to force small molecules and blood plasma into the Bowman's capsule and out of the capillaries.

Hydrostatic pressure pushes water, electrolytes, glucose, amino acids, and other small molecules past the capillary walls and into the Bowman's capsule as blood passes through the glomerular capillaries. The filtration barrier, which is made up of the basement membrane, glomerular endothelium, and podocytes, allows substances that are dissolved in blood plasma to pass through. This filtered fluid is known as the glomerular filtrate.

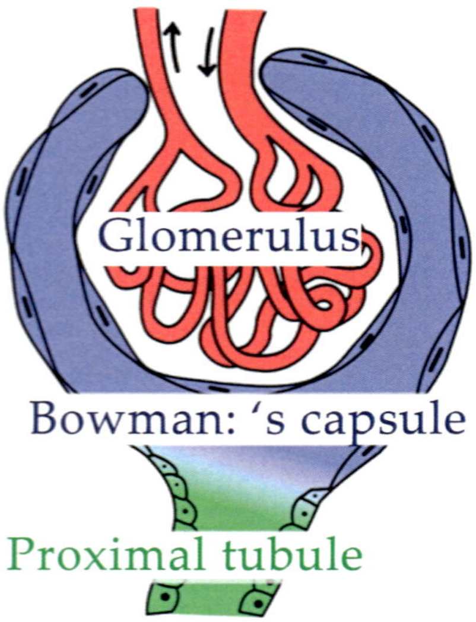

Source: *By Mikael Häggström - Public Domain, CC0, https://commons.wikimedia.org/w/index.php?curid=85695850.*

The rate at which blood is filtered by the glomerulus is measured by the glomerular filtration rate (GFR), which is a crucial sign of kidney function. It is controlled by a number of variables, such as the glomerulus's blood pressure, the surface area that can be filtered, and the permeability of the filtration barrier.

Summary

- Renal function refers to the vital role played by the kidneys in maintaining homeostasis within the body by regulating fluid balance, electrolyte levels, and acid-base equilibrium, as well as removing metabolic waste products from the bloodstream.
- Urine is an ultrafiltrate of plasma with selected solutes reabsorbed, other solutes secreted, and the final water volume determined by the body's state of hydration.
- Osmolality is the concentration of a solution expressed in osmoles of solute particles per kilogram of solvent.
- Specific gravity (SG) is another expression of solute concentration that relates the density of urine to the density of an equal volume of pure water.
- A fluid deprivation test evaluates the ability of renal tubular cells to selectively absorb and secrete solutes. In other words, it assesses the renal concentrating ability of the kidneys.
- For the kidneys to remove metabolic wastes and selectively reabsorb solutes and water, they require adequate renal plasma flow (RPF) through the glomeruli.
- A clearance test can aid in the evaluation of glomerular filtration, tubular reabsorption, and tubular secretion and in determining renal blood flow.
- Glomerular changes are evidenced by a urine albumin excretion that exceeds 30 mg/day (or 20 µg/min). Screening for microalbuminuria can be performed using a random, timed, or 24-hour urine collection.
- The renal tubules actively secrete acids in response to changes in the acid-base equilibrium of the body.
- Renal disease in its diverse forms can lead to bodily deficits or excesses of water, sodium, potassium, and magnesium, and also to protein deficits occasioned by great losses of protein in the urine.

References

1. Alpern, R. J., & Hebert, S. C. (Eds.). (2008). *Seldin and Giebisch's the Kidney: Physiology and Pathophysiology* (4th ed.). Amsterdam: Academic Press.
2. American Diabetes Association. (2004). Nephropathy in diabetes (position statement). *Diabetes Care, 27*(Suppl 1), S79–S83.
3. Boga, M. S., & Sönmez, M. G. (2019). Long-term renal function following zero ischemia partial nephrectomy. *Research Reports in Urology, 11*, 43–52.
4. Boothby, W. M. (1921). Nomogram to determine body surface area. *Boston Medical and Surgical Journal, 185*, 337.
5. Coresh, J., & Stevens, L. A. (2006). Kidney function estimating equations: Where do we stand? *Current Opinion in Nephrology and Hypertension, 15*, 276–284.
6. Damiati, S. (2019). A Pilot Study to Assess Kidney Functions and Toxic Dimethyl-arginines as Risk Biomarkers in Women with Low Vitamin D Levels. *Journal of Medical Biochemistry, 38*(2), 145–152.

7. Dustan, H., & Corcoran, A. (1955). Functional interpretation of renal tests. *Medical Clinics of North America, 39*, 947–956.

8. Gai, Z., Wang, T., Visentin, M., Kullak-Ublick, G. A., Fu, X., & Wang, Z. (2019). Lipid Accumulation and Chronic Kidney Disease. *Nutrients, 2019 Mar 28;11(4):722.*

9. Hounkpatin, H. O., Fraser, S. D. S., Glidewell, L., Blakeman, T., Lewington, A., & Roderick, P. J. (2019). Predicting Risk of Recurrent Acute Kidney Injury: A Systematic Review. *Nephron, 142*(2), 83–90.

10. Kamianowska, M., Szczepański, M., & Wasilewska, A. (2019). Tubular and Glomerular Biomarkers of Acute Kidney Injury in Newborns. *Current Drug Metabolism, 20*(5), 332–349.

11. Laterza, O. F., Price, C. P., & Scott, M. G. (2002). Cystatin C: An improved estimator of glomerular filtration rate? *Clinical Chemistry, 48*, 699–707.

12. Lennon, E. J., Lemann, J., & Litzow, J. R. (1966). The effect of diet and stool composition on the net external acid balance of normal subjects. *Journal of Clinical Investigation, 45*, 1601–1607.

13. Levey, A. S., Coresh, J., Balk, E., et al. (2003). National Kidney Foundation practice guideline for chronic kidney disease evaluation, classification, and stratification. *Annals of Internal Medicine, 139*, 137–147.

14. Levey, A. S., Stevens, L. A., Schmid, C. H., et al. (2009). A new equation to estimate glomerular filtration rate. *Annals of Internal Medicine, 150*, 604–612.

15. Miller, B. F., & Winkler, A. W. (1938). The renal excretion of endogenous creatinine in man: Comparison with exogenous creatinine and inulin. *Journal of Clinical Investigation, 17*, 31–40.

16. Myers, G. L., Miller, W. G., Coresh, J., et al. (2006). National Kidney Disease Education Program Laboratory Working Group: Recommendations for improving serum creatinine measurement: A report from the Laboratory Working Group of the National Kidney Disease Education Program. *Clinical Chemistry, 52*, 5–18.

17. Nwose, E. U., Obianke, J., Richards, R. S., Bwitit, P. T., & Igumbor, E. O. (2019). Prevalence and correlations of hepatorenal functions in diabetes and cardiovascular disease among stratified adults. *Acta Biomedica, 90*(1), 97–103.

18. Okoro, R. N., & Farate, V. T. (2019). The use of nephrotoxic drugs in patients with chronic kidney disease. *International Journal of Clinical Pharmacy, 41*(3), 767–775.

19. Pincus, M. R., Bock, J. L., & Bluth, M. H. (2011). Evaluation of renal function, water, electrolytes, and acid-base balance. In R. A. McPherson & J. Ben-Ezra (Eds.), *Clinical Diagnosis and Management by Laboratory Methods* (22nd ed.). Philadelphia: Saunders.

20. Poggio, E. D., Wang, X., Greene, T., et al. (2005). Performance of the modification of diet in renal disease and Cockcroft-Gault equations in the estimation of GFR in health and in chronic kidney disease. *Journal of the American Society of Nephrology, 16*, 459–466.

21. Pucci, L., Triscornia, S., Lucchesi, D., et al. (2007). Cystatin C and estimates of renal function: Searching for a better measure of kidney function in diabetes patients. *Clinical Chemistry, 53*, 480–488.

22. Rock, R. C., Walker, W. G., & Jennings, C. D. (1987). Nitrogen metabolites and renal function. In N. W. Tietz (Ed.), *Fundamentals of Clinical Chemistry* (3rd ed.). Philadelphia: W.B. Saunders.

23. Rodríguez-Cubillo, B., Carnero-Alcázar, M., Cobiella-Carnicer, J., Rodríguez-Moreno, A., Alswies,

A., Velo-Plaza, M., Pérez-Camargo, D., Sánchez Fructuoso, A., & Maroto-Castellanos, L. (2019). Impact of postoperative acute kidney failure in long-term survival after heart valve surgery. *Interactive Cardiovascular and Thoracic Surgery, 29*(1), 35–42.

24. Wiles, K., Bramham, K., Seed, P. T., Nelson-Piercy, C., Lightstone, L., & Chappell, L. C. (2019). Serum Creatinine in Pregnancy: A Systematic Review. *Kidney International Reports, 4*(3), 408–419.

Chapter

URINE EXAMINATION

4

Contents

Introduction

Urinalysis has been used for several thousand years and was the first laboratory test conducted in medicine. Urinalysis is still a highly effective method for getting vital data for medical diagnostics today. Since urine is an unstable fluid, as soon as it is void, changes in its composition start to occur. Therefore, handling, storage, and collection are crucial for preserving the integrity of this specimen. Urine can be identified in a laboratory setting based on its physical characteristics, chemical makeup, and microscopical analysis. A description of the urine's color, odor, clarity, volume, and specific gravity is part of the physical examination. Urine can be chemically examined to determine the presence of leukocyte esterase, ketone bodies, nitrites, protein, glucose, bilirubin, urobilinogen, and blood cells. In conclusion, microscopic analysis comprises the identification of crystals, cells, molds, and microbes.

Orientation and Directional Terms

Term	Definition	Illustration
Blood cells	Blood cells are cells that circulate throughout the body in blood, a life-sustaining fluid. The three main types of blood cells are red blood cells, white blood cells, and platelets.	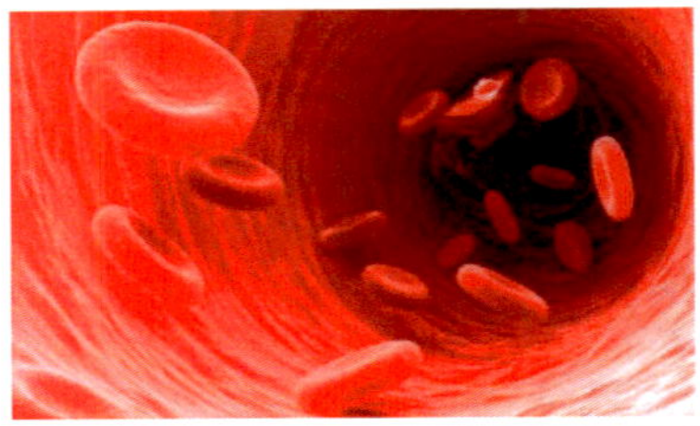
Ketones	Fat is metabolized into ketones, which are eliminated via urine. Large amounts of ketones in the urine may indicate diabetic ketoacidosis, a diet low in sugars and carbohydrates or starvation.	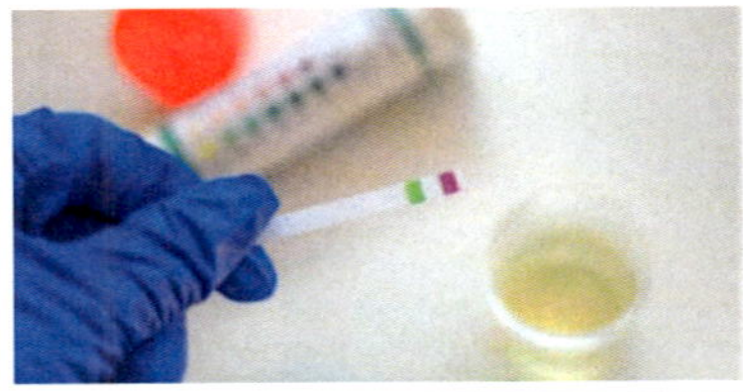
Nitrites	Bacteria that cause a urinary tract infection (UTI) possess an enzyme that converts nitrates to nitrites. Thus, urinary nitrites indicate a UTI.	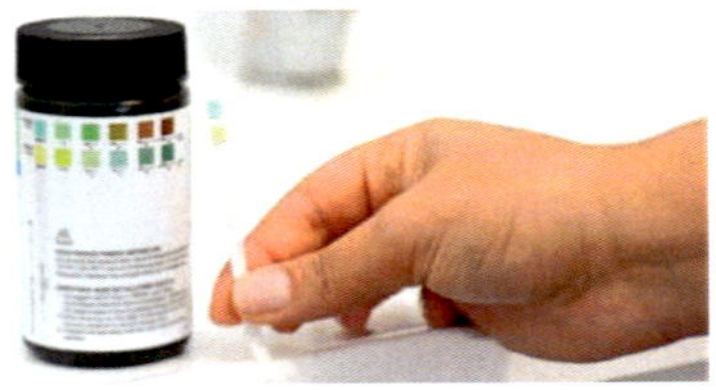
Urinalysis	Urinalysis is a panel of medical tests that includes a physical examination of the urine, chemical evaluation using urine test strips, and microscopic examination.	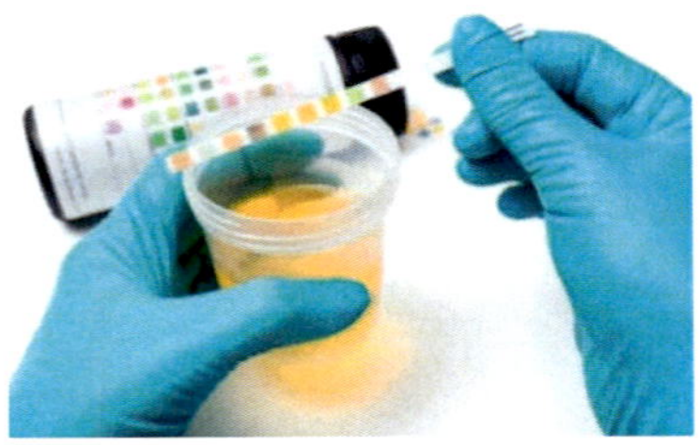
Urine color	Urine color can appear different after eating certain foods or taking medication, therefore in most cases, changes to urine color are not of clinical concern. Nonetheless, changes in urine color may be a sign of a health condition, like a UTI, kidney stones or liver inflammation.	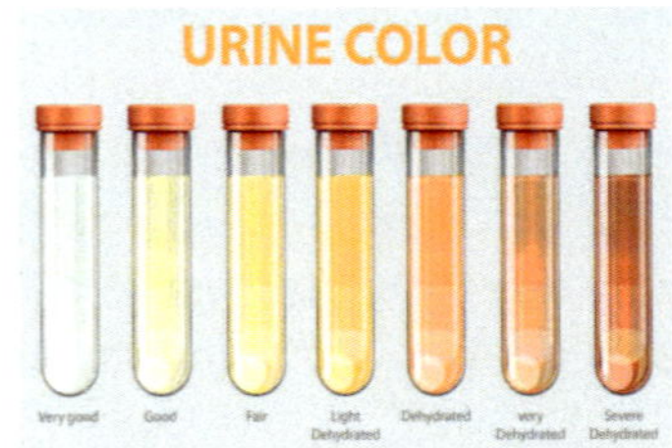
Urobilinogen	Urobilinogen is a colorless pigment produced in the gut from the metabolism of bilirubin. Some is excreted in feces, and the rest is reabsorbed and excreted in the urine. In obstructive jaundice, bilirubin does not reach the bowel, and urinary excretion of urobilinogen is diminished.	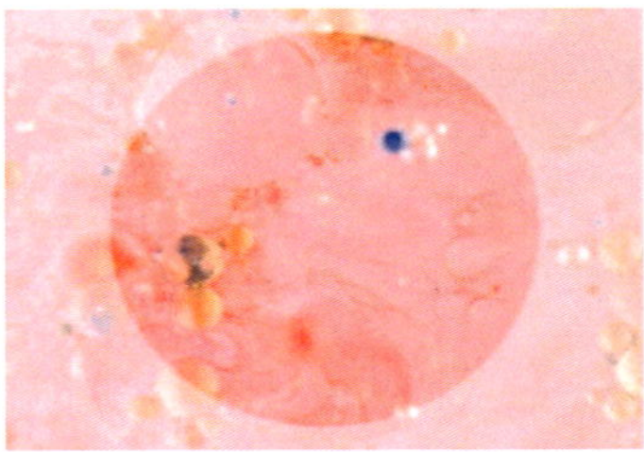

4.1. History of the Urinalysis

Urinalysis was the first test conducted in a laboratory for medical purposes, and it has been utilized for over 6,000 years by many different societies. Urine collection flasks were once a symbol of medicine, much like the caduceus is today, because the field is so intricate. Urine changed physically in different disease states, and Sumerian and Babylonian physicians were well aware of this. They used urine along with other physical examination components to diagnose and treat illnesses. Egyptians recorded the frequency and retention of urine, demonstrating their awareness of its significance. Although it is argued that they were unaware of the kidneys' physiological function in producing urine, they still left them in place during mummification procedures because they considered them to be sacred organs. Given that black ants were drawn to urine, Hindus connected diabetes mellitus (DM) with the sweet taste of urine.

Chemical evaluation of urine really began when alchemists started their quest to purify its various components, though numerous publications have emerged throughout history teaching doctors how to interpret various findings. Roulle discovered urea in 1771, and Matthew Dobson provided evidence in the 18th century that glucose was the cause of the sweetness in DM urine. Hippocrates accurately defined urine as a filtrate of blood, one of the four humors of the body along with yellow bile, black bile, and phlegm. He also reflected that "One can obtain considerable information concerning the general trends by examining the urine." The field of kidney research was pioneered by an English physician named Richard Bright in the early to mid-1800s, and he is renowned as the "father of nephrology." Furthermore, in the urine of a multiple myeloma patient, Henry Bence Jones identified the first tumor markers, lambda and kappa light chains, through a systematic analysis of the chemical makeup of both healthy and diseased urine. Urinalysis remains an effective method for obtaining vital data for medical diagnostics even in the modern era (Fuller et al., 2001; Hanno et al., 2001; Kaplan, 2002; Bain, 2015; Mundt and Shanahan, 2016; Brunzel, 2018).

4.2. Urine Collection/ Transportation/Storage

Since urine is an unstable fluid, as soon as it is void, changes in its composition start to occur. To reduce the possibility of tampered test results, it is crucial to gather, preserve, and transport specimens in an appropriate manner. Since it is the most concentrated and contains traces of substances, the first void, also known as "morning urine," is frequently collected. It also sheds light on the kidneys' capacity for concentration.

To reduce the possibility of contamination, patients should be given clear instructions when it comes to collecting specimens. Before urinating, the male patient should be told to clean his glans penis and retract his foreskin, if one is present. The female patient should use a similar technique to clean the urethral meatus and labia. The patient should start urinating, collecting the specimen by inserting the container midstream in the urine flow. The patient can finish urinating in the bed pan or toilet after the container is full, and then cap it, being careful not to contaminate the rim or lid.

Urine samples are unstable, especially the formed elements (cells, casts, and crystals), so it's important to evaluate them soon after collection. Compared to the chemical components of urine, which remain more stable provided bacterial growth is inhibited—for example, by refrigeration—these are more labile. Urine should be kept at room temperature for no more than two hours, with minimal exposure to light or complete darkness. If you need to store something for a longer period of time, you can slow down the decomposition process by keeping it at 4°C for up to 24 hours. Urinalysis specimens should not be used that are more than 24 hours old.

Urine sample collection must be done appropriately and correctly for urine analysis to yield reliable results.

4.2.1. First Morning Urine

For most urine tests, the first urine of the morning works best. Urine collection should ideally be preceded by at least eight hours spent supine. Urine in the morning has more acidity and concentration. It works particularly well for urine chemical analysis. Exercise, diet, and fluid intake already have an impact on urine collected later.

The urine flow in the middle is meant for inspection. Every time, bacteria and cells from the area surrounding the outer urethra contaminate the first stream. As a result, the patient pees in the toilet for the first part of the urine flow and collects the second urine stream in the collection container for analysis. Urine may occasionally be collected via bladder catheterization or suprapubic puncture.

Exams should be avoided in women from the time just before menstruation until the end of the period. For the majority of qualitative and semi-quantitative urine chemical test strip analyses, stabilizing additives are not necessary. Urine should be preserved or kept in a refrigerator if the examination cannot be completed in the two hours following collection.

4.2.2. Second Morning Urine

Two to four hours after the initial urination, the sample is soaked. Exercise and the amount of food and liquids consumed already influence its composition. For quantitative measurements of the urine's creatinine content, the second morning urine is generally advised.

4.2.3. Random Urine Sample

When fresh urine is collected, it is labeled as a random urine sample since the patient's preparation is typically unknown, as are the collection time and volume. For severe circumstances, it is feasible. A multitude of errors can arise from urine analysis.

4.2.4. Time Collection of Urine

Urine should be collected periodically to assess the clearance of various analytes and for quantitative analyses. Urine collection can be done for one to three hours or for twelve to twenty-four hours. Sometimes, urine is collected for eight hours at night, e.g., to assess albuminuria. The test results heavily depend on the accuracy of the collection. Finding the urine's creatinine concentration is a rough way to verify the accuracy of the urine collection process.

Urine is collected and stored in clean, dark, and cool containers, sometimes with a preservative added.

By emptying the bladder and timing the collection, it is possible to begin at any time of day. On the other hand, between six and seven in the morning is the ideal time for a 24-hour collection. The patient has to urinate before any urine is collected; this part is not collected yet. All of the urine is gathered after that. Prior to using the stool, the patient needs to be told to urinate in the collection container. Urinating the entire contents of the bladder into a collection container completes urine collection in precisely twenty-four hours.

The exact time of the start and end of the collection (to the nearest minute) as well as the precise volume of urine collected are recorded, and at least 5 milliliters of an average sample are typically sent to the laboratory after the urine is measured and thoroughly mixed (Fuller et al., 2001; Hanno et al., 2001; Kaplan, 2002; Bain, 2015; Mundt and Shanahan, 2016; Brunzel, 2018)

4.3. Physical Examination of Urine

The physical examination of urine includes evaluating its color, odor, foam, and clarity, as well as measuring its pH, relative specific gravity, and osmolality. In addition, functional examinations require measuring the volume of urine produced in a specific time period.

4.3.1. Volume of Urine

Diet and alcohol consumption have a significant impact on the amount of urine produced each day (diuresis). Volumes that are either 500 milliliters or more per 24 hours are regarded as pathological.

4.3.1.1. Oliguria and Anuria

Urine volumes under 400 milliliters per day should be treated as oliguria, and those under 100 milliliters per day as anuria.

Anuria and oliguria are the two main signs of renal failure. One of the reasons could be dehydration from either consuming too little water or losing too much of it through perspiration and diarrhea. In addition to water retention (oedemas and transsudates in body cavities), primary damage to the renal parenchyma may also be the cause of a low diuresis.

A mechanical obstruction of the urinary tract (prostatic hypertrophy, wedged concrement, pelvic tumors) can also cause oliguria or anuria. Urine retention is the term used to describe the situation if the obstruction is below the bladder.

4.3.1.2. Polyuria

A rise in daily diuresis above 2,500 ml is referred to as polyuria.

There are two types of polyurethane states:

- **Polyuria Caused by Water Diuresis:** A decrease in tubular water resorption in the distal portion of the nephron causes water diuresis. Osmotically active substances are excreted and reabsorbed by the tubules within normal bounds. The osmolality of urine is lower than that of serum. Less than 250 mmol/kg H_2O is always the case. Physiologically, water diuresis occurs when the body absorbs more water or, for example, when anti-diuretin secretion is inadequate (diabetes insipidus).
- **Polyuria Caused by Osmotic Diuresis:** It is caused either by increased filtration of osmotically active substances due to their increased osmotic concentration in the ECT (e.g., hyperglycemia) or by their reduced tubular resorption. Unabsorbed osmotically active substances "bind" water to each other and the result is a reduction in their tubular resorption. Urine osmolality is higher than 250 mmol/kg H_2O. Osmotic diuresis is characteristic, for example, of diabetes mellitus or polyuric phase of kidney failure or is result of diuretics.

4.3.2. Color of Urine

The amber color of fresh urine is a result of certain bilirubinoids, particularly urobilin. The concentration and volume of urine, which are influenced by fluid intake and extrarenal output, determine the coloration's intensity. Urine produced in the morning usually has a darker color due to its higher concentration. Discoloration may result from the ingestion of specific exogenous substances or certain pathological conditions (e.g., rhubarb, and beetroot). The natural pigment urobilin, formerly known as urochrome, is linear tetrapyrrole generated from heme breakdown and is responsible for the typical yellow color of urine. Alpha-1-microglobulin also contributes a yellow/brown tint. In cases of vitamin supplementation, additional yellow coloring may be attributed to riboflavin. Individual differences in hydration status, food, medication, and other factors all affect the color of urine. Hemoglobin, erythrocytes, myoglobin, fuscin, porphyrin, aniline dye, beets, or menstrual contamination can all cause red urine. Melanin, methemoglobin, or homogentisic acid can all cause black urine. Pseudomonas infections, as well as the presence of indicans or chlorophyll, can cause green urine. Lastly, urine that has an excess of porphyrins in it will appear blue-purple in color. Analysis for serum and urinary mtDNA and UACR, eGFR, parameters of podocyte damage (synaptopodin and podocalyxin), and PT dysfunction (KIM-1 and NAG).

Parameter	Variable	R^2	Coef β	p
Urinary mtDNA	UACR	0.255	0.0036	<0.001
eGFR	0.474	−0.210	<0.001	
Synaptopodin/creat	0.307	0.064	<0.001	
Podocalyxin/creat	0.546	0.015	<0.001	
KIM-1/creat	0.499	0.011	<0.001	
NAG/creat	0.466	0.392	<0.001	
Serum mtDNA	UACR	0.228	−0.004	<0.001
eGFR	0.460	0.232	<0.001	
Synaptopodin/creat	0.252	−0.067	<0.001	
Podocalyxin/creat	0.422	−0.0156	<0.001	
KIM-1/creat	0.388	−0.011	<0.001	
NAG/creat	0.419	−0.4287	<0.001	

mtDNA: mitochondrial DNA; UACR: urine albumin/creatinine ratio; eGFR: estimated glomerular filtration rate; KIM-1/creat: urinary kidney injury molecule-1/creatinine ratio; NAG/creat: N-acetyl-β-(D)-glucosaminidase/creatinine ratio.

Source: Petrica L, Vlad A, Gadalean F, Muntean DM, Vlad D, Dumitrascu V, Bob F, Milas O, Suteanu-Simulescu A, Glavan M, et al. Mitochondrial DNA Changes in Blood and Urine Display a Specific Signature in Relation to Inflammation in Normoalbuminuric Diabetic Kidney Disease in Type 2 Diabetes Mellitus Patients. International Journal of Molecular Sciences. 2023; 24(12):9803. https://doi.org/10.3390/ijms24129803.

4.3.3. Odor

Urine frequently has an ammoniacal odor due to a high ammonium ion content, depending on pH; however, odor varies with diet and medication. Foods with distinct smells include garlic, onions, and asparagus. Strong urine odors are linked to infections or specimens that have been exposed to extreme temperatures. Other scents to be aware of include the sweet smell of acetone in diabetic ketoacidosis, the smell of "burnt sugar" in maple syrup urine disease, and the smell of honey in diabetic ketoacidosis.

Urine must be analyzed using fresh samples because urine that has been left out in the light for extended periods of time can lose some of its components and change in smell. Urine with certain disease states has a distinct odor (Figure 4.1).

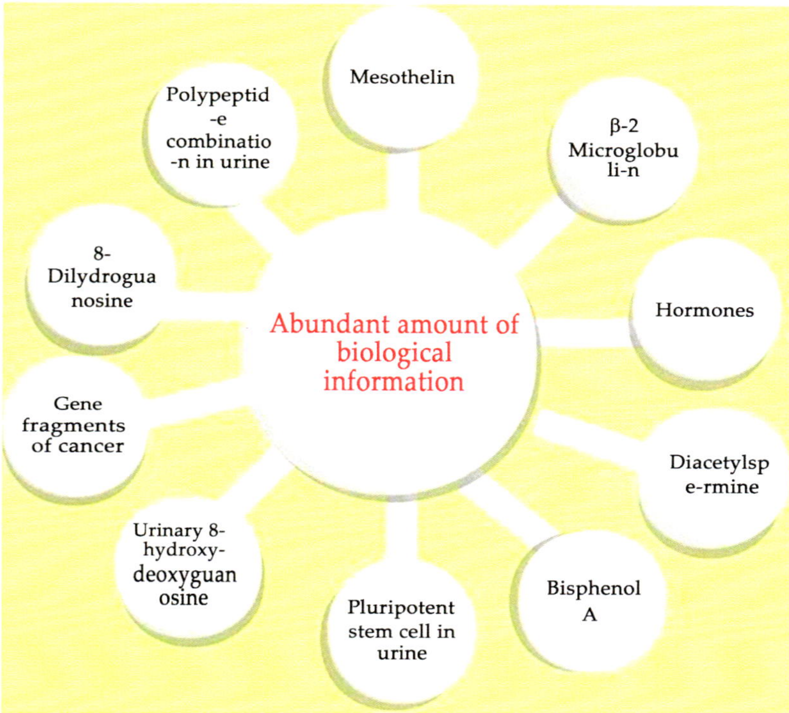

Figure 4.1. *Urine smell analysis.*

Source: Zhang Z, Liu J, Cheng Y, Chen J, Zhao H and Ren X (2022) Urine Analysis has a Very Broad Prospect in the Future. Front. Anal. Sci. 1:812301. doi: 10.3389/frans.2021.812301.

4.3.4. Foam of Urine

Normal urine produces little, white foam that dissipates fast. Proteinuria is characterized by a more prevalent, colorless, and persistent foam. Urine foam becomes yellow to yellow-brown when bilirubin is present.

4.3.5. Turbidity of Urine

Typically, fresh urine is transparent. Prolonged standing produces turbidity, which is caused by epithelium and has no pathological significance. The presence of bacteria, leukocytes, lipids, phosphates, carbonates, uric acid, leucine, tyrosine, and oxalates can all result in turbidity in fresh urine. It can be identified through microscopy or chemical analysis.

4.3.6. Relative Specific Gravity

All dissolved substances excreted into urine have mass concentrations that determine their relative specific gravity, formerly known as relative density. It is dependent on both the quantity and molecular mass of the dissolved particles, in contrast to osmolality. Density is influenced by high-molecular-weight compounds more so than electrolytes. Urine's relative specific gravity rises when there is noticeable proteinuria or glucoseuria. The urinary relative specific gravity increases by 0.003 with 10 g/l of protein and 0.004 with 10 g/l of glucose. Temperature also has a significant impact on the relative specific gravity of pee.

The range of the 24-hour specific gravity of urine under physiological conditions is 1.015 to 1.025. The maximum values that can be achieved in the dilution and concentration tests are 1.003 and 1.040, respectively.

Ordinarily, the higher is the volume of urine, the lower is its specific gravity (diluted urine); and vice versa, i.e. in low diuresis the specific gravity of urine increases. But, in diabetes mellitus a high volume of urine with a high specific gravity is produced.

The specific gravity makes it possible to evaluate the kidneys' capacity for concentration. Values greater than 1.020 signify optimal renal function and the kidney's capacity to eliminate surplus solutes. Urine with a high concentration indicates a significant drop in the amount of blood in circulation (Table 4.1).

Table 4.1. Changes in Relative Specific Gravity of Urine

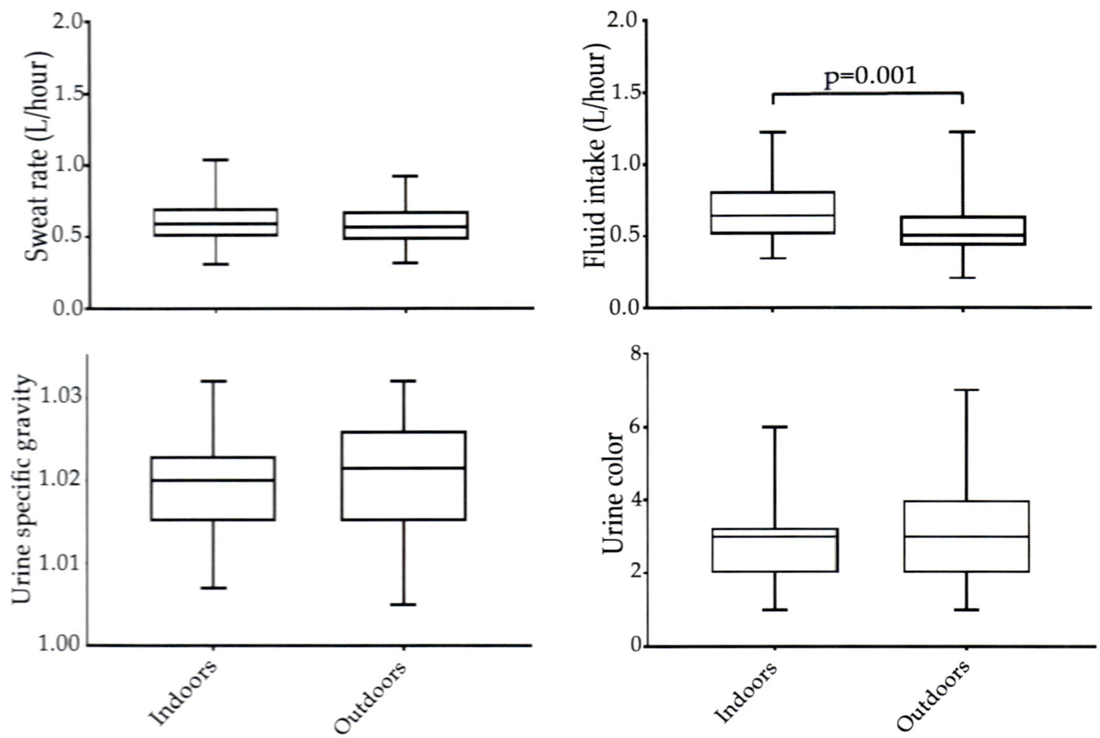

Term	Value of relative specific gravity	Causes
Eusthenuria	1.020 – 1.040	
Hypersthenuria	↑ 1.040	• dehydration • glucosuria • proteinuria
Hyposthenuria	↓1.020	• diabetes insipidus • hyperhydration • renal failure • diuretic drugs
Isosthenuria	= 1.010	• severe kidney damage

Figure 4.2 lists a few variations in the relative specific gravity.

Source: Olzinski S, Beaumont J, Toledo M, Yudell A, Johnston CS, Wardenaar FC. Hydration Status and Fluid Needs of Division I Female Collegiate Athletes Exercising Indoors and Outdoors. Sports. 2019; 7(7):155. https://doi.org/10.3390/sports7070155.

Hyposthenuria is the inability of the kidney to concentrate urine. To eliminate the same quantity of solutes, the patient needs to drink more water. Serum that is excessively diluted may indicate a kidney-related impairment, such as diabetes insipidus (insufficient ADH), or adverse drug reactions. When polyuria and hyposthenuria coexist, the renal tubular system is damaged but glomerular filtration is largely unaffected. Isosthenuria is a grave indicator of renal damage. Urine with the same specific gravity as the glomerular filtrate is eliminated by the kidneys, which are no longer able to concentrate or dilute. At about 1.010, the relative specific gravity is consistently low. When isosthenuria and oliguria are found simultaneously, it is indicative of severe renal insufficiency. Proteinuria or glycosuria leads to hypersthenuria, an elevation of the urine's relative specific gravity.

4.3.6.1. Estimation of the Relative Specific Gravity of Urine

One can use a refractometer, test strips, or urinometer to estimate the relative specific gravity of urine.

- **Urinometer:** A simple tool for estimating urine's specific gravity is a urine gravity tester. Because 15°C roughly corresponds to the temperature of urine standing an hour at room temperature, most commonly used urinometers are calibrated for this temperature. The values must be adjusted when used at different temperatures: 0.001 is added for every 3 °C above the calibrated temperature, and vice versa. For this test, a urine sample with a minimum volume of 10 to 15 milliliters is required.
- **Refractometer**: Refractometers use the index of light refraction to calculate the density of urine. It has various benefits over a urinometer, including the need for no temperature adjustment and the ability to examine just one or two drops of pee.
- **Diagnostic Strips**: A suitable polyelectrolyte functioning as an ion exchanger and bromthymol blue serving as an acid-base indicator are both present in the strip indication zone. The exchange of urine cations, particularly Na^+, K^+, and NH_4^+, for the polyelectrolyte's H^+ ions in the indication zone is the basis for the diagnostic strip's

operation. The weakly buffered acid-base indicator, which was initially in alkaline (unprotonated) form, is acidified by the released H^+. Acidification alters the color of bromthymol blue. The insensitivity to the presence of urine substances that aren't electrolytic, like proteins, glucose, urea, creatinine, and some others, is a drawback of this system.

4.3.7. Osmolality of Urine

When drinking regular amounts of water, the normal range for urinary osmolality is 300–900 mmol/kg. The kidney's capacity for dilution and concentration determines the osmolality of urine. The maximum concentration and maximal dilution are 50 and 1200 mmol/kg, respectively, respectively, the extreme values. Urine is considered isoosmolal if its osmolality is approximately equal to that of blood. Likewise, urine with hypoosmolality has a lower osmolality than blood, i.e., less than 290 mmol/kg, whereas urine that is hyperosmolal has an osmolality that is higher than blood.

The final urine is thought to be formed from an isoosmolal glomerular filtrate, to which the renal tubules either add or remove clear water, also referred to as solute-free water.

The amount of the solute-free water can be determined as its clearance. In order to explain this term, let's define first a clearance of osmotically active substances (osmolal clearance):

$$Cl_{osm} = \frac{U_{osm} \cdot V}{P_{osm}} \quad ,$$

Where;

Cl_{osm} = osmolal clearance in ml/s

V = volume of urine in ml/s

U_{osm} = osmolal concentration of urine in mmol/kg of water

P_{osm} = osmolal concentration of blood plasma in mmol/kg of water

If the primitive urine has the same osmolality as plasma and the contribution of proteins to plasma osmolality is neglected, the volume of filtered primitive urine must be equal to the clearance of osmotically active substances Cl_{osm}.

The clearance of solute-free water is the difference between the actual volume of the final urine excreted per unit of time, and the osmolal clearance:

$$Cl_{H2O} = V - Cl_{osm},$$

Where;

$Cl_{H_2}O$ = clearance of solute-free water in ml/s

Cl_{osm} = osmolal clearance in ml/s

V = volume of urine in ml/s

The final urine is more osmotically concentrated if there is a negative clearance of solute-free water, which indicates that part of the solute-free water has been absorbed from the primitive urine. In contrast, when blood plasma is diluted with the solute-free water, a positive clearance of the solute-free water indicates the production of a hypoosmolal urine. The range of physiological values is –0.027–-0.007 ml/s.

To prevent hyponatremia, the kidney can excrete a large volume of water that is free of solutes. In contrast, water excretion is restricted and solutes exit the body in small amounts when water is scarce.

4.3.7.1. Examination of Kidney Concentration Ability

One of the earliest indications of renal diseases

is a disruption in the kidney's capacity to concentrate. This is how it is looked at:

- An early morning urine sample's osmolality is first determined. When the osmolality value is more than 600 mmol/kg, it suggests a good ability to concentrate and does not require additional testing.
- The ability of the distal renal tubule and collection ductule to respond to adiuretin (vasopressin) by producing concentrated urine is indicated by the adiuretin test. Following an overnight liquid withdrawal, a patient is given 10 µg (2 drops) of 1-deamino-8-D-arginine vasopressin (DDAV), a synthetic vasopressin analog that has a stronger antidiuretic effect and a suppressed ability to produce other pharmacological effects. The osmolality of each urine sample is then measured after the patient collects urine at intervals of one hour. The test can be stopped if the osmolality in any sample is higher than the reference value. This indicates a good concentration ability. Urine and blood samples are collected at the same time and used to estimate serum osmolality. The osmotic index (U_{osm}/S_{osm}), which is derived from the values of urine and serum osmolality, offers more precise information on the renal concentration ability than urine osmolality alone (Figure 4.3).

Urine osmolality testing under different durations of liquid withdrawal is an additional option. These days, its use is rare.

Diseases affecting the renal tubules and intersticium, which disrupt the medullar concentration gradient, are the main causes of impaired kidney concentration ability. It is then reduced to e.g., in insipidus diabetes.

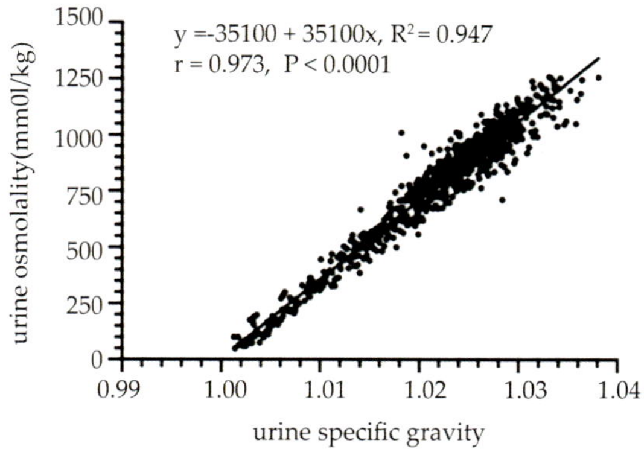

Figure 4.3. *Relationship between urine specific gravity and urine osmolality.*

Source: Feng Y, Fang G, Qu C, Cui S, Geng X, Gao D, Qin F and Zhao J (2022) Validation of urine colour L*a*b* for assessing hydration amongst athletes. Front. Nutr. 9:997189. doi: 10.3389/fnut.2022.997189.

Following a large volume of liquid intake, the kidney's capacity to dilute substances can also be examined. An osmolality of less than serum in urine is produced by the kidneys, as demonstrated by the test (Fuller et al., 2001; Hanno et al., 2001; Kaplan, 2002; Bain, 2015; Mundt and Shanahan, 2016; Brunzel, 2018).

4.3.7.2. Estimation of Osmolality

- **Osmometer:** For accurate measurement of osmolality the osmometers are used. These devices are based on the fact that dissolved substances lead to modification of some solvent properties, such as:
  - o decreased freezing point (cryoscopic principle),
  - o increased boiling point of solution (ebulioscopic principle),

- o decreased pressure of solvent vapors above the solution.

Changes of these variables depend on concentration of osmotically active substances and can be measured by the osmometers with a high precision. Typically, a decrease in freezing point is measured. One mole of particles dissolved in 1 kg of water renders its freezing point 1.86°C lower.

- **Approximately by Calculation Based on Molar Concentrations of Na^+, K^+, NH_4^+ and Urea in Urine:**

Urine osmolality = 2([Na^+] + [K^+] + [NH_4^+]) + [urea].

This calculation fails if the urine contains a high concentration of other substances, which are physiologically present in orders of magnitude lower amounts - for example, with significant glycosuria or ketonuria.

- **Approximately by Calculation from Relative Specific Gravity:**
  - o Procedure for urine not containing protein or sugar:
    - § last two digits from the value of relative gravity are multiplied by a factor 33
    - § example: relative gravity of urine = 1.019 → 19 x 33 = 627 mmol/kg
  - o Procedure for urine containing protein or sugar:
    - § the value of relative gravity is first corrected
      - in presence of protein, from the specific gravity 0.003 is subtracted for each 10 g/l of protein
      - in presence of glucose from the specific gravity 0.004 is subtracted for each 10 g/l of glucose
    - § last two digits from the corrected value of relative gravity are then multiplied by a factor 33

4.3.8. pH of Urine

The kidney is the organ that regulates the acid-base balance through the excretion or retention of H^+. At first, the pH of glomerular filtrate is the same as that of plasma. After that, as it passes through the renal tubular system, it becomes more acidic. H^+ is eliminated and hydrogen carbonates are absorbed in the proximal tubule. H^+ is secreted by a proton pump and K^+ is exchanged for H^+ in the distal portions of the nephrone.

Since free protons make up a very small percentage of urine when compared to other ions, we can conclude that the kidneys remove H^+ in two ways:

- bound to the anions present, e.g., to phosphates (conversion of hydrogen phosphate to dihydrogen phosphate)

$$H^+ + HPO_4^{2-} \longrightarrow H_2PO_4^-$$

- or anions of some organic acids. This portion is designated as titratable acidity; under normal condition it represents 10-30 mmol/24 hours. It can be determined by titration of urine with sodium hydroxide (0.1 mol/l) to pH 7.4.
- as ammonium cation, which constitutes the most significant system.

$$H^+ + NH_3 \longrightarrow NH_4^+$$

The amount of NH_4^+ excreted in the urine is between 30-50 mmol/24hours.

The normal range of a urine's pH is 5 to 6; the extreme values are 4 to 8. Abnormally high or low pH levels may indicate improper urine sample collection.

The pH of urine depends on:

- **Diet:** In a healthy individual, diet composition has the biggest impact on urine pH. Urine gets alkaline from a lacto-vegetarian diet. On the other hand, acidification is associated with a diet high in protein (meat).
- **Acid-base Equilibrium:** Urine pH is a pathological indicator of acid-base imbalances. pH variations in urine are an indication of the kidneys' corrective and compensatory function. While alkaliuria is the initial stage of compensating for respiratory and correcting metabolic alkalosis, aciduria is the outcome of correcting metabolic and respiratory acidosis. On the other hand, the excretion of alkaline urine in alkalosis and acidic urine in acidosis is limited to mild disorders and healthy kidneys. As of right now, aciduria and ketonuria point to starvation. When diabetes mellitus decompensates, aciduria, ketonuria, and glycosuria are frequently present in combination.

Permanently alkaline urine pH may indicate:

- Infection of the kidneys or urinary tract with urease-producing bacteria. Enzymatic hydrolysis of urea produces ammonia, which alkalizes the urine. The situation is similar for bacterially contaminated urine, in which the bacteria multiplied during a longer period of storage.

$$H_2N\text{-}CO\text{-}NH_2 + H_2O \xrightarrow{\text{urease}} 2NH_3 + CO_2$$
$$NH_3 + H_2O \rightarrow NH_4^+ + OH^-$$

- Renal tubular acidosis, distal type. It is a disorder of renal tubular cells in which the distal tubulus is unable to excrete protons.

Urolithiasis and urinary infections are the two conditions for which the measurement of urine pH is most helpful in diagnosis and treatment. Urinary concrements may develop as a result of long-term changes in urine pH.

The concrements in acidic urine are typically made of calcium oxalate, though they can also easily come from uric acid. Urine can be alkalized to a pH above 7.0 to gradually dissolve uric acid crystals and stop them from forming in the first place. A pH that is acidic also encourages cystine precipitation.

When urine is alkaline, the stones are composed of phosphates. When the pH level is over 7.0, struvite ($MgNH_4PO_4 \cdot 6H_2O$), calcium phosphate, and calcium carbonate will precipitate out of the solution.

4.3.8.1. Estimation of the pH of Urine

The urinary pH must always be estimated in fresh urine.

- Diagnostic strips are frequently used to estimate the pH of urine. A combination of appropriate acid-base indicators can be found in the pH indication zone. Two substances are usually used to detect pH in the range of 5 to 9, changing from orange (acid pH) to green or even blue (alkaline pH). These compounds are methyl red and bromthymol blue. It is possible to measure pH with an accuracy of 0.5 pH units.

- pH meters are used.

4.3.8.2. Examination of Acidification Ability of the Kidney

Measuring the pH of a urine sample taken early in the morning is the fundamental test used to evaluate the renal acidification capacity. After the sample is collected, it must be completed right away, and using a pH meter is advised. The urine's pH in the early morning is less than 6.0 in a healthy adult. If no contraindications apply, a higher value is suggestive of an acidification ability disorder (e.g., severe restriction of kidney function), it is recommended to conduct an acidification test following an $NH_4ClorCaCl_2$ load (in patients with impaired liver function). The patient is given ammonium chloride (2 mmol per kg of body weight); three hours later, three one-hour urine collections are conducted. Each sample's pH is determined as soon as it is collected. The pH of the urine during such a test should be less than 5.5, indicating intact renal acidification ability.

Patients with the distal form of renal tubular acidosis experience disturbances in their ability to acidify, which is brought on by the distal tubule's incapacity to expel H^+.

When the acidification test yields no useful information, the kidney's capacity for alkalization is assessed after sodium hydrogen carbonate is administered orally or intravenously (Fuller et al., 2001; Hanno et al., 2001; Kaplan, 2002; Bain, 2015; Mundt and Shanahan, 2016; Brunzel, 2018).

4.4. Chemical Examination of Urine

In clinical medicine, it is frequently important to understand specific urine chemical properties. Reagent strips and tablets can be used for a variety of semiquantitative and qualitative tests. Quantitative techniques can be employed to measure protein, electrolytes, and porphyrins.

A reagent strip is a thin plastic band that is 4-6 mm wide and 11–12 cm long, and it is attached to a linear sequence of absorbent pads. Multiple tests can be conducted at the same time because each pad contains the necessary ingredients for a distinct reaction. The methodology of reagent strips involves several intricate chemical reactions. The pad changes color to indicate a reaction, which can then be interpreted by comparing the result to the manufacturer's color chart. This can be accomplished visually, but since everyone perceives color differently, photometric techniques with equipment supplied by the manufacturer are recommended. It's crucial to use controls, comprehend the benefits and drawbacks of each test, and test the urine as soon as possible when using reagent strips. When there are variations in sensitivity and specificity between dipstick methods and specimen pigments obscure the colors obtained on reagent pads, tablets and chemical tests are utilized to verify the results.

Urine is routinely chemically examined using qualitative tests for bile pigments, protein, glucose, hemoglobin, and ketone bodies. The majority of these substances are also found in the urine of healthy people, albeit in trace amounts that are not picked up by standard testing. Urine samples from various pathological conditions have higher concentrations of them.

4.4.1. Test Tube Reactions

Previously, colored or precipitating reactions were carried out using "wet chemistry," were employed to identify the pathologic elements of urine in test tubes (Figure 4.4).

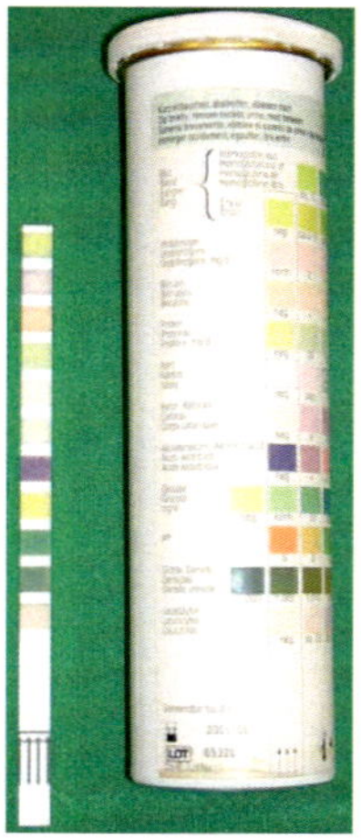

Figure 4.4. *Urine analysis.*

Source: By Uwe Gille - Own work, CC BY-SA 3.0, https://commons.wikimedia.org/w/index.php?curid=901510.

4.4.2. Test Strips

The diagnostic test strips allow for the immediate identification of pathological urine components in the patient's bed or in the doctor's consultation area. The strips are made up of one or more indication zones attached to a plastic support. Applications of a liquid analytic reagent on appropriate absorbents (e.g., specialized filter paper), and allowed it to air dry. There are several varieties of diagnostic strips available, including monofunctional, polyfunctional, and strips for specific tests.

Basic indication zones for semiquantitative estimation of a single urine component are present in monofunctional strips. Polyfunctional strips allow for the simultaneous measurement of multiple biochemical parameters because they have multiple indication zones. They are intended for use in scenarios where gathering as much data as possible about the patient's health status is beneficial, like in different screening exams.

Two or more indication zones selected for screening for or examining a particular disease are included in strips intended for specialized examinations. For instance, ketone bodies and glucose are tested for in diabetes mellitus screening strips; blood, protein, pH, and nitrite are tested for in renal disease strips; bilirubin and urobilinogen are tested for in hepatic disease strips.

The following urine parameters can be determined using test strips:

- protein
- glucose
- ketone bodies
- bilirubin
- urobilinogen
- hemoglobin, erythrocytes
- ascorbic acid
- leukocytes
- pH
- density

Test-strip detection reactions are primarily based on the same principles as traditional test-tube reactions.

4.4.2.1. Protein

Urinary proteins originate in the urinary tract and plasma and are normally only present in trace amounts, up to approximately 150 mg/24 h or 10 mg/dL. Small globulins make up the remaining plasma proteins, with albumin making up around one-third of the total. Small plasma proteins typically pass through the glomerulus and are reabsorbed in large quantities by a process mediated by receptors, leaving behind trace amounts in the urine. Similar processes are used to deal with the minute amounts of albumin that pass through the glomerulus; only a small amount is eliminated in urine. About one-third of the total protein that is typically lost is made up of the Tamm-Horsfall glycoprotein, which is secreted by the tubular cells.

Three patterns of proteinuria can be distinguished: glomerular, tubular, and overflow. When proteins like albumin and transferrin, which are typically retained in the plasma, cross the glomerulus in greater quantities, the result is the glomerular pattern. Low serum albumin from severe glomerular leakage can cause elevated serum lipids and generalized edema. It is noted that protein excretion exceeds 3.0–3.5 g/dL. Since tubular function is normal, small serum proteins are still reabsorbed, and their concentration in urine does not change. Because the tubular cells cannot reabsorb low-molecular-weight proteins, they are excreted more frequently, which is a characteristic of the tubular pattern. Numerous tubular diseases, including Fanconi's syndrome, Wilson's disease, and pyelonephritis, exhibit this pattern. Proteinuria in the tubular pattern is about 1-2 g/day, which is lower than in the glomerular pattern. Lastly, very high concentrations of small proteins in the plasma can cause overflow proteinuria when they surpass the tubular cells' capacity to reabsorb them through the glomerulus. In addition to causing the excretion of these proteins in the urine, this damages the tubular cells, as evidenced by the tubular cell casts that are visible in the patients' sediment. Up to 80% of patients with multiple myeloma excrete Bence Jones proteins, which are immunoglobulin light chains. Because the reagent strip methodology is most sensitive to albumin, these proteins might not be detected; therefore, electrophoresis or immunoelectrophoresis is needed. As a result of the excessive workload, the tubular cells undergo degeneration, inclusion formation, and shedding. The term "myeloma kidney" refers to the damaged kidney in these patients.

In healthy subjects, urine albumin excretion is typically less than 30 mg/day. Microalbuminuria, the term for increases in urine albumin excretion to 30–300 mg/day, is commonly used to describe the risk of renal disease progression and glomerular injury, especially in diabetes mellitus. A number of physiological conditions, such as intense exercise, fever, hypothermia, emotional distress, congestive heart failure, and dehydration, can also result in the excretion of urine albumin. This is a temporary condition known as "functional proteinuria" that goes away with time and supportive care.

The proteinurea dipstick test makes use of the fact that proteins act as hydrogen ion acceptors at fixed pH levels, changing the color of some dyes. Depending on the manufacturer, the sensitivity of this method varies from 6 to 30 mg/dL. Since albumin is the protein that this test is most sensitive to, it is crucial to perform a confirmatory test, such as the sulfosalicylic acid (SSA) precipitation method, to find out whether other proteins are present. Alkaline urine that has been heavily buffered can cause false positive results.

The urine supernatant and SSA reagent are combined in the SSA method, mixed by inversion, and left to stand at room temperature for ten minutes. The specimen is mixed once more by inversion and examined in direct light after ten minutes. Precipitation reaction concentration values in milligrams per deciliter that correlate to a range of protein standards, or a negative, trace, 1+, 2+, 3+, and 4+ scale based on different protocols, can be used to grade the reaction. The sensitivity ranges from 5 to 20 mg/dL. When the acid precipitates nonproteins (e.g., proteins), false positive SSA results may arise (e.g., radioactive dyes, and specific medications). Urine that is very alkaline and neutralizes the SSA can produce false negative results.

4.4.2.2. Hemoglobin, Red Blood Cells

The peroxidase activity of hemoglobin serves as the foundation for identifying the presence of red blood cells or hemoglobin in urine.

Hemoglobin catalyzes the oxidation of a chromogen to yield a blue-colored product when peroxide is present. Since myoglobin can execute the same reaction, it's critical to distinguish between the two using immunochemical testing and electrophoresis when in doubt. Ascorbic acid and highly concentrated or acidic urine can cause false negative results by obstructing the complete lysing of the red blood cells.

Up to five RBCs per microliter can be found in normal urine, but dipstick methodology cannot detect this. Hematuria is the result of bleeding anywhere from the glomerulus to the urethra and can be brought on by a number of conditions, such as renal calculi, glomerulonephritis, pyelonephritis, bladder and kidney tumors, and bleeding disorders associated with the use of anticoagulants. Positive outcomes are the norm rather than the exception for women who are menstruating. Although much less common, hemoglobinuria can result from poisoning, severe burns, trauma, or transfusion reactions. Moreover, RBC lysis in the urinary tract may be the cause. Muscle trauma and crush injuries are linked to myoglobinuria.

4.4.2.3. Glucose

Urine occasionally contains trace amounts of glucose, particularly after a meal high in carbohydrates. Under normal circumstances, there is not much glucose in the urine because it is largely reabsorbed in the tubules and freely filtered through the glomerular basement membrane. When blood glucose levels rise above 180 mg/dL, which is higher than the tubular capacity for reabsorption, glycosuria is typically identified. One common clinical cause of glycosuria is diabetes mellitus. In these patients, the glomerular ultrafiltrate shows an increase in blood glucose concentration due to an absence of insulin. This causes the tubular cells' reabsorption capacity to be exceeded, which results in its excretion. In addition, disorders affecting the liver, kidneys, endocrine system, central nervous system, and general metabolic issues like starvation and obesity can cause glycosuria. Glycosuria can also result from birth control tablets and diuretics. The two-step enzymatic reaction used in the dipstick method is caused by the enzyme glucose oxidase, which changes glucose into gluconic acid and hydrogen peroxide, which oxidize chromogen and cause a color shift. The range of results from 1+ to 4+ is contingent upon the glucose concentration in the sample, which can range from 100 to 2000 mg/dL. Although it is less sensitive and less specific than the reagent strip method, Bayer Diagnostics also offers a copper reaction in tablet form that can detect other reducing sugars like galactose, lactose, and pentose. The copper sulfate methodology must be used to screen for galactosemia, an inherited metabolic disorder that prevents the newborn from converting galactose into glucose, to prevent the development of cataract formation, hepatic dysfunction, and mental retardation in these patients due to the buildup of toxic intermediates.

4.4.2.4. Ketone Bodies

As a consequence of incomplete fat metabolism, keto bodies are a sign of a gluconeogenic metabolic state, which can be brought on by starvation, low-carb diets, feverish illnesses, or uncontrolled diabetes mellitus. These substances—beta-hydroxybutyric acid, acetoacetic acid, and acetone—are released into the bloodstream by the liver and utilized as an energy source by other bodily tissues. Nevertheless, a portion of these compounds are also filtered by the kidneys and eliminated as urine (ketonuria). The nitroprusside reaction, which produces a violet-colored product when sodium nitroferricyanide and glycine react with acetoacetate and acetone at an alkaline pH, is the mechanism used in the reagent strip test. Similar steps are taken by the Multistix system, which only looks for acetoacetic acid and yields a pinkish-maroon chemical. False positive results can happen when certain hypertension medications are combined with phthaleins, high concentrations of phenyl ketones, 8-hydroxyquinoline, or L-dopa metabolites (Figure 4.5).

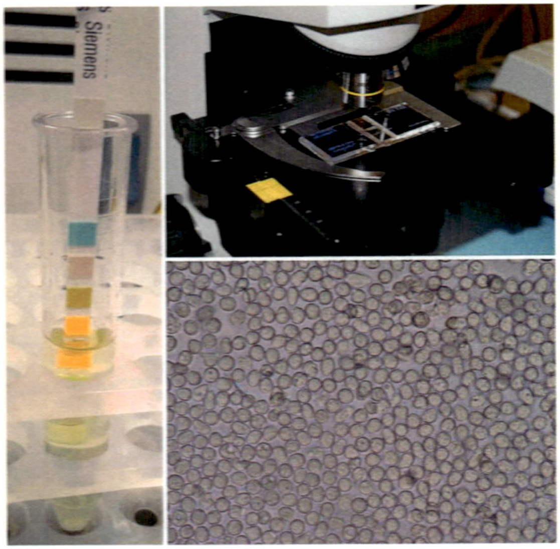

Figure 4.5. *Collage showing the procedure of urinalysis. Left: A urine test strip is immersed into the sample. Top right: A urine sample is about to be examined under a phase-contrast microscope using a Neubauer counting chamber. The urine is under the cover slide, in the upper segment formed by the H-shaped grooves.*

Source: By User: Spicy, User: Stevenfruitsmaak, User: Bobjgalindo - Source files: File: Dipstick urinalysis.jpg by User: Spicy (own work, CC-BY-SA 4.0) File:Urinary phase-contrast microscopy.jpg by User: Stevenfruitsmaak (GFDL/CC-BY-3.0) File:Pyuria2.JPG by User: Bobjgalindo (GFDL/CC-BY-SA)Images cropped and made into a collage by uploader., CC BY-SA 4.0, https://commons.wikimedia.org/w/index.php?curid=120522728.

4.4.2.5. Bilirubin

The reticuloendothelial system's RBC senescence produces bilirubin as a byproduct. The reticuloendothelial cells transform hemoglobin into unconjugated bilirubin, which is subsequently released into the bloodstream. After that, it binds reversibly to albumin, which transports it to the liver where hepatocytes extract it through an active transport process mediated by carriers. Bilirubin and glucuronic acid are conjugated in the hepatocytes to create a compound that is soluble in water. This conjugated bilirubin is excreted by the liver as bile and travels to the small intestine. The flora in the digestive tract reduces bilirubin to urobilinogen by converting it back to its unconjugated form. Following a major reduction in urobilinogen to stercobilinogen, both substances undergo oxidation in the large intestine to produce urobilins and stercobilins. 20% or so of the urobilinogen is excreted back into the gall bladder by the liver after being reabsorbed into the enterohepatic circulation. A tiny quantity stays in the bloodstream and is sent to the kidney for elimination from the body. Although conjugated bilirubin is normally present in urine in small amounts (~0.02 mg/dL), dipsticks cannot detect it. In most cases, bilirubinuria indicates either intrinsic or extrinsic bilary obstruction, as well as liver dysfunction (e.g., gallstones, pancreatic carcinomas in the head) as well as Rotor and Dubin-Johnson types of congenital hyperbilirubinemia.

The foundation of dipstick methods is the coupling reaction between bilirubin and a diazotized aniline dye, which produces a purplish azobilirubin compound. Certain medications, like pyridium, can cause false positive results by masking the results with a similar color at the low pH of the reagent pad. If urine is not tested right away or is not stored properly, bilirubin will change into unreactive biliverdin and lead to false negative results. To verify the results, another approach that uses comparable dyes but is more sensitive is the tablet method.

4.4.2.6. Urobilinogen

The intestine's bacteria use bilirubin for metabolism to produce urobilinogen. A portion of it is reabsorbed and transported by enterohepatic circulation to the liver, where the majority is reexcreted in bile, even though the majority is eliminated in feces. The kidneys then filter the remaining urobilinogen, which, if it is present in greater quantities, shows up in urine. Random urine samples containing 0–1 mg/dL reveal that normal individuals can excrete up to 4 mg daily. Serum and urine urobilinogen levels can be elevated in patients with severe liver disease, such as cirrhosis or hepatitis because they are unable to reuptake urobilinogen. Hemolytic disease patients may exhibit similar symptoms.

The Ehrlich reaction is utilized in the reagent strip method for urobilinogen detection. Urobilinogen is combined with dimethylaminobenzaldehyde in an acid buffer, resulting in a tan to orange-colored compound. However, false positive results may be seen with certain compounds such as porphobilinogen, sulfonamides, and aminosalicylic acid. On the other hand, false negative results can occur if urine is exposed to daylight, causing urobilinogen to degrade. Additionally, formaldehyde and high nitrite levels can also lead to false negative results.

A novel and precise technique for detecting urobilinogen involves utilizing a diazonium salt in an acid buffer. When using the Chemstrip dipstick from Roche Diagnostics, the presence of urobilinogen in excess is indicated by the production of a red azo dye color. Other compounds besides urobilinogen do not result in a color change on the pad.

4.4.2.7. Ascorbic Acid

Because ascorbic acid (vitamin C) has strong reducing properties that impact the estimation of other analytes in urine, it is investigated. Specifically, it obstructs direct reduction reactions involving hydrogen peroxide and breaks down diazonium salts.

Phosphomolybdenic acid is used in the ascorbic acid detection principle; when combined with ascorbic acid, it reduces to molybdenum blue. Since ascorbic acid and other strong reducing agents would react similarly, the test is not specific to ascorbic acid.

4.4.2.8. Leukocytes

The basis for the diagnostic strip's chemical leukocyte detection is the presence of esterase enzymes in granulocytes. When an ester of indoxylcarbonic acid is hydrolyzed by the esterase to indoxyl, it combines with a stable diazonium salt to produce the corresponding azo dye (Figure 4.6).

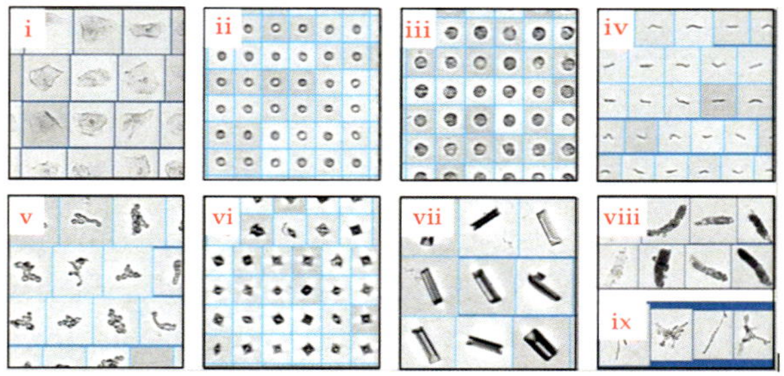

Figure 4.6. *Microscopic view of various elements of the urine; (i) squamous epithelial cells, (ii) red blood cells, (iii) white blood cells, (iv) bacteria, (v) yeast, (vi) calcium oxalate crystals, (vii) triple phosphate crystals, (viii) granular casts, and (ix) yeast with pseudohyphae.*

Source: By Lehmann R. - Lehmann R. From bedside to bench-practical considerations to avoid pre-analytical pitfalls and assess sample quality for high-resolution metabolomics and lipidomics analyses of body fluids. Anal Bioanal Chem. 2021 Sep;413(22):5567-5585. doi: 10.1007/s00216-021-03450-0. Epub 2021 Jun 22. PMID: 34159398; PMCID: PMC8410705., CC BY 4.0, https://commons.wikimedia.org/w/index.php?curid=120285373.

The color of the strip zone changes to pink or violet in a positive reaction, and to creamy yellow in a normal (negative) reaction. The microscopic analysis of urine sediment cannot be replaced by the chemical demonstration of leukocytes. Nevertheless, the biochemical analysis can also detect lysed leukocytes (e.g., in hypotonic urine), something that microscopy cannot achieve.

Leukocyturia typically indicates inflammation of the kidneys or urinary tract. Urinary tract infections caused by bacteria account for the majority of positive results. It is advised to conduct a microbiological analysis, urine sediment analysis, proteinuria, hematuria, and nitrituria examination in the event of a positive leukocyte test.

4.4.2.9. Nitrite (Indirect Detection of Bacteria)

Nitrites are not present in normal urine. Some bacteria, especially those classified as gram-negative, have the capacity to convert urine's natural nitrates to nitrites. Examples of these bacteria include Proteus, Klebsiella, *Escherichia coli*, and staphylococci. The Griess reaction is triggered by nitrites in the strips used for the indirect detection of bacteriuria. Its basic idea is the diazotation of sulfanilic acid with nitrites, which is created when bacteria reduce nitrates in urine and yield a diazonium salt. After that, azo-coupling occurs, producing a pink or even violet color.

Urine collected in the morning is the only urine sample that has to be tested for nitrites because only then does the urine remain in the bladder long enough for bacteria to convert nitrates to nitrites. Eating vegetables the day before an exam is another suggestion as they contain nitrates.

Urinary nitrite testing that is positive indicates bacteriuria; a negative result does not rule it out. The indirect evidence of bacteriuria is only preliminary and does not replace microbiological examination.

4.4.2.10. pH

The main organs in the body that control the acid-base balance are the kidneys, lungs, and blood buffers. Urine pH can range from 4.5 to 8, but because acid formation is so common, most people's urine has a slightly acidic pH. This isn't the case after a meal during the "alkaline tide," when the stomach's parietal cells release bicarbonate into the interstitial fluid and blood, which the kidneys then excrete, along with hydrochloric acid for digestion. Patients with high-protein diets and specific fruit allergies, as well as those with metabolic or respiratory acidosis and certain medication regimens, may exhibit acidic urine. Patients who follow a vegetarian diet, have respiratory or metabolic alkalosis, have renal tubular acidosis, or are on certain medications have been observed to have alkaline urine. Over time, the breakdown of urea and the growth of bacteria will cause urine left at room temperature to become more alkaline by releasing ammonia.

4.4.2.11. Density

The ratio of urine density to water density is referred to as relative urine density. The difference between the relative density of urine and the density of water (in kg/l) is negligible because the density of water is nearly equal to 1 kg/l. kg · m -3 is the density in the SI system. Since the sample's density is a relative quantity, it can be expressed as a dimensionless number in relation to the density of water.

- **Determination of Urine Density:** Using diagnostic strips, urine density is indirectly calculated from cation concentrations. The indicator zone of the strip contains a suitable polyelectrolyte as an ion exchanger and the acid-base indicator bromothymol blue. The principle of diagnostic strips is based on the exchange of cations from urine, especially Na^+, K^+, NH_4^+, H^+ polyelectrolyte ions in the indication zone. The released H^+ acidifies the weakly buffered acid-base indicator, which is in alkaline form. The color of bromothymol blue changes in tandem with acidification. The disadvantage is that the examination with diagnostic strips does not take into account non-electrolyte substances such as glucose, proteins, urea, creatinine etc.

4.4.3. Procedure for Urine Examination with Test Strips

Remove only the strips that you need to use right away, then replace the remaining strips in the tube. Never put your bare hand near the strip indication zones. The strips should be kept between +2 and +30°C in a dark, dry area, securely sealed in their original containers with a desiccant. When analyzing a urine sample, immerse the strip completely—that is, for two to three seconds—into the urine. After that, remove the strip and touch the sample container's walls to wipe away any extra urine. To prevent reagents from different reaction zones from mixing, keep the strip horizontal. Aim for the color changes that occur after the suggested incubation period, which is typically 60 seconds for leukocytes and 120 seconds for other cultures. The can be:

- Subjective by comparing colors.
- Objective by intensity measurement

4.4.4. Simple Analysis of Inborn Errors of Metabolism

There are multiple steps involved in the biochemical investigation of inborn errors in the metabolism of amino acids. Usually, screening comes first. Screening investigations are a set of basic tests based on different principles that are conducted on blood or urine samples. Some of these tests are performed on all newborns in obstetrics departments.

Although there should be very little possibility of a false negative result, a good screening test may frequently yield a false positive result. Any screening reaction that tests positive does not result in a diagnosis at this time; instead, it prompts additional, in-depth testing.

Screening tests for amino acid inborn errors include:

1. Simple chemical reactions
2. Chromatographic methods
3. Indicator papers
4. Bacterial inhibition tests

4.4.4.1. Selected Simple Chemical Reactions in Urine

1. **Fölling' Tests:** A traditional test for identifying newborns with phenylketonuria is a reaction with ferric chloride. A green complex is produced when ferric chloride and phenylpyruvate are combined in the patient's urine. But other substances also react with Fe^{3+} to form colored complexes.

   One of the most significant cases of inborn errors of amino acids in medicine is hyperphenylalaninemia, also known as phenylketonuria. The condition known as phenylketonuria is brought on by a complete failure of the hydroxylation process, which normally involves the presence of oxygen and tetrahydrobiopterin as a coenzyme and is catalyzed by phenylalanine-4-monooxygenase (phenylalanine-4-hydroxylase). The blood contains phenylalanine accumulation. This drug's pathologic metabolites, phenylpyruvate, phenyllactate, and phenylacetate, are excreted more readily through the urine. The Fölling's test, which involves a reaction with $FeCl_3$, can be used to demonstrate phenylpyruvate. Phenylketonuria causes severe, irreversible brain damage and mental retardation if it is not identified soon after birth. However, if phenylalanine intake is restricted early in life, the harm can be completely avoided and the child's development can continue normally.

2. **Brand's Test with Sodium Nitroprusside:** Reaction of sodium nitroprusside with sulfhydryl compounds (e.g., cysteine, homocysteine) yields rose or purple-red complex products:

$$[Fe^{II}(CN)_5NO]^{2-} + S^{2-} \rightarrow [Fe^{II}(CN)_5NOS]^{4-}$$

Since disulfides (cystine and homocystine) do not react, alkaline sodium cyanide must first be used to reduce them to free sulfhydryls.

One of the inborn errors brought on by a disruption in the kidney and gut's ability to transport amino acids is cystinuria. It is brought on by a malfunction in the renal tubules and digestive tract's epithelial cells' ability to transport cystine, lysine, arginine, and ornithine in reverse. Increased excretion of all the mentioned amino acids in the urine is revealed by biochemical tests. The main clinical symptom is cystine urolithiasis, which is brought on by cystine's low solubility in water. The Brand's test using sodium nitroprusside can be used to show whether cystine is present in urine.

3. **Dinitrophenylhydrazine Test for Ketoaciduria:** In an acidic medium, 2,4-dinitrophenylhydrazine combines with 2-oxo acids, also known as α-keto acids, to generate hydrazone precipitates. A positive test results in increased excretion of other ketone bodies or keto acids in the urine.

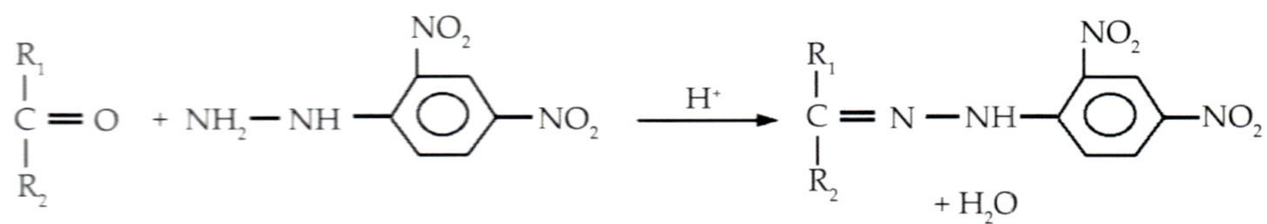

A malfunction in the enzyme system executing the oxidative decarboxylation of branched-chain α-ketoacids leads to leucinosis, also known as maple syrup urine disease. The serum has high concentrations of isoleucine, valine, and leucine. Urine excretes 10-100 times more oxo-acids than normal due to the transamination of these amino acids (2-oxoisovalerate, 2-oxo-3-methylvalerate, and 2-oxoisocapronate). The reaction between urine and 2,4-dinitrophenylhydrazine can be used to illustrate the presence of oxoacids (Fuller et al., 2001; Hanno et al., 2001; Kaplan, 2002; Bain, 2015; Mundt and Shanahan, 2016; Brunzel, 2018).

4.5. Microscopic Examination of Urine

The third step in a standard urinalysis is a microscopic inspection of the urinary sediment. Through centrifugation, all of the insoluble components of urine are separated and examined under a microscope. While some contend that microscopic examination ought to be carried out on each specimen, the majority of laboratory professionals concur that it is a crucial part of assessing patients who exhibit symptoms. Standardized bright-field microscopy remains the most widely used technique even though there are a number of microscopic procedures available for the examination of sediment. An increasing number of automated particle analyzers are being used to assess unspun urine as a preliminary screen for formed elements.

Urinary sediment analysis is not regarded as a standard screening procedure. It is carried out in the indications listed below:

- chemical analysis finds some pathological components in the urine, especially blood, protein, nitrite,
- the strip test for leukocytes is positive,
- clinical signs point to a disease of kidney or urinary tract,
- control examination of patients with nephrologic or urologic diseases.

Urine sediment is examined under a microscope to look for corpuscular elements, and flow cytometry is also used these days to look into this matter.

4.5.1. Introductory Examination

Erythrocytes, leukocytes, and bacteriuria—the latter indirectly through the presence of nitrite—can all be detected by the test strips. A positive result with the strip calls for additional microscopic analysis. Although the strips cannot take the place of microscopy, their appropriate use can reduce the number of requests for needless, time-consuming microscopic examinations. The strips remain functional even in cases where the urine's high pH or low osmolality, extended storage times, or elevated room temperature cause the cellular components to break down. Even though the urine sediment test results are negative, the test strip reveals the presence of broken-down leukocytes and/or erythrocytes. After being released from the cells, the pseudoperoxidase activity of hemoglobin or leukocytic esterase activity can last for several hours.

4.5.2. Microscopic Examination Procedure

- **Urine Sample Preparation:** The middle flow of the first or second morning urine is the best sample to use for microscopic analysis of urinary sediment. Because the cellular components in the first morning sample may have been harmed or degraded, it is advised to collect urine in the second morning. Additionally, because of their lysis, low urine osmolality and an overall alkaline pH reduce the occurrence of corpuscular elements.

It is essential to process a new urine sample within an hour of collection to examine urinary sediment. After thoroughly mixing the material, 5 or 10 milliliters are measured and added to a centrifugation test tube. It is centrifuged for five minutes at 400 g, or at most 4°C. After that, 9 out of 10 of the supernatant is carefully discarded, leaving a sediment suspension that is 10 times more concentrated than the urine in the beginning. After that, the sediment can be examined under a phase-contrast microscope or stained before being examined under a microscope.

- Staining Procedure
    1. 50 µl of staining solution (Alcian Blue and Pyronine B in ratio 1:1) is combined with 0.5 ml of sediment suspension and gently mixed.
    2. After five minutes 13 µl of stained sediment is transferred

on the microscopic slide and covered with a coverslip 18 x 18 mm (higher volume of the sample can be taken with the corresponding size of the coverslip).

4.5.3. Possibilities of Microscopic Examination

First, a lower magnification of 100–200x is used for examination to assess the distribution of elements and identify rare particles like casts and epithelial cells. Then, at least ten randomly selected visual fields are counted for corpuscular elements, and the magnification is changed to 400x. The mean number of particles in 1 µl of urine is the result, which is recalculated based on the initial urine volume. The use of Bürker's chamber allows for a more precise count of the elements.

Bright-field microscopy and the phase contrast technique are used for the microscopic examination of urine sediment; in some rare circumstances, polarization filter microscopy may also be used.

- **Bright-Field Light Microscopy:** A basic understanding of light microscopy facilitates the preparation and identification of pathologic elements. Certain elements, like hyaline casts and bacteria, can evade detection when viewed under a bright-field light microscope without staining; additionally, it can be exceedingly challenging to accurately identify leukocytes, macrophages, and renal tubular cells. Thus, it is advised to use supravital staining, which brings out specific details of cellular structures. The staining of a wet, unfixed preparation in which some cells may still be alive is referred to as "supravital." These days, the most widely recommended stain is Sternheimer's, which uses the blue and red color contrast offered by Pyronine B and Alcian Blue, respectively. Because Alcian Blue has a strong affinity for mucopolysaccharides, it stains the surface of cells as well as other materials, whereas Pyronine B enters cells and primarily colors the cytosol.
- **Phase Contrast Microscopy:** It is an effective method for quickly assessing unstained preparations. Phase contrast allows for a more thorough analysis of the sediment, particularly in identifying leukocytes, casts, crystals, and the differentiation of red blood cells, including changes in the shape of their membranes. An enhanced contrast, made possible by a phase shift in the light wave of some rays, allows for a better representation of details.
- **Polarization Filter Microscopy:** It works well for more accurate crystal and lipid body identification.

4.5.4. Components of Urinary Sediment and Their Evaluation

Urinary sediment is used to evaluate both non-organ components, like crystals, and organ components, which are primarily represented by cells and casts. Microorganisms are also observed, and different artifacts may also appear.

4.5.4.1. Corpuscular Elements in Urinary Sediment

- **Leukocytes**
    - o Most frequently found

granulocytes are polymorphonuclear. They have granular cytoplasm and resemble orbicular cells with an average diameter of 10 μm. The nucleus is divided, but it frequently experiences degenerative changes that make it harder to tell it apart from the cytoplasm. Sometimes it is not well stained; when it is, the staining is intensely blue, whereas the cytoplasm is reddish-brown. Urine's osmolality has an effect on granulocyte appearance. They group together frequently. Granulocytes are suggestive of urinary tract infections; if they are also present in conjunction with erythrocytes, this may also indicate glomerulopathy. Leukocytes and bacteria are found together in approximately half of the cases.

- Urine contamination (vaginal secretion, failing to sample the middle flow of urine) can also result in a false positive result for leukocytes.
- The presence of lymphocytes in the urine is typically linked to kidney transplant rejection, transient viral infections, and chronic inflammation of the kidneys. The distinctive feature of a lymphocyte is its uniform nucleus with a thin cytoplasmic border. Their smooth cytoplasm and high nucleus-to-cytoplasm ratio are the best indicators of their differentiation from renal tubular cells.
- Macrophages are occasionally observed in the sediment as well. They occur in urinary tract infections rather frequently.
- Physiological values: roughly < 5 leukocytes/visual field

≤10leukocytes/1μlurine

- **Erythrocytes**
  - Red blood cells in the urine are typically an indication of kidney or urinary tract disease.
  - Leukocytes are larger than erythrocytes. Their appearance is that of non-nucleated discoid bodies with an average diameter of roughly 6 μm. Their size reduces as the urine's osmolality rises; at low osmolality, however, they swell and may decompose. Low hemoglobin levels make them hard to identify and give the appearance of erythrocyte "ghosts."
  - Urinary red blood cell appearance can provide information about where they come from; most notably, it can determine whether the red blood cell source is subrenal (bleeding into the urinary tract) or renal (passing through the glomerular membrane). Serious damage to the glomerular membrane allows erythrocytes as well as proteins to enter the filtrate. However, an erythrocyte's shape and structure are changed when it passes through the glomerular membrane. Dysmorphic

erythrocytes are those that exhibit deformations from the typical discoid shape. Some may resemble “tires” and are referred to as annular erythrocytes; others may have “blebs” formed by their membranes and are referred to as acanthocytes in this instance. Renal glomeruli are specifically impacted by a notable fraction of dysmorphic erythrocytes. It is definitely glomerular hematuria if more than 80% of the erythrocytes in the urine have dysmorphic features; proteinuria is also detected at the same time. On the other hand, if over 80% of the red blood cells in the sediment have an isomorphic (normal shape) appearance, the cause of the non-glomerular hematuria is bleeding into the urinary tract e.g., urolithiasis, kidney/urinary tract tumors. Proteinuria is not linked to hematuria that starts in the urinary tract. A microscopic examination using phase contrast is necessary for the accurate identification of dysmorphic erythrocytes.

- It is always necessary to determine the cause of hematuria; in particular, a tumor or a severe glomerulopathy (glomerulonephritis) need to be ruled out.
- Admixture of menstrual blood, anticoagulant medication therapy, and intense physical labor can also result in an elevated count of red blood cells in the urine sediment.
- Physiologicalvalues: roughly < 5 erythrocytes/visual field

  <5erythrocyte/1µlurine

4.5.4.2. Epithelial Cells

They come from epithelial lining of renal tubuli or the urinary tract.

- **Renal Tubular Cells**
  - o When they appear in urine sediment, it is always a pathological sign of serious kidney damage, especially when it comes to the tubules (acute tubular necrosis, acute interstitial nephritis). The average diameter of renal tubular cells is 13 µm, making them slightly larger than leukocytes. They have a round, irregularly polygonal, cubic or faceted shape, and smooth, round nuclei without nucleoli. The cells are typically not found in the center of the cell and appear dark blue in stained samples. In the stained sample, their cytoplasm is granular and red. Though they often arrive separately, they can also form casts or clusters.
  - o In unstained preparation the renal tubular cells are difficult to distinguish from transitional epithelial cells. Therefore, in clinical laboratory practice sometimes the descriptive term ‘small round epithelial cells’ is used. They can even be confused with leukocytes.
- **Transitional Epithelial Cells**
  - o They come from the transitional epithelium that lines the urinary tract, either

in the deeper or superficial layers. It is impossible to pinpoint the specific area of the urinary tract where they originate.

- o Findings of cells from superficial layers occur rather frequently. They have ovoid or round nuclei that are centered or slightly eccentric and have nucleoli that are visible. Less than in tubular cells, the cytoplasm is primarily covered in fine granulations, which are mostly confined to the cell's periphery and infrequently perinuclear. They have an average diameter of roughly 30 µm. The presence of these cells typically indicates a lower urinary tract infection, particularly in cases where leukocytes are also detected. They can, however, even be found in the urine of healthy people.
- o Deeper layers' cells are smaller than those at the surface (17 µm on average diameter), and their shapes vary greatly, ranging from ovoid to G. form of a tail-equipped cell, a club, or a hammer. Typically, two nuclei are found in a cell. Patients with urothelial carcinomas or urinary tract infections have these cells in their urine.

- **Squamous Epithelial Cells:**
  - o These are the biggest cells in the urine sediment, with an average diameter of 55 µm. They are rectangular or polygonal in shape, have small nuclei, and have an abundance of cytoplasm. The number of them varies depending on the method used to collect urine samples, and they originate from the vagina or urethra. They have no diagnostic value and are typically detected in women's urine when the urine collection technique is subpar. (Figure 4.7).

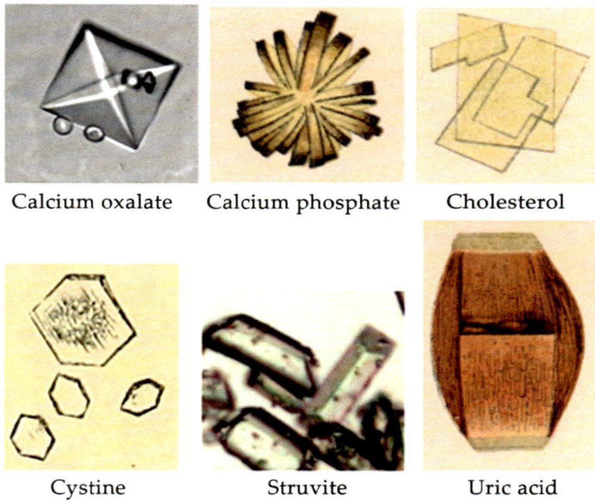

Figure 4.7. *Crystals.*

Source: *By Mikael Häggström, M.D. Author info- Reusing images- Conflicts of interest:NoneMikael Häggström, M.D.- using source images by multiple authors (see above). - Source images used:By Julius Klinkhardt (Public Domain)By SuSanA Secretariat (Creative Commons Attribution 4.0 International license)By Lionel S. Beale (Public Domain)By Julius Klinkhardt (Public Domain) By Julius Klinkhardt (Public Domain)By Sienes Bailo P, Santamaría González M, Izquierdo Álvarez S, Lahoz Alonso R, Serrano Frago P, and Bancalero Flores JL (Creative Commons Attribution 4.0 International license), CC BY 4.0, https://commons.wikimedia.org/w/index.php?curid=135084284.*

4.5.4.3 Tumor Cells

- Urine can contain tumor cells released from the kidney, urinary tract, and accessory organ tumors, such as prostate tumors. A typical example of this type of cell has a nucleus that is noticeably asymmetrical and relatively large in relation to the cytoplasm. Tumor cell detection in urine sediment is challenging unless the preparation is stained (Fuller et al., 2001; Hanno et al., 2001; Kaplan, 2002; Bain, 2015; Mundt and Shanahan, 2016; Brunzel, 2018)

4.5.4.4. Casts

Casts are cylindrical formations that start in the kidney's distal tubules and collection ductules. The Tamm-Horsfall protein, which is made by tubular epithelial cells and protects their surface, makes up the cast matrix. The Tamm-Horsfall protein can polymerize and create casts of tubular lumen in response to specific circumstances, such as low pH, high osmolality, or high protein concentration. These casts can then be released into urine and examined under a microscope in a urine sediment preparation. Other elements such as leukocytes, erythrocytes, kidney cells, pigments (bilirubin, hemoglobin), crystals, and plasmatic proteins can be added during the cast formation process. The only components of the urine sediment that can be positively identified as originating from the kidney as opposed to the urinary tract are the casts. Morphology of casts depends on the shape of tubuli in which they have formed. If the tubulus where the cast originates is dilated due to atrophy or obstruction, the resulting cast is markedly wide. Wide casts are a telltale sign of kidney failure.

The casts are classified as:

- Cell-free:
  - o hyaline
  - o granular
  - o wax
  - o fat
- Cellular (more than one third of cast surface consists of cells):
  - o erythrocytic
  - o leukocytic
  - o epithelial
  - o bacterial

A pathologic process in the kidney is indicated by the presence of cellular casts in the urine sediment.

Table 4.2. Urinary Casts

Type	Main causes
Acellular casts	
Hyaline	Nonspecific
Granular	Exercise or dehydration Acute tubular necrosis
Waxy	Advanced chronic kidney disease
Fatty	Various types of tubulointerstitial disorders, in large numbers, strongly suggest nephrotic syndrome.
Pigment	Acute kidney injury secondary to hemolysis or rhabdomyolysis Acute tubular necrosis

Cellular casts	
Red blood cell	Glomerulonephritis
White blood cell casts	Pyelonephritis or other type of tubulointerstitial inflammation Proliferative glomerulonephritis
Epithelial cell casts	Acute tubular injury Glomerulonephritis Nephrotic syndrome

Source: https://en.wikipedia.org/wiki/Urinary_cast.

4.5.4.5. Microorganisms

The presence of microorganisms in the urine sediment is clinically significant when the specimen is properly collected. Microbiology should examine specimens containing bacteria, fungi, parasites, or cells infected with viruses to confirm and categorize the pathogen.

- **Bacteria:** Urine usually contains no bacteria at all. It is a pathologic finding if they are found in fresh urine. It goes without saying that the presence of bacteria in the urine may also be the result of contamination occurring during or after sample collection, since bacteria can multiply quickly in storage. They appear as tiny, moving coccoid or rod-like objects under a microscope, in contrast to all the other sedimentary elements.
- **Yeast:** The yeast cells have an oval shape, vary greatly in size, and are slightly smaller than erythrocytes. They group together or form chains. Yeast cells are frequently found in the urine sediment of diabetic patients, patients undergoing immunosuppressive therapy, and occasionally as a result of antibiotic administration.
- **Trichomonads:** These are spherical or oval-shaped protozoan organisms with multiple flagella and jerky, fast movements when they're living. If there is also vaginal inflammation, or colpitis, this is a common finding in urine sediment.

4.5.4.6. Crystals

Urine collected in the early morning hours must be examined for crystals right away. It is not appropriate to overestimate the frequency of crystal appearance in the urine sediment. Their development may simply be the consequence of urine's brief oversaturation, e.g., because of eating a diet high in oxalates or urates. Crystals can also form in vitro when a urine sample cools down or changes pH. The clinical significance of crystals found in these conditions is negligible. Urinary tract infections frequently result in the presence of crystals of ammonium magnesium phosphate in alkaline urine and uric acid or amorphous urates in acidic urine.

Nonetheless, there is some benefit to crystal detection in urolithiasis patients. Their presence can provide insight into the types of concrements that form in the urinary tract, but the discovery of a specific type of crystal in sediment does not necessarily indicate that the urinary tract contains concrements with the same chemical makeup. Repeated crystal detection is useful, especially when patients with recurrent urolithiasis or those who have had surgical removal of a concrement are being monitored.

The diagnosis of cystinuria is supported by the identification of hexagonal crystals of cystine. A high urine pH and ammonium-magnesium phosphate crystals suggest the possibility of struvite concrements.

The presence of crystalline calcium oxalate in large quantities is indicative of ethylene glycol intoxication; otherwise, calcium oxalate crystals are frequently found, particularly in individuals who consume a high-plant diet, and they are not connected to the development of concrements.

Uric acid crystals in acute urate nephropathy are another example of a useful discovery. Serious liver diseases are associated with the formation of leucine and tyrosine crystals. Some medications can also crystallize in the urine, particularly when taken excessively, when dehydrated, or when the albumin level is low.

- **Lipids:** As plasmatic lipoproteins, lipids can pass through damaged glomerular membranes and into urine. Lipiduria is indicative of severe kidney damage and is always associated with heavy proteinuria due to the larger particles of plasma lipoproteins than plasma proteins. Lipids can show up in the urine as clusters or as free droplets; in this instance, the presence of lipids may also be the result of rectal suppositories contaminating the urine. Cellular degeneration is indicated by the presence of lipid inclusions inside the cells. Subsequently, lipids may also manifest as fat casts and cholesterol crystals in the urine.
- **Other Findings:**
  - o In the urinary sediment, we can also notice motile spermatozoa with a long thin flagellum, mucus and fibrin fibers and various contaminating formations, such as fibers of toilet paper or various textiles.

4.5.5. Quantitative Examination of Urinary Sediment According to Hamburger

According to Hamburger, if indicated, the urinary sediment can be quantitatively examined; it essentially measures the rate at which erythrocytes, leukocytes, and casts are excreted into urine.

Urine is collected for three hours by the patient. The maximum deviation of ± 30 minutes is acceptable during the collection period and needs to be factored in when making calculations. After the urine collection is finished, the entire volume of urine is delivered to the laboratory in less than an hour, along with information on the exact start and end times of the collection period (down to the minute). Counting erythrocytes, leukocytes, and casts in five sizable Bürker's chamber squares is part of the laboratory examination.

- **Physiological Values:**

Erythrocytes	upto2000/minute, i.e., 33Ery/s
Leukocytes	upto4000/minute, i.e., 67Leu/s
Casts	upto60-70/minute, i.e., 1cast/s

4.5.6. Automatic Examination of Urinary Sediment

As of right now, there are devices for automatically analyzing urine sediment. They use digital imaging of particles or flow cytometry as their foundation. A laboratory method called flow cytometry can measure a vast range of parameters in a large number of particles. This advanced equipment has primarily been used in hematological laboratories, but more and more people are realizing how helpful it can be for the laborious and subject to subjectivity urine sediment examination process.

The cell suspension passes through a tiny capillary after the examined particles, or cells, are labeled with different fluorophores. A light beam—typically a laser beam—is encountered by the particles as they pass through the capillary. In addition to exciting the fluorescent labels on the cells, the particles scatter the laser's light. Typically, three parameters are measured: side scatter, which provides information about the inner structure of the analyzed particles; fluorescence of the labels used; and forward scatter, which is directly proportional to cell size.

Using flow cytometry, the examination of cells and other components of the urine sediment can be done entirely automatically.

4.5.6.1. Procedure

- The urine sample is mixed, aspirated into the instrument (0.8 ml), diluted and its conductivity is recorded.
- Automated staining of urinary elements with two different fluorescent dyes follows. Phenanthridine dye stains nucleic acids (orange fluorescence). The other employed stain is a carbocyanine dye that visualizes negatively charged cell membranes, nuclear membranes and mitochondria (green fluorescence).
- The stained particles encounter a laser beam that is both scattered and absorbed resulting in excitation of fluorophores. Identification and counting of elements is based on evaluation of fluorescent signal from both dyes together with measurement of light scatter and electric impedance of the cell suspension.

All urinary cellular components, including bacteria, leukocytes, erythrocytes, and epithelial cells, can be found using a flow cytometer. Furthermore, it has the ability to distinguish between a few clinically relevant entities, like isomorphic or dysmorphic erythrocytes. It accurately reports the presence of pathologic casts; however, additional microscopic examination is required to obtain more details. It also discovers crystalline formations, but it doesn't tell us what kind they are—that has to be determined once more through microscopic analysis. Trichomonads are not detectable by the flow cytometer.

The quantity of bacteria, flat epithelia, erythrocytes, leukocytes, and casts is expressed as a number of elements/ 1 ul.

Using the diagnostic strips assessed with the reflection photometer, it is possible to "cross check" the results of the flow cytometer with chemical analysis to improve the accuracy of the urine sediment. According to reports, there is an 80–90% agreement between flow cytometry and microscopy, and a 72–96% agreement with diagnostic strips. Flow cytometry greatly reduces the need for microscopic analyses, enhances examination accuracy, and makes result standardization easier.

4.5.6.2. Digital Particle Sensing

An injection of an uncentrifuged urine sample is made into a planar cuvette in this automatic urine sediment analysis method. Urine particles are scanned with a digital camera several times, and the images are compared with a database included in the device software based on the particles' size, shape, and structure (Figure 4.8).

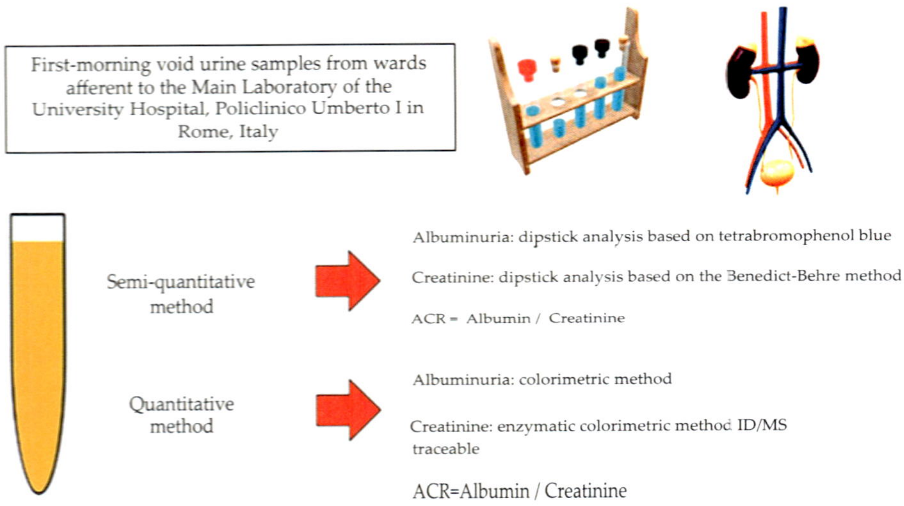

Figure 4.8. *An example of automated urine analysis.*

Source: *Terracina S, Pallaria A, Lucarelli M, Angeloni A, De Angelis A, Ceci FM, Caronti B, Francati S, Blaconà G, Fiore M, et al. Urine Dipstick Analysis on Automated Platforms: Is a Reliable Screening Tool for Proteinuria? An Experience from Umberto I Hospital in Rome. Biomedicines. 2023; 11(4):1174. https://doi.org/10.3390/biomedicines11041174.*

1. Urine Test Reference Values

- Chemical examination
  - pH 5–7.
  - Relative density 1,016–1,022.
  - Protein upto 0.3g/l.
  - Glucose negative.
  - Ketone bodies negative.
  - Bilirubin negative.
  - Urobilinogen 3,2–16μmol/l.
  - Blood upto 5/μl.
  - Leukocytes upto 10/μl.
  - Nitrite negative.
- Sediment (quantitative)
  - Erythrocytes<33/s.
  - Leukocytes<67/s.
  - Cylinders<1/s, only hyaline.

(Simerville et al., 2005)

A Closer Look

Results of Chemical Examination of Urine and Urinary Sediment in Urinary Tract Infections

If a urinary tract infection is suspected, we examine the urine chemically and evaluate the urinary sediment, among other things. In indicated cases, we also use urine culture tests with evidence of antibiotic susceptibility.

1. **Chemical Examination of Urine:** In the chemical examination of urine, we can find a number of abnormalities in urinary tract infections:
   - **Alkali Uria:** Some bacteria (e.g., *Pseudomonas*, *Klebsiella*) break down urea into ammonia by the enzyme urease. This alkalizes the urine. Therefore, we should always think about a urinary tract infection if the pH of the urine is higher than 6.5. However, more acidic urine does not rule out a urinary tract infection.
   - **Nitrites**: In particular, gram-negative bacteria (mainly *E. coli*, *Proteus*, *Klebsiella*, *Aerobacter*) can reduce nitrates to nitrites. Nitrite detection is thus an indirect sign of bacteriuria. This test is very specific, but its sensitivity is only around 50%.
   - **Hematuria:** It is detectable in most urinary tract infections. The presence of peroxidases in bacteriuria can also cause a positive blood test for urine. Unfortunately, the test is not very specific.
   - **Leukocyturia:** It also accompanies a large proportion of urinary tract infections. Quantitative examination of urinary sediment is more sensitive than chemical examination of urine.
   - **Proteinuria:** The amount of protein in the urine in urinary tract infections varies from concentrations that cannot be determined by basic techniques to values around 2 g / l.
   - **Other Findings in Chemical Examination of Urine:** In urinary tract infections, false positives of bilirubin, urobilinogen and ketone bodies are often false.

It follows that the result of a chemical urine test can be very abundant in urinary tract infections. On the other hand, we also encounter bacteriuria with a completely normal chemical finding. Therefore, any combination of results between these two extremes is compatible with the diagnosis of urinary tract infection. However, the following applies:

- If there are positive nitrites, the urinary tract infection is almost certain (specificity> 95%). Quite often, however, in a urinary tract infection, nitrites remain negative (sensitivity around 50%).
- In 98% of urinary tract infections, at least one of the parameters of hematuria, leukocyturia, nitrites, proteinuria is positive. With the exception of nitrites, however,

the finding is often caused by another cause and urinary tract infection must therefore be confirmed by further examination (microscopically and by culture).

2. **Sediment Examination:** Higher erythrocyte and leukocyte counts are usually found in urinary sediment for urinary tract infections; in these parameters, the sediment examination is more sensitive than the chemical examination. Furthermore, there are usually higher numbers of epithelial cells corresponding to the site of inflammation, and of course we find a larger number of bacteria.

Summary

- Urine is an unstable fluid, and changes to its composition begin to take place as soon as it is voided. It is, therefore, important to properly collect, store, and transport specimens to minimize the risk of altered test results. Often the first void or "morning urine" is collected because it is most concentrated, and trace amounts of substances can be detected. Furthermore, it provides an insight to the kidneys' concentrating abilities.
- Urine is usually obtained by spontaneous micturition. The actual urine collection is performed after thorough washing and drying of the external urethral orifice. Urine in a clean, dry, closable container that contains no detergent or disinfectant residues that distort the results of the chemical analysis. The middle urine flow is intended for examination. The first stream is always contaminated with cells and bacteria from around the outer urethra.
- A random urine sample is a label for fresh urine collection without knowledge of collection time and volume, and details of patient preparation are not usually known. It is possible for acute conditions. Urine analysis can be fraught with a number of errors.
- The physical urine examination consists of the assessment of urine color, its smell, foam and turbidity; and also measurements of its pH, relative specific gravity and osmolality. For functional examinations, estimation of the volume of urine per defined period of time is necessary.
- The routine chemical examination of urine involves qualitative tests for protein, glucose, hemoglobin, ketone bodies and bile pigments. These components are mostly present in urine from healthy individuals as well but in tiny amounts undetectable by routine tests. Various pathological conditions increase their concentration in urine.
- Urinary proteins are normally present only in trace amounts, up to about 150 mg/24 h or 10 mg/dL, and originate in the plasma and urinary tract. Albumin is about a third of the total, while the remaining plasma proteins are small globulins.
- Small amounts of glucose may be present in urine, especially after a meal containing a high concentration of carbohydrates. Glucose is freely filtered through the glomerular basement membrane and is mostly reabsorbed in the tubules, so under normal circumstances, little is found in the urine.
- Ketone bodies are a byproduct of incomplete fat metabolism indicative of a gluconeogenic metabolic state that can occur with starvation, low-carbohydrate diets, febrile illness, or uncontrolled diabetes mellitus. These compounds, acetoacetic acid, acetone, and beta-hydroxy-butyric acid, are released into the blood by the liver and are used by other tissues of the body as an energy source; however, some are also filtered by the kidneys and excreted in urine (ketonuria).
- Bilirubin is a byproduct of RBC senescence in the reticuloendothelial system. Hemoglobin is converted to unconjugated bilirubin, which is then released into the bloodstream by the reticuloendothelial cells. It then becomes reversibly bound to albumin, which carries it to the liver where hepatocytes remove it by a carrier-mediated active transport.

- Urobilinogen is a product of bilirubin metabolism by bacteria in the intestine. Though most of it is excreted in feces, some of it is reabsorbed and carried by enterohepatic circulation to the liver where the majority is reexcreted in bile. The remaining urobilinogen is then filtered by the kidneys and appears in urine if increased in amount.
- Microscopic examination of the urinary sediment is the third part of routine urinalysis. All nonsoluble components of urine are isolated through centrifugation and are observed under the microscope. Although it has been argued that microscopic examination should be performed on every specimen, most laboratorians agree that it is an essential component in the evaluation of symptomatic patients.

References

1. Bain, B. J. (2015). *Blood Cells: A Practical Guide* (5th ed.). John Wiley & Sons. ISBN 978-1-118-81733-9.
2. Brunzel, N. A. (2018). *Fundamentals of Urine and Body Fluid Analysis* (4th ed.). Elsevier. ISBN 978-0-323-37479-8.
3. Clarke, W., & Palmer-Toy, D. E. (2002). Clinical chemistry of urine, pleural effusions, and ascites. In K. D. Lewandrowski (Ed.), *Clinical Chemistry: Laboratory Management and Clinical Correlations* (pp. 849–864). Philadelphia: Lippincott Williams & Wilkins.
4. Fuller, C. E., Threatte, G. A., & Henry, J. B. (2001). Basic Examination of Urine. In J. B. Henry (Ed.), *Clinical Diagnosis and Management by Laboratory Methods* (20th ed., pp. 367–402). Philadelphia: WB Saunders.
5. Hanno, P. M., Wein, A. J., & Malkowicz, S. B. (2001). *Clinical Manual of Urology* (3rd ed.). New York: McGraw-Hill.
6. Kaplan, L. A., Pesce, A. J., & Kazmierczak, S. (2003). *Clinical Chemistry: Theory, Analysis, Correlation* (4th ed.). St. Louis: Mosby.
7. Liang, S. L., & Clark, W. (2006). *Professional Practice in Clinical Chemistry*. Washington, DC: AAAC Press.
8. McClatchey, K. D. (2002). *Clinical Laboratory Medicine* (2nd ed.). Philadelphia: Lippincott Williams & Wilkins.
9. Mundt, L. A., & Shanahan, K. (2016). *Graff's Textbook of Urinalysis and Body Fluids* (3rd ed.). Wolters Kluwer. ISBN 978-1-4963-2016-2.
10. Sharp, V. J. A., Antes, L. M., Sanders, M. L., & Lockwood, G. M. (2020). *Urine Tests: A Case-Based Guide to Clinical Evaluation and Application*. Springer. ISBN 978-3-030-29138-9.
11. Simerville, J. A., Maxted, W. C., & Pahira, J. J. (2005). Urinalysis: A Comprehensive Review. *American Family Physician, 71*, 1153–1162.

Chapter

5

RENAL AND METABOLIC DISEASE

Contents

Introduction

Renal disease, commonly referred to as kidney disease, is any illness that affects the kidneys' structure or functionality. Nephritis is an inflammatory kidney disease that can be classified into multiple types based on the site of inflammation. Blood tests can be used to diagnose inflammation. Nephrosis is a kidney disease that is not inflammatory. Nephrotic syndrome and nephritic syndrome are conditions that can result from nephrosis and nephritis, respectively. Kidney disease often results in a partial loss of kidney function and can lead to kidney failure, which is the total loss of kidney function. Dialysis or a kidney transplant are the only available treatments for kidney failure, which is referred to as the end-stage of kidney disease. Long-lasting renal abnormalities (of a functional or structural nature) lasting longer than three months are referred to as chronic kidney disease. Acute kidney disease, also known as acute kidney injury, is characterized by a sharp decline in kidney function that lasts for seven days. Roughly one in eight Americans suffered from chronic kidney disease in 2007. As a result of this rising rate, by 2021 it is predicted that 1 in 7 Americans will have CKD.

Orientation and Directional Terms

Term	Definition	Illustration
Nephritis	Nephritis is a condition in which the tissues in the kidney become inflamed and have problems filtering waste from the blood. Nephritis may be caused by infection, inflammatory conditions (such as lupus), certain genetic conditions, and other diseases or conditions.	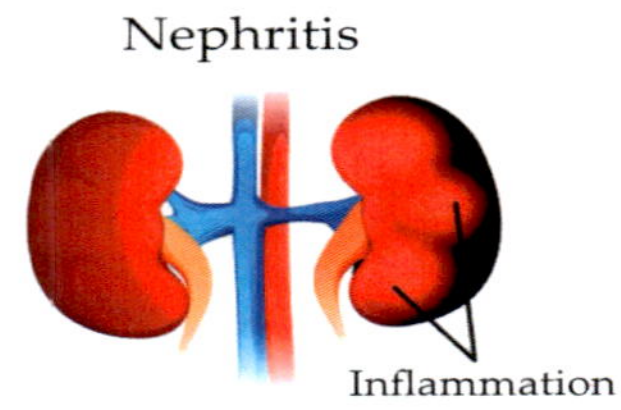
Glomerulonephritis	Glomerulonephritis is inflammation and damage to the filtering part of the kidneys (glomerulus). It can come on quickly or over a longer period of time. Toxins, metabolic wastes and excess fluid are not properly filtered into the urine. Instead, they build up in the body causing swelling and fatigue	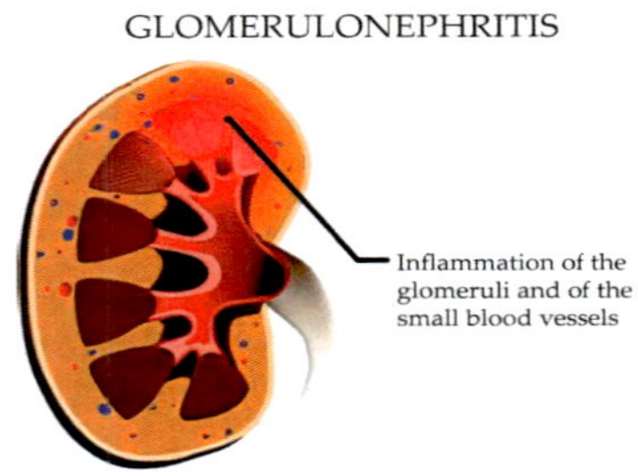
Systemic lupus erythematosus (SLE)	Systemic lupus erythematosus (SLE), is the most common type of lupus. SLE is an autoimmune disease in which the immune system attacks its own tissues, causing widespread	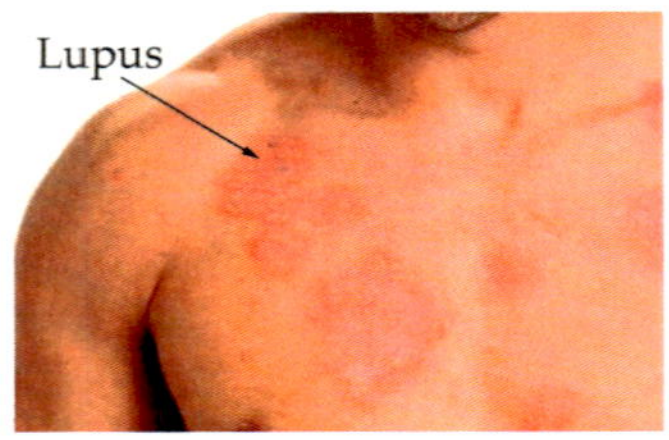
Diabetic nephropathy	Diabetic nephropathy is a serious complication of type 1 diabetes and type 2 diabetes. It's also called diabetic kidney disease.	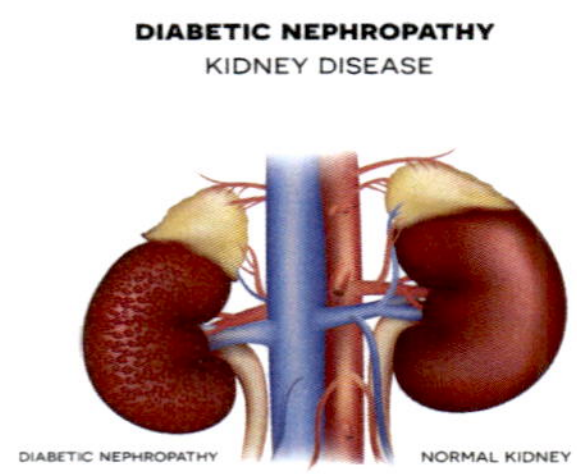
Amyloidosis	Amyloidosis is a rare disease that occurs when a protein called amyloid builds up in organs. This amyloid buildup can make the organs not work properly. Organs that may be affected include the heart, kidneys, liver, spleen, nervous system and digestive tract.	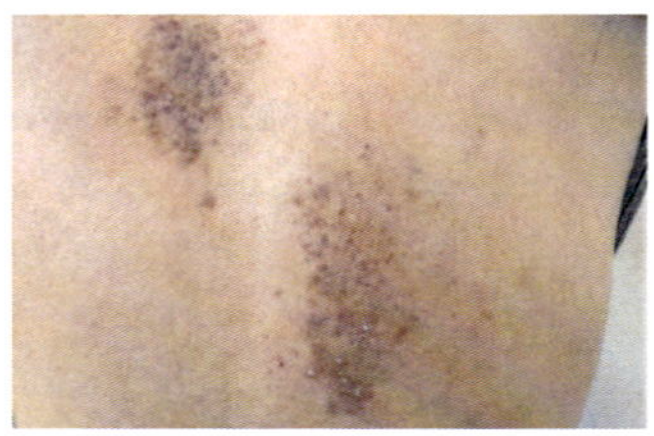

5.1. Glomerular Disease

The ability of the kidneys to keep certain substances in the bloodstream balanced is diminished by glomerular disease. Normally, red blood cells and protein remain in the bloodstream while toxins are filtered out of the bloodstream and eliminated in the urine. Red blood cells and protein may be eliminated into the urine in individuals with glomerular disease, but toxins may stay in the body. (Figure 5.1).

Glomerular disease can be isolated (i.e., affect only the kidney) or it can be linked to an underlying illness such as diabetes, lupus, or specific infections that affect other organ systems. Acute glomerular disease is a type of glomerular disease that appears suddenly, while chronic glomerular disease develops gradually over years. The type and cause of glomerular disease determine how it should be treated.

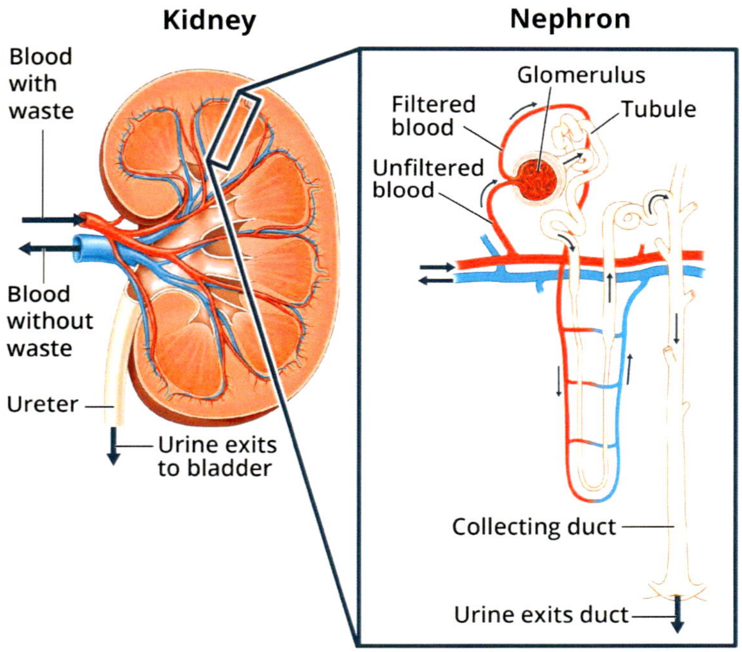

Figure 5.1. *As blood passes through healthy kidneys, the glomeruli filter out waste products and allow the blood to keep the cells and proteins the body needs.*

Source: https://www.niddk.nih.gov/health-information/kidney-disease/glomerular-disease.

5.1.1. Types of Glomerular Disease

Nephrotic and nephritic are the two main forms of glomerular disease, though there are some conditions where the two can coexist.

5.1.1.1. Nephritic

Hematuria, or blood in the urine, is the main symptom of glomerulonephritis, a type of nephritic disease. Proteinuria and renal function impairment may not be very noticeable in less severe cases of the disease. Actually, glomerulonephritis may not cause any symptoms, and a patient's condition might go undiagnosed until a routine urinalysis reveals the presence of blood and protein. Individuals with more advanced nephritic disease frequently have impaired kidney function in addition to hematuria. High protein levels in the urine may also indicate high blood pressure or edema, or swelling in the lower limbs. Examples of conditions that may cause glomerulonephritis include:

- Immunoglobulin A (IgA) nephropathy
- Lupus
- Vasculitis
- Certain bacterial and viral infections (postinfectious glomerulonephritis)
- Mixed cryoglobulinemia
- Membranoproliferative glomerulonephritis
- Alport syndrome
- IgA vasculitis (Henoch-Schönlein purpura)
- C3 glomerulopathy

5.1.1.2. Nephrotic Syndrome

Nephrotic syndrome patients often have little to no blood in their urine (hematuria), but they also have proteinuria (the presence of protein in the urine). As nephrotic syndrome worsens, kidney function might deteriorate.

Examples of conditions that may cause nephrotic syndrome include:

- Minimal change disease
- Focal segmental glomerulosclerosis
- Membranous nephropathy (including lupus)
- Diabetic kidney disease
- Postinfectious glomerulonephritis (later stage)
- IgA nephropathy
- Primary amyloidosis or the related disorder light chain deposition disease

5.1.2. Symptoms of Glomerular Disease

The type of damage to your glomeruli determines the symptoms of glomerular disease. While some people with more severe damage may have more obvious symptoms, some people with less damage may have few or none at all.

Symptoms can include:

- High blood pressure, which may develop or get worse.
- Swelling. Also called edema, swelling can affect many parts of your body including your hands, ankles, legs, and around your eyes.
- Weight gain. As fluid builds up in your body, your weight can increase.
- Proteinuria. Too much protein in your urine, called proteinuria, can cause bubbles or foam to appear in your urine.
- Blood in your urine. Also called hematuria, blood in the urine can make your urine look pink or cola-colored. The blood can usually only be seen under a microscope.

5.1.3. Causes Glomerular Disease

The following are the main causes of glomerular disease:

- One kind of kidney disease brought on by diabetes is diabetic kidney disease. High blood glucose, or blood sugar, levels over years can harm your glomeruli.

- A condition known as focal segmental glomerulosclerosis (FSGS) NIH external link results in the formation of scar tissue in certain glomeruli in your kidneys. Numerous factors can contribute to FSGS, such as genetics, autoimmune disorders, and conditions like obesity and sleep apnea that increase pressure in the glomeruli.
- Systemic lupus erythematosus, or lupus, is the cause of lupus nephritis, a kidney disease NIH external link. An autoimmune condition that affects numerous body parts is lupus. Antibodies may accumulate in your glomeruli as a result of the disease, resulting in inflammation that may impair kidney function and eventually cause scarring.
- Membranous nephropathy (NIH external link) is a condition where antibodies accumulate in the glomerular basement membrane, a section of the kidney. Your glomeruli may consequently thicken and inflame. Infections, cancer, and autoimmune disorders are a few possible causes.
- IgA nephropathy, also known as Berger's disease, is an autoimmune condition in which your glomeruli become inflamed and damaged due to an accumulation of the antibody immunoglobulin A (IgA).
- Also known as nil disease, minimal change disease (NIH external link). Your glomeruli will change as a result of this kidney disease, and these changes will only be visible under an electron microscope, which is an extremely strong microscope.
- Goodpasture's disease, also known as anti-GBM, is an autoimmune condition in which your glomeruli are attacked by antibodies, resulting in inflammation and damage. Your lungs may also be impacted by the illness.

5.1.4. Pathogenesis of Glomerular Diseases

Glomerular diseases can present as a range of clinical syndromes, with varying degrees of severity. They are thought to be the consequence of inherited or acquired disorders. Occasionally, patients present with rapidly progressing glomerulonephritis, a dangerous condition that, if left untreated, can progress to advanced or end-stage kidney disease. The assessment of renal histopathology in conjunction with the traits of the clinical syndrome continues to be the foundation for precise diagnosis and evidence-based care. Significant advancements have been made in this field over the last ten years, particularly concerning the etiology and pathophysiology of these illnesses. The autoimmune basis of glomerulonephritis is linked to genetic risk factors and environmental stimuli that trigger immune-mediated glomerular injury. New information has emerged regarding molecular mechanisms, genetic associations, and immunologically-mediated forms of glomerulonephritis. In this section, studies using animal models have played a major role in bolstering a translational model that explains how immune responses mediate the glomerular lesion, which renal pathologists detect in the biopsy specimen. Numerous researchers have hypothesized and presented the idea that the majority of glomerulonephritis forms are related to immune responses to self-antigens and infectious agents.

Complement and toll-like receptors are thought to be involved in these immune responses, and resident glomerular cells and monocytes are activated to cause inflammatory reactions in the glomeruli. Red blood cells and proteins from the blood space (glomerular capillary lumen) can pass through multiple lesions in the glomerular filtration barrier and end up in the urine. Therefore, one of the most prevalent clinical signs of glomerular diseases, such as lupus nephritis, ANCA-vasculitis, and IgA nephropathy (IgAN), is microscopic hematuria, either with or without proteinuria. Although some nephrologists view microscopic hematuria as a benign finding stemming from prior damage, clinicians with extensive training in glomerular diseases view persistent hematuria as an indication of ongoing disease activity.

However, since it has been demonstrated to be independently linked to the advancement of renal disease in patients with IgAN, the significance of microhematuria in the onset of glomerular diseases and progressive kidney damage has recently drawn increased attention. In patients with primary membranous nephropathy (MN), a higher level of initial hematuria was a remarkable predictor of relapse, whereas the degree and persistence of microscopic hematuria were independently linked to the advancement of kidney disease. 80% of patients with primary MN have nephrotic-range proteinuria at presentation, 20% have subnephrotic proteinuria, and approximately 50 to 60% of patients have microhematuria. During follow-up, patients with idiopathic MN and persistent hematuria had significantly higher risks of kidney disease progression than those without persistent hematuria. As previously mentioned, damage to the glomerular filtration barrier structure results in glomerular hematuria. Leukocytes and other infiltrating inflammatory cells may release metalloproteinases and reactive oxygen species in patients with glomerular inflammation, increasing the risk of glomerular basement membrane rupture. Conversely, chronic glomerular hematuria can lead to renal damage by inducing oxidative stress from the iron and hemoglobin released into renal tubular cells from broken erythrocytes. Nonetheless, when compared to patients who still had microhematuria, hematuria remission was independently linked to a 37% lower risk of renal failure. Therefore, although its precise relationship with end-stage kidney disease or death and histopathological findings needs to be clarified in prospective studies, hematuria diminution may be a predictor of renal survival for patients with primary MN.

In 442 patents with biopsy-proven MN, the function of tertiary lymphoid organs (TLOs) in the pathogenesis of the disease and its clinical correlations with it were investigated. It was discovered that these patients' kidney tissue frequently contained TLOs, which are structures made up of accumulated lymphoid cells. The clinical picture severity and the TLO density were correlated, meaning that an increase in TLOs was associated with a worsening of the disease. Anti-phospholipase A2 receptor autoantibodies were more common in the blood of patients with TLOs, whereas patients without TLOs had a much higher chance of achieving total remission.

When compared to proliferative classes of renal involvement, lupus MN, a type of secondary form of this disease that accounts for 10–20% of all cases of lupus nephritis, is generally associated with a better patient and renal survival. A report of 27 patients with pure lupus MN highlighted the favorable prognosis that is linked to the type of lupus glomerulopathy. All of the patients had eGFRs greater than 60 ml/min/1.73 m^2, had very good long-term renal survival, and were followed for a median of 77 months.

Prognosis is still a critical concern for all patients with glomerular disorders, but it is especially important for those with IgAN because patients may present with different clinical and histopathological pictures depending on how severe their condition is. In this regard, Dong discovered that arterial-arteriolar sclerosis was an independent risk factor for the progression of IgAN and was associated with the composite outcome of >50% reduction in estimated glomerular filtration rate, end-stage kidney disease, or death after studying 1,424 patients with IgAN. These results were correlated with the severity of arterial-arteriolar sclerosis, and a trend suggesting that it could function as a separate risk marker for the advancement of IgAN was observed.

Wang Y-N et al. demonstrated that patients with IgAN had a higher frequency of hyperhomocysteinemia than those with other types of glomerular disease. The proportion of global glomerulosclerosis, the proportion of ischemia-originated glomerular sclerosis, and the severity of tubular atrophy/interstitial fibrosis are among the histopathologic features of IgAN that have been linked to the homocysteine/eGFR ratio. Significantly, this ratio was a separate risk factor for the occurrence of chronic kidney disease progression.

Lastly, a study addressed pregnancy, which is a significant factor for people with glomerular disease. Women who have glomerular disease may be more susceptible to infertility, early menopause, and unfavorable pregnancy outcomes. Marinaki et al describe the results of 22 glomerular disease patients who became pregnant. Prior to conception, all patients had maintained renal function and were in either complete or partial remission. Only 6.9 and 6.7 percent of cases involved disease relapse and preeclampsia, respectively, while 23% involved preterm births. The low incidence of adverse events overall emphasizes how crucial it is to ensure disease quiescence before conception (Couser and Johnson, 2014; O'Shaughnessy et al., 2017; Khalighi et al., 2018; Mariani et al., 2019; Satoskar et al., 2020).

5.2. Acute Glomerulonephritis

Only diabetes and hypertension are more significant causes of renal impairment than glomerulonephritis, which accounts for 10–15% of end-stage renal failure cases in the United States. We have chosen to address glomerular diseases that can manifest as nephritic syndrome, which includes hematuria, proteinuria, and decreased renal function along with hypertension, fluid overload, and edema, when characterizing acute glomerulonephritis. Their pathology entails cellular proliferation and intraglomerular inflammation, resulting in days to weeks of secondary renal impairment. This definition does not include glomerular diseases like minimal change disease, membranous nephropathy, and focal segmental glomerulosclerosis that can impair renal function over time but do not involve cell proliferation or nephritic presentations. Primary glomerulonephritis (like IgA nephropathy or post-streptococcal glomerulonephritis) is a disease that is almost exclusively limited to the kidneys, whereas secondary glomerulonephritis is associated with a more diffuse form of inflammation (like systemic lupus erythematosus or systemic vasculitis). It is critical to diagnose glomerulonephritis as soon as possible because patients with hypertension, even mildly impaired renal function, and abnormalities in their urine can quickly lose their kidney function if treatment is delayed.

While the etiology of glomerulonephritis remains largely unknown, inflammation is believed to be autoimmune-mediated and to involve both the humoral and cellular immune systems. In every instance, a distinct initial stimulus (arising from one of a minimum of four distinct mechanisms) is succeeded by an identical sequence of inflammatory and subsequently fibrotic events. Patients with anti-glomerular basement membrane disease generate antibodies that directly interact with the glomerulus and lung's specialized basement membranes. Antibodies to an exogenous streptococcal antigen that was inserted into the glomerulus during infection rather than an endogenous antigen are produced in post-streptococcal glomerulonephritis. The antigen-antibody response happens both in situ in the glomerulus and systemically with subsequent complex trapping in the kidney in systemic lupus erythematosus and IgA nephropathy. Ultimately, it is believed that cellular rather than humoral immune responses are triggered in the glomerulonephritis associated with small vessel vasculitis. As a result, inflammation that often starts in organs far from the kidney eventually causes a renal influx of T-cells and macrophages as crescentic glomerulonephritis develops.

Activation of the complement and coagulation cascades, along with the production of proinflammatory cytokines, are common inflammatory pathways that ensue from whatever the initial events may be. Complement component activation causes inflammatory cells to chemotactic signals and cells to lyse (through the membrane attack complex). The deposit of fibrin is the result of the coagulation cascade. Acute glomerular crescent formation is caused by the cellular proliferation of parietal epithelial cells in Bowman's space combined with an influx of inflammatory cells like neutrophils and macrophages. The release of cytokines causes the glomerular cells to become activated, and an alteration in the phenotype of endogenous cells leads to the proliferation of cells, excessive production of oxidants and proteases, and the deposition of extracellular matrix, which is followed by fibrosis. These processes may be induced by factors like transforming growth factor beta and platelet-derived growth factor. It's also crucial if apoptosis, the regular process that permits inflammation to subside, fails. Last but not least, during a chronic phase of damage, changes in hemodynamics cause intraglomerular hypertension and hyperfiltration, which in turn cause glomerular sclerosis and chronic interstitial damage to develop. Therefore, what starts out as an inflammatory process that may go away can instead lead to fibrosis and permanent scarring. This dynamic picture may help to explain why even acute renal failure can be expected to resolve spontaneously in post-streptococcal glomerulonephritis, where antigen is rapidly cleared. On the other hand, antigens cannot be eliminated in hepatitis C associated mesangiocapillary glomerulonephritis (MCGN), a condition where renal damage may worsen over time due to persistent viral infection.

Changes brought on by inflammation, proliferation, and fibrosis may have distinct effects on different kidney cells or may lead to more widespread alterations with distinct patterns that produce a range of clinical manifestations. Renal biopsies are essential for making a diagnosis and providing prognostic information by separating chronically scarred non-viable kidneys that do not warrant the risks of potentially toxic therapy from acutely damaging kidneys that can be repaired. Even though the current treatments are, at best, rudimentary, we hope to develop more targeted therapies in the future as we gain a better understanding of the pathological events that lead to acute damage and the inevitable decline in renal function that results from it.

5.2.1. Post-infectious Endocapillary Glomerulonephritis

The most well-known instance of endocapillary glomerulonephritis, which is the most prevalent type of acute glomerulonephritis that can result from various bacterial, viral, fungal, and parasitic infections, is post-streptococcal glomerulonephritis. While streptococcal infections continue to be a major cause of acute renal failure in developing nations, endocarditis following intravenous drug abuse is increasingly linked to this pattern of glomerular injury in Europe and the USA. Children with post-streptococcal glomerulonephritis typically have a male predominance. It can occur one to twelve weeks after the original infection and can be followed by pharyngitis (usually in winter) or skin infections (usually in summer) caused by a β-hemolytic nephritogenic strain of streptococcus, usually type 12. Up to 15% of infected individuals may experience symptoms, however many of them are subclinical and resolve on their own. The classic nephritic picture of swollen eyelids, facial edema, hypertension, and dark, scant urine with microscopic hematuria and proteinuria is present in the most severely affected children.

When a streptococcal component is deposited in the glomerulus during infection, the pathology is similar to that of a planted antigen. The host's subsequent generation of antibodies results in the formation of in situ immune complexes, which change the glomerular basement membrane's permeability and permit the deposition of more pre-formed immune complexes. Furthermore, streptococcal antigen can directly activate complement, which attracts inflammatory cells, or it can cross-react with glomerular structures. A diffuse proliferative glomerulonephritis, specifically affecting mesangial and endothelial cells, is brought on by immune deposits. Immunostaining reveals C3 along capillary walls and in the mesangium, accompanied by IgG.

Since many nephritogenic strains do not produce streptolysin, serology may reveal elevated anti-streptolysin antibody titers; however, its absence does not rule out the diagnosis. Acutely, low C3 levels with normal C4 levels (caused by activation of an alternate pathway) should have returned to normal in two months.

5.2.2. Mesangioproliferative Glomerulonephritis/ IgA Nephropathy

Globally, IgA nephropathy is the most prevalent type of glomerulonephritide. As a result, even though only 4–13% of patients have acute nephritis (micro-or macroscopic hematuria is the more common presentation), this still amounts to a sizable number of cases. Peak manifestation occurs in the second and third decades, with a 2:1 male preponderance and occasional attacks following infection, especially pharyngitis. Geographically, the disease varies greatly; it is more common in Asia and the Western Pacific region (where it accounts for half of primary glomerular disease in Japan), but it is uncommon in black populations.

IgA nephropathy is a type of glomerulonephritis characterized by mesangial proliferation, with deposits of IgA, IgG, and IgM in the mesangium. Electron microscopy reveals dense deposits in the mesangium. The condition is caused by the deposition of polymeric IgA1 in the kidneys due to overproduction and impaired clearance, possibly triggered by infection. Abnormal glycosylation of IgA can lead to the formation of immune complexes that target the mesangium. While 50% of patients have elevated IgA levels in their serum, complement levels remain normal as complement activation is confined to the kidneys.

5.2.3. Henoch-Schönlein Purpura

The kidney damage seen in Henoch-Schönlein purpura (HSP) closely resembles that of the more severe forms of IgA nephropathy. However, as a type of small vessel vasculitis, HSP also exhibits systemic symptoms such as a purplish rash primarily on the lower limbs, arthritis or joint pain, and abdominal discomfort often accompanied by rectal bleeding. This condition typically affects individuals under the age of 20. While renal issues may not be present initially, they become more common over time, especially in older children with persistent rash and abdominal pain. Adults can also develop kidney problems with HSP, which tends to have a poorer outcome. The most common renal symptoms include blood and protein in the urine, with about 8% of patients experiencing acute nephritis and up to 29% showing both nephritic and nephrotic features.

Immune complexes containing IgA are also present in the systemic circulation of HSP patients, although they are larger than those found in IgA disease. Although capillary wall staining for IgA is also common, mesangial deposition of IgA is typically observed. In HSP, there is a higher prevalence of leucocytoclastic vasculitis, fibrin deposition, and glomerular crescents. It is believed that minute variations in the IgA complexes of HSP cause increased leucocyte stimulation, which in turn causes the extrarenal manifestations and small vessel vasculitis that characterize HSP.

5.2.4. Rapidly Progressive Glomerulonephritis (RPGN)

The most dangerous type of glomerulonephritides are those that progress quickly, as they can completely destroy renal function in a matter of days. The histological discovery of extensive crescents, which affect more than 50% of glomeruli and are caused by a proliferation of parietal epithelial cells, mononuclear phagocytes, and possibly fibroblasts in Bowman's capsule, unites the various causes, despite their heterogeneity. There are three main categories of causes, each with unique manifestations, courses of action, and outcomes.

About 50% of RPGN is caused by pauci-immune glomerulonephritis, which is primarily caused by small vessel vasculitides. Its incidence is about 2 per 100,000 people annually, peaks in the sixth decade, and is distributed equally among all sexes. Idiopathic crescentic glomerulonephritis is a type of disease that only affects the kidneys. Wegener's granulomatosis and microscopic polyangiitis are two conditions where the disease is linked to widespread systemic inflammation. Weight loss and a general feeling of being unwell often precede overt presentation, with specific illness-related features appearing later. In just 50% of cases, pulmonary symptoms associated with microscopic polyangiitis are caused by non-granulomatous arteriolar vasculitis and capillaritis. Other symptoms include cutaneous (palpable purpura), neurological (mononeuritis multiplex), or gastrointestinal vasculitis in addition to renal failure. In contrast, Wegener's granulomatosis is primarily characterized by pulmonary manifestations, including cavitating lung lesions visible on radiography, upper respiratory tract involvement (deafness, nasal cartilage collapse, sinusitis), and lower respiratory tract involvement (pulmonary hemorrhage due to granulomatous vasculitis).

A diffuse or focal proliferative glomerulonephritis with large crescents is revealed by the biopsy. Although direct immunoglobulin deposition in the glomerulus is not believed to play a significant role in the pathogenesis of vasculitis, research on the subject is still focused on this area (hence the term pauci-immune). On a serological level, however, the presence of antineutrophil cytoplasmic antibodies (ANCA) links these illnesses in approximately 90% of cases. In Wegener's disease, antibody staining is typically perinucleur in pattern and directed against myeloperoxidase, whereas in microscopic polyangiitis, it is typically directed against the neutrophil cytoplasm with an antigen specificity for proteinase 3 on ELISA. It is still debatable whether ANCA directly causes small vessel vasculitis; instead, experimental data suggests that T cells, macrophages, and neutrophils play roles in the disease's etiology.

In a European Caucasian population, anti-glomerular basement membrane disease (RPGN) accounts for 10–20% of cases, with a frequency of 0.5 cases per million per year. There are two peaks to the disease: the first occurs in the third decade and is predominantly affecting men, and the second occurs in the sixth and seventh decades and affects both sexes equally. When the condition is referred to as Goodpasture's disease, associated lung involvement is more common in young men, whereas isolated kidney involvement is more common in older patients. Compared to vasculitides, there is a lower incidence of a prodrome of weight loss and malaise. Patients typically present with acute renal failure or hemoptysis as a result of lung involvement. Smokers, people with fluid overload, and people with ongoing infections are more likely to experience hemoptysis (the latter also makes the kidney damage more severe). The most frequent cause of death in the early stages of the disease is lung hemorrhage, which should be suspected if there is hemoptysis or if a chest radiograph demonstrates alveolar shadowing that is unrestricted by anatomical fissures and sparing of the upper zones. A temporary increase in the transfer factor during pulmonary function testing could be an indication of acute hemorrhage.

Antibodies that bind the alpha 3 chain of type 4 collagen, which is present in the kidney and lung's specialized basement membranes, are the cause of anti-glomerular basement membrane disease. A previously normal kidney can develop 100% crescents in as little as five days. Initially, histology may show a focal segmental glomerulonephritis with necrosis and interstitial inflammation. However, the condition will quickly progress to show widespread crescent formation with all crescents at the same stage of evolution. IgG antibodies (which are occasionally linked to C3) are linearly deposited along the glomerular basement membrane as visible by immunofluorescence. Antiglomerular basement membrane antibodies are positive in serology, however, ANCA antibodies are also found in 20–30% of patients. These patients have a better prognosis for their kidneys than those who only have antiglomerular basement membrane antibodies; this could be because the antiglomerular basement membrane antibodies are a secondary reaction to the damaged basement membrane, and the patients actually have vasculitis. These patients exhibit clinical behaviors more similar to those of vasculitis, such as lethargy, malaise, and weight loss.

30 to 40% of cases of RPGN are caused by a variety of diverse conditions in which immune complex deposition or other causes of basement membrane damage, such as accelerated hypertension, are linked to renal damage. Pathology is often an aggressive form of glomerulonephritis, often associated with a more benign course (e.g., IgA nephropathy, post-streptococcal glomerulonephritis), with complex histology including crescent formation and extensive inflammation. It is also observed in conjunction with multisystem diseases like systemic lupus erythematosus or following infections like endocarditis and shunt nephritis.

5.2.5. Mesangiocapillary Glomerulonephritis; Also Known as Membranoproliferative Glomerulonephritis

Since a subtype of MCGN type I has been linked to chronic hepatitis C infection, interest in this uncommon form of glomerulonephritis has increased. Although nephrotic syndrome is the typical initial presentation of MCGN, acute nephritis occurs in 16–30% of cases. The disease can be further classified into types I and II. The idiopathic forms of the disease are primarily seen in children and young adults; type II cases typically present at a younger age (15 years ±11 years) than type I cases (24 years ±16 years), with a slight preponderance of female cases. Certain characteristics of Type I MCGN are similar to those of lupus nephritis, and endocarditis and infected arteriovenous shunts also present with a similar histological appearance. Patients with type II MCGN may also have a partial lypodystrophy, which makes their faces appear extremely gaunt.

Recent research has revealed that a sizable percentage of type I MCGN cases that were previously classified as idiopathic are actually related to chronic hepatitis C infection, of which 20–25% will manifest as acute nephritis. The prevalence of hepatitis C-associated renal disease varies by country. While it is more common in Italy and Japan, where it can account for up to 60% of cases of membranoproliferative glomerulonephritis, it is less common in the USA, where it only accounts for 10% to 20% of cases, and it has not been observed much in France. Patients with mild biochemical abnormalities and subclinical liver disease present 10-15 years after middle-aged infection. Cryoglobulinaemia, or cold precipitable mixed immunoglobulins made up of polyclonal IgG, rheumatoid factor, and monoclonal IgM, is frequently associated with renal disease. Along with lower limb ulceration and Raynaud's disease, patients also experience polyarthralgia, anemia, peripheral neuropathy, malaise, and a purpuric rash. Rarely, the cardiovascular or gastrointestinal systems are also impacted by vasculitis.

While low C4 concentrations are linked to the activation of the classical complement pathway in idiopathic type I MCGN, low C3 and the presence of the C3 nephritic factor—an antibody that permanently activates the complement cascade—are indicative of the activation of the alternative pathway in MCGN type II. Along with low levels of classical complement component, patients with hepatitis C-associated MCGN also have positive antihepatitis C antibodies and hepatitis C RNA on polymerase chain reaction. Additionally, 70% of them may have positive results for rheumatoid factor, 70% for antinuclear antibodies, and 75% for cryoglobulins.

Although the exact cause of MCGN is unknown, mesangial cells in particular are likely to undergo rapid cell proliferation. Histologically, both types exhibit mesangial expansion and thickening of the capillary walls (along with a decrease in the capillary lumina). In the case of MCGN type I, this thickening and classic tramline effect are partially caused by cellular proliferation extending between the capillary basement membranes. Both types of MCGN exhibit mesangial and capillary loop deposition of C3, but only type I MCGN exhibits immunoglobulin deposition in conjunction with this. Based on results from electron microscopy, the different types are distinguished: type I disease is characterized by subendothelial immune deposits in the glomerular basement membrane, whereas type II disease is characterized by dense intramembranous deposits in the glomerular, tubular, and vascular basement membranes (the nature of these deposits in type II disease is unknown but does explain its alternative name, dense deposit disease). It is believed that intracapillary deposits in type I MCGN associated with hepatitis C result from the precipitation of the cryoglobulins themselves.

5.2.6. Lupus Nephritis

Systemic lupus erythematosus involving the kidneys can manifest as acute nephritis, nephrotic syndrome, proteinuria, or hematuria. Although it usually happens within five years and maybe the initial presentation leading to a definitive diagnosis, it is rarely the first sign of systemic lupus. In the months preceding presentation, patients—mostly women in their 20s and 30s with a preponderance of black ethnicity—will typically have experienced arthralgia or arthritis, skin rashes, pericarditis, and lethargy. Since lupus nephritis is more likely than other glomerulonephritises to change and evolve over time, a repeat biopsy and, if necessary, more aggressive treatment should be initiated in a patient whose initial glomerular lesion was benign. This is because a new presentation of acute glomerulonephritis should prompt this action. Low complement levels and high titers of antinuclear and anti-double-stranded DNA antibodies can be beneficial during a nephritic flare-up, though changes in these markers frequently occur months before glomerular inflammation actually occurs.

Immune complex deposition, whereby antigen-antibody complexes form systemically or in situ and subsequently trigger the inflammatory cascade, is at least partially responsible for the pathology. Additionally, positively charged nuclear histone antigens can attach to the glomerular basement membrane, changing its permeability and function. These antigens can also act as planted targets for anti-DNA antibodies.

Patients with focal and diffuse proliferative glomerulonephritis, or World Health Organization (WHO) classes III and IV lupus nephritis (class I, which is normal kidney function, and class II, which is mesangial proliferation, do not present as acute glomerulonephritis), are known to have acute glomerulonephritis in lupus. Less than 50% of glomeruli in class III lupus nephritis (focal proliferative glomerulonephritis) have proliferation in the mesangial and endocapillary areas. These patients occasionally have nephritis, hematuria, and proteinuria. The more aggressive class IV diffuse proliferative glomerulonephritis, in which mesangial and endocapillary hypercellularity affect over 50% of glomeruli with additional necrosis and possibly crescent formation, is more frequently linked to nephritic syndrome and renal impairment. Under light microscopy, subendothelial deposits appear as a wire loop-like thickening of the basement membrane. Subendothelial and mesangial regions exhibit broad granular deposition of IgG, IgA, IgM, and complement, as demonstrated by immunofluorescence.

5.2.7. Treatment of Glomerulonephritis

There are two approaches to treating acute glomerulonephritis. While supportive care, such as dialysis and blood pressure management, is often life-saving, it does not aim to reverse the underlying pathology. Certain treatments, which are frequently extremely toxic and rely on non-specific suppression of the entire immune system, are intended to prevent and reverse glomerular inflammation and ultimately preserve renal function. They run the risk of deadly infections right away as well as cancer and reproductive toxicity down the road. It is important to choose patients for such therapies whose kidney recovery is unlikely to happen on its own but whose potential reversibility justifies the potential for toxicity. Based on this, we go over current treatments and, if applicable, explain why they are used. Clinical trials are being conducted on a number of these treatments as well as more recent ones to identify the best course of action.

It is impossible to overstate the value of supportive therapies for acute glomerulonephritis. Controlling hyperkalemia, uremia, and fluid overload through dialysis when needed, as well as maintaining strict blood pressure control and using diuretics appropriately, can literally save lives. For any patient left with even mild renal impairment or proteinuria, blood pressure control is essential not only in the short term but also down the road. Angiotensin-converting enzyme (ACE) inhibitors have a special place in this regard because of their additional antiproteinuric and antifibrotic effects.

Supportive therapy alone will be adequate in the majority of post-streptococcal glomerulonephritis cases where inflammation does resolve spontaneously, with improved renal function observed in 95% of patients between four and 14 days after the initial acute failure. While hematuria may last for six months and mild proteinuria may still be present in a small percentage of patients even at ten years of age, serum creatinine usually returns to baseline levels in four weeks on average. Seldom do hematuria and proteinuria last a long time and are accompanied by increasing blood pressure and deteriorating kidney function. Reversing the underlying causes of glomerular inflammation is necessary for most other causes of glomerulonephritis to preserve renal function.

Since the precise immunological mechanisms causing IgA nephropathy are unknown, treating the condition is very challenging. Regular review may be sufficient for patients who present acutely with macroscopic hematuria but with normal blood pressure and renal function. Again, blood pressure control and careful fluid management are critical for patients who follow a more accelerated clinical course. With anecdotal reports of success with mycophenolate mofetil, cyclophosphamide and pulsed steroids, and intravenous immunoglobulin, acute inflammation on biopsy may justify the use of immunosuppressives. ACE inhibitor use is becoming more and more significant in the more chronic phase, for both hypertensive and non-hypertensive patients with proteinuria (>1 g/24 hours). These medications slow the typical decline in glomerular filtration rate and lower the degree of proteinuria.

Estimating the prognosis for patients who present acutely with IgA nephropathy is challenging. Adverse prognostic features include hypertension, impaired renal function, and severe proteinuria at presentation. A study found that a patient had only a 20% chance of independent renal function seven years later if they had both elevated creatinine (>150 μmol/l) and proteinuria (>1 g/24 hours). The prognosis for patients with HSP is predicted by their clinical presentation; 15% of patients with nephritis eventually experience end-stage renal failure, while up to 50% of patients with a combined nephritic and nephrotic picture ultimately require renal replacement therapy.

Without treatment, rapidly progressing glomerulonephritis can permanently damage renal function in a matter of days. The use of considerably toxic therapies in an effort to maintain independent renal function is therefore justified by these risks. High-dose steroids and cyclophosphamide are used in anti-glomerular basement membrane disease to inhibit B-cell production of antiglomerular basement membrane antibodies, while additional plasma exchange is used to eliminate any existing antibodies during the two weeks prior to the the effects of cyclophosphamide becoming apparent. Although the pathophysiology of renal vasculitis (Wegener's and microscopic polyangiitis) is much less understood, comparable treatment regimens attempt to inhibit both T-cell and B-cell activity.

Few patients with antiglomerular basement membrane disease who present with serum creatinine greater than 600 μmol/l and require dialysis will ever regain independent renal function unless treatment is promptly initiated. 80% of patients with a creatinine less than 600 μmol/l can expect improvements in renal function with aggressive cytotoxic treatment and plasma exchange, usually evident within days of beginning treatment. Even people whose kidneys are irreversibly damaged may undergo plasma exchange in an effort to treat pulmonary hemorrhage.

When RPGN is positive for ANCA, the prognosis is better than when antiglomerular basement membrane disease is present. Even 75% of patients who initially required renal support may recover renal function with aggressive treatment that includes steroids, cyclophosphamide, and plasma exchange at least five times if they are dialysis dependent. At five years, 80% of these patients will still be dialysis-independent. In cases of ANCA-positive vasculitis-related pulmonary hemorrhage, plasma exchange is also utilized. Recent trial results have shown that many of these patients can be safely switched to an oral azathioprine regimen after a three-month initial induction with steroids and cyclophosphamide.

The degree of glomerular inflammation in immune complex RPGN determines the prognosis, and underlying pathology is the focus of treatment. The clinical course of the rare cases of genuinely idiopathic immune complex RPGN seems to be comparable to that of pauci-immune RPGN, and immunosuppressive treatments akin to those employed in ANCA-positive disease may be suitable.

The pathophysiology of idiopathic MCGN is still unknown, and blood pressure control becomes more crucial in the absence of effective specific treatment. Aspirin and dipyridamole have been used with some success to try and limit the platelet activation linked to cellular proliferation, and steroid treatment may have a role in pediatrics. Rarely, Type II MCGN responds poorly to traditional treatments. Renal survival at 10 years is 60% in cases of truly idiopathic MCGN type I; this percentage is likely lower in cases of MCGN type II.

Complex treatment is required for MCGN patients who have hepatitis C. Alpha-interferon and ribavirin control of viral load should be most effective if virus-containing immune complexes are thought to be the cause of the disease. Although this has shown some success with improvements in mild MCGN, relapse of viral load after stopping treatment is frequently observed. On the other hand, immunosuppressives may be the most effective means of controlling the inflammatory aspect of a lesion in cases of more severe renal damage, despite the possibility of viral activation. Therefore, pulsed methylprednisolone would be used by some nephrologists to treat an aggressive nephritic flare, followed by three to six months of tapered oral steroids. When the illness is very active, oral cyclophosphamide is administered for two months. While proteinuria responds much more slowly to such treatments for cryoglobulinaemic vasculitis, extrarenal manifestations improve rapidly; in over 85% of patients, the plasma creatinine decreases in less than a week. Long-term immunosuppression is not warranted, and opinions on plasma exchange are still divided. End-stage renal failure affects about 10% of patients with kidney disease related to hepatitis C. Only some of the pathology of lupus nephritis is known, making treatment extremely difficult. Renal disease is a disease that frequently affects young women, so the risks must be evaluated against the potential infertility brought on by immunosuppressive treatment plans. Renal biopsy is essential because, in the event of an acute nephritic flare, it's critical to identify the kidneys that are irreparably damaged and scarred from those that may benefit from intensive immunosuppression. An approximate 85% remission rate was observed in a recent study of patients with type IV lupus nephritis who received intravenous cyclophosphamide and pulsed monthly methylprednisolone. Following six months of monthly induction therapy, additional quarterly doses of pulsed cyclophosphamide also decreased the rate of relapse that followed. Mycophenolate mofetil in acute flare-ups and intravenous immunoglobulin (which solubilizes immune complexes or blocks

Fc receptors to stop the inflammatory cascade) may also have a role in refractory cases. According to the most recent data, 70–85% of patients with type III and IV lupus nephritis will still have independent renal function after five years if they receive their current course of treatment. Hypertension, black race, and recurrent acute nephritic flares are poor prognostic indicators.

Currently, the only treatments available for glomerulonephritis, a significant cause of renal failure, are potentially harmful and non-specific. With faster diagnosis times and more knowledge about pathology, we have to hope that things will get better. With further research, we may be able to completely prevent certain glomerulonephritides, such as MCGN, by successfully immunizing against hepatitis C or by developing treatments to prevent the formation of immune complexes in systemic lupus erythematosus. Drugs that target cell signaling that causes proliferation and subsequent fibrosis, or that disrupt complement or cytokine cascades to combat inflammation, may be developed for patients with glomerulonephritis. The numerous cases of chronic renal failure brought on by these illnesses cannot be avoided until then (Couser and Johnson, 2014; O'Shaughnessy et al., 2017; Khalighi et al., 2018; Mariani et al., 2019; Satoskar et al., 2020).

5.3. Pathogenesis of Kidney Disease in Systemic Lupus Erythematosus

5.3.1. Pathogenic Autoantibodies in Lupus Glomerulonephritis

Antinuclear antibody detection in serum is one of the most common laboratory tests used to diagnose SLE. Anti-Sm antibodies have a strong correlation with lupus nephritis, and anti-dsDNA antibodies are thought to be a hallmark of SLE. Passive transfer of anti-DNA antibodies has not been able to replicate the disease lupus nephritis, nor can all anti-dsDNA antibodies deposit in the kidney. Anti-DNA antibodies' capacity to cause glomerulonephritis and transient proteinuria in mice has been linked to their cross-reactivity with glomerular antigens like laminin and alpha-actinin. It has previously been reported that positively charged nucleosomes are deposited on the glomerular basement membrane (GBM) and serve as targets for autoantibodies. Rekvig and colleagues have shown in a recent series of articles that NZB/W F1 mice, who are susceptible to lupus and proteinuria, exhibit electron-dense deposits. These deposits, known as oligo-nucleosomes and identified by anti-dsDNA reactive monoclonal antibodies, are the result of inefficient apoptotic material fragmentation and clearance in the renal glomerulus. Furthermore, the authors present proof that, in contrast to serum anti-DNA antibodies, the antibodies eluted from the kidneys of nephritic mice have a higher affinity for DNA. These antibodies only react with the electron-dense deposits; they do not react with the laminin or alpha actinin-containing tissues in the vicinity. The pathogenic potential of anti-DNA antibodies was found to be determined by the accumulation of chromatin fragments on the glomerular basement membrane and high-affinity antibodies to nucleosomal DNA, not by cross-reactivity to glomerular proteins. A limitation of these investigations is that the mice did not exhibit glomerular electron-dense deposits until 26 weeks of age, at which point they developed severe proteinuria suggestive of a well-established lupus glomerulonephritis. Furthermore, more evidence is needed to support the anti-DNA antibodies' monospecificity. Therefore, it is still unknown what characteristics of autoantibodies in immune complex deposits cause the disease to start. Furthermore, these findings contradict the research in NZM2328. Antinuclear or anti-dsDNA antibodies are not necessary for lupus glomerulonephritis, as demonstrated by Lc4 mice that develop glomerular immune complex deposits and fatal lupus glomerulonephritis in the absence of these antibodies in serum or in IgG eluted from kidney homogenates.

Studies using patient samples also cast doubt on the necessity of anti-DNA or antinuclear antibodies in lupus glomerulonephritis. Twenty-five lupus patients' kidney tissue extruded during autopsy was used to screen immunoglobulin against a panel of fourteen distinct antigens, which included histones, chromatin, collagen-like regions of C1q complement, Sm, SSA, and SSB. In the various samples, the cumulative reactivity to all of these antigens varied from 0 to 41 points 3 percent of the total IgG eluted from the corresponding kidneys. Hence, a significant portion of renal IgG responds to unidentified antigens. Potential cross-reactivity to other antigens, such as binding to blocking agents like bovine serum albumin, which is a well-known feature of lupus sera in ELISAs, further complicates this. Indeed, serum from lupus patients and mice reacts with multiple antigens, as demonstrated by glomerular proteome arrays. A more accurate indicator of the disease might be the identification of antigen clusters from the glomerular proteome that patient sera have identified. Another study found that 15–26% of 200 monoclonal antibodies produced by isolating single IgG+ memory B cells from four lupus patients and one healthy control were polyreactive against a variety of antigens, including insulin, ssDNA, dsDNA, and LPS. Remarkably, the autoreactivity of the memory IgG+ B cells did not significantly differ between the patients and controls, suggesting that polyreactive autoantibody populations are a common occurrence in all people. This, however, can be explained by the growing understanding of the polyreactivity of many B and T cell receptors.

5.3.2. Autoreactive T Cells and Lupus Glomerulonephritis

Given that SLE is characterized by autoantibodies with multiple specificities, it makes sense that research on the function of B cells and autoantibodies has dominated the understanding of both lupus glomerulonephritis and SLE in general. T cells were primarily thought to be useful in helping B cells produce autoantibodies. Over the last few years, the emphasis has shifted from T cells' involvement in lupus glomerulonephritis to their function as effectors mediating tissue injury.

Numerous methods provide evidence for the significance of T cells as effectors in lupus glomerulonephritis. The first method was based on the discovery that renal disease exists in MRL/lpr mice with B cells expressing a B cell receptor transgene but no circulating Ig. The research demonstrated that, even in the absence of circulating Ig, MRL/lpr mice expressing a surface transgenic B cell receptor to 4-hydroxy-3-nitrophenyl develop a distinct renal disease marked by glomerular sclerosis and interstitial inflammation. Secondly, despite a decrease in glomerular immune complex deposits, NZB/W F1 mice with established chronic glomerulonephritis that were given CTLA4Ig and a suboptimal dose of cyclophosphamide demonstrated a notable delay in mortality. Therefore, preventing CTLA4Ig-induced T cell activation may stop the disease from progressing. Thus, blocking T cell activation by CTLA4Ig could prevent disease progression. This reaffirms the original observation by Wofsy et al. that anti-T cell antibody therapy of NZB/WF1 mice reduced glomerular inflammation, severe proteinuria and early mortality. In NZM2328 mice, early immune complex deposits and acute proliferative glomerulonephritis was associated with glomerular and peri-glomerular T cell infiltration. In addition, MHC II positive, CD11c dendritic cells were seen in the glomeruli. This was accompanied by an increased frequency of CD4+ T cell activation in the regional lymph nodes. All these findings suggest a local T cell response in kidney and regional lymph nodes early in the disease process.

Distinct patterns of gene expression with disease progression are revealed by a careful examination of the kinetics of inflammatory cell migration and chemokine expression in the NZB/W F1 kidneys collected at different ages. As was previously mentioned, glomerular antigen-reactive T cells in the renal cortex induce peri-glomerular inflammation, which in turn increases macrophage infiltration. The periglomerular T cell infiltrate is probably what draws the inflammatory macrophages to the renal interstitium.

Numerous studies conducted recently have examined the pathogenic potential of various subsets of CD4+ T cells. Th1 cytokines (IL12 and IFN gamma) are more highly expressed in the kidneys of nephritic NZM2328 mice. According to a recent study, NZM2328 mice lacking TNF receptors 1 and 2 had a higher death rate. Renal disease developed more quickly in the TNF receptor-deficient mice, and their activated CD4+ cells displayed a Th17 gene profile. Thus, Th17 T cells may also play a role in the development of lupus glomerulonephritis, in addition to Th1 T cells. In addition to IFN gamma and IL13, laser microdissection of glomerular, periglomerular, and perivascular infiltrates in MRL/lpr mice also revealed elevated IL17 expression. This is corroborated by the Crispin et al. study that demonstrated an increased production of IL17 by double negative T cells and kidney invasion in SLE patients. Garrett-Sinha et al. reviewed additional research that may point to a Th17 cell role in SLE. The spleens of BXSB-yaa mice have been found to contain the follicular helper T cell subsets that are defined as IL21-producing CD4 + inducible T cell costimulator (ICOS) + cells. In a different investigation, MRL/lpr mice deficient in ICOS exhibit a marked decrease in IgG autoantibody but only a slight decrease in glomerulonephritis. It is unknown how these subsets function in renal disease.

5.3.3. Pathogenic Contribution of End-organ Responses

One of the first indications of renal involvement in SLE is the deposition of glomerular immune complex. Chemokines such as MCP-1 and RANTES are then produced in the glomeruli of MRL/lpr mice, mainly by mesangial cells. Mesangial expansion and cellular infiltration into the glomeruli are the hallmarks of acute proliferative glomerulonephritis, which is caused by the first stimulation of mesangial cells. This may develop into severe persistent proteinuria, life-threatening renal failure, and chronic glomerulonephritis, which is characterized by glomerulosclerosis, interstitial fibrosis, and tubular atrophy. As we have shown before, acute glomerulonephritis in NZM2328 mice does not always lead to chronic glomerulonephritis. A subgroup of patients also exhibits this absence of disease progression. NZM2328 mice were used for microarray analyses looking for glomerular gene expression patterns at various stages of glomerulonephritis to look into the molecular alterations linked to progressive glomerular disease.

Four distinct clusters based on transcriptional profiles could be identified: normal, acute, transitional, and chronic glomerulonephritis. Myeloid cell markers and inflammatory chemokines and cytokines dominated acute glomerulonephritis. The stage of chronic glomerulonephritis was marked by increased genes involved in tissue remodeling and repair, as well as glomerular fibrosis and sclerosis. Progression of renal dysfunction and severe proteinuria are linked to chronic glomerulonephritis. A stage of transitional glomerulonephritis was identified employing micro-array analysis, which revealed elevated expression of seven genes: matrix metalopeptidase (Mmp10); transforming growth factor beta (TGFβ2); insulin-like growth factor binding protein (igfbp2); and lipocalin (Lcn2). The last common pathway that appears to cause fibrosis and irreversible glomerular damage, which ultimately leads to end-stage renal disease, is the activation of TGF beta signaling. This pathway offers new targets for therapeutic intervention, as seen in Figure 5.2.

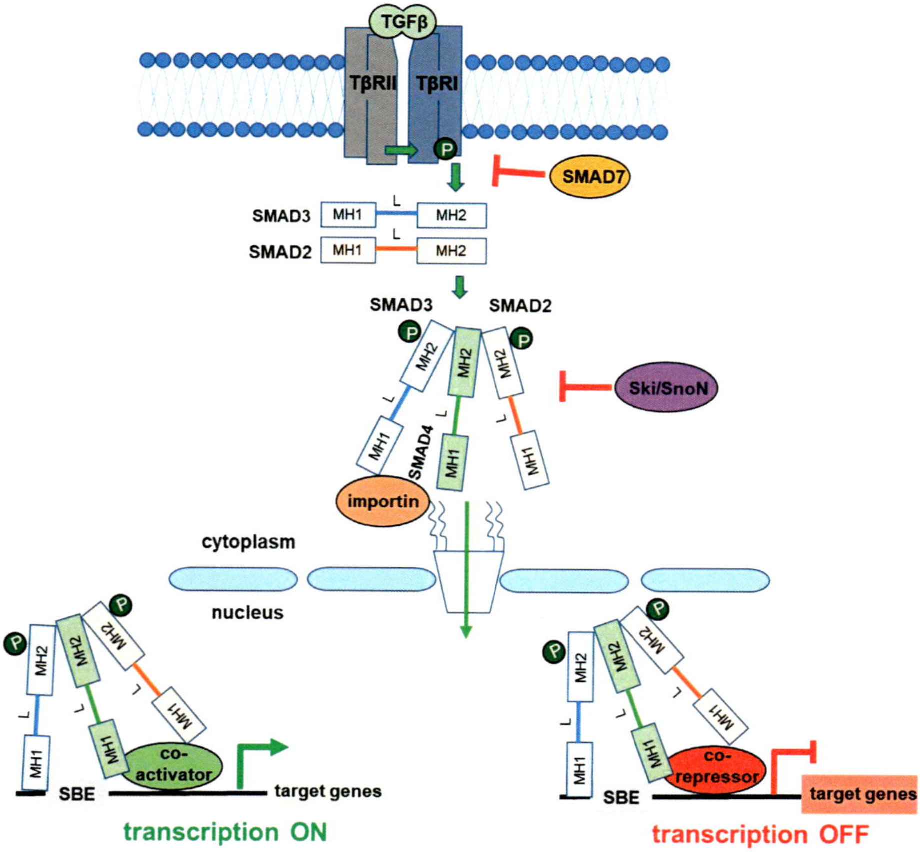

Figure 5.2. *A schematic showing the TGF beta signaling pathway and its interaction with other molecules like PDGF, CD44 and cyclins through transcription factor Egr-1.*

Source: Papoutsoglou P, Louis C, Coulouarn C. Transforming Growth Factor-Beta (TGFβ) Signaling Pathway in Cholangiocarcinoma. Cells. 2019; 8(9):960. https://doi.org/10.3390/cells8090960.

5.3.4. Genetic Control of End-organ Damage

Genes controlling susceptibility to SLE have been identified and mapped using murine models of spontaneous SLE. Using (C57L/J × NZM2328)F1 × NZM2328 backcross mice, we studied NZM2328 and found specific genetic intervals that dictate susceptibility to three distinct phenotypes: proteinuria and acute glomerulonephritis (Agnz1 on chromosome 1 and Agnz2 on chromosome 17), chronic glomerulonephritis and proteinuria (Cgnz1 on chromosome 1), and autoantibodies against nuclear and dsDNA (Adaz1 on chromosome 4). Congenic mice were produced on a genetic background susceptible to lupus (NZM2328) that carried lupus-resistant C57L/J chromosomal segments on chromosomes 1 and 4. The NZM2328. Unlike NZM2328, C57Lc1 did not develop autoantibodies or fatal glomerulonephritis. Despite not producing antinuclear or anti-dsDNA autoantibodies, C57Lc4 passed away from severe renal failure and lupus glomerulonephritis. These traits are present in the NZM2328 congenic mouse strains. NZM2328 and C57Lc1. C57Lc4, in turn, validated the preliminary genetic mapping research. These investigations demonstrate a distinct genetic susceptibility separation between lupus glomerulonephritis and antinuclear anti-dsDNA autoantibodies.

To determine the genes governing the development of chronic glomerulonephritis, NZM2328 was used to create new congenic lines. Cross Lc1 × NZM2328. An 8 Mb C57L/J chromosome 1 fragment with the Cgnz1 locus on an NZM2328 genetic background is present in one of these lines, R27. The Agnz1 locus, which is from the parental lupus-prone strain NZM2328, was not replaced. Both antinuclear and anti-dsDNA antibodies did not develop in the R27 mice. Acute proliferative glomerulonephritis and glomerular immune complexes were observed in all R27 mice. Notably, no renal failure occurred in any of the 12-month-old R27 mice. This offers genetic support for the theory that the genetic regulation of acute and chronic glomerulonephritis differs. This underlines even more how crucial organ resistance is in dictating how immune complex-mediated renal disease turns out. Therefore, chronic glomerulonephritis need not develop from acute glomerulonephritis.

Genes for complement receptor 2 and Fc inhibitory receptors may not be essential in end-organ damage, according to recent research in R27 mice (Ge and Fu,). B6 was used to identify Ly108, the lupus gene, in the R27 region. mice with Sle1. Given that autoantibody formation is addressed by Sle1 on the B6 background, Ly108 probably plays a role in the production of antinucleosome antibodies. Research is being done on additional R27 region genes that might influence end organ responses.

5.4. Mechanisms of Glomerulosclerosis in Diabetic Nephropathy

Numerous mechanisms contribute to the progression of diabetic nephropathy to end-stage kidney disease, but none are more significant than the slow, unstoppable scarring of the renal glomerulus, or glomerulosclerosis. To develop effective therapies and preventative measures, numerous studies conducted over the years have attempted to elucidate the molecular mechanisms that lead to this chronic sclerosing condition. The general knowledge of the pathogenic factors leading to this significant aspect of diabetic nephropathy has significantly improved over the last few years. Extracellular matrix (ECM) protein buildup in the mesangial interstitial space causes glomerulosclerosis in diabetic nephropathy, which leads to fibrosis shown as diffuse or nodular alterations. The most frequently found matrix proteins are fibronectin and collagen types I, III, and IV. These build up as a result of decreased degradation by mesangial matrix metalloproteinases and increased synthesis by mesangial cells. Two decades prior, Mauer et al. showed that measurements of mesangial expansion significantly predicted the clinical signs of diabetic nephropathy, establishing the direct connection between mesangial matrix expansion and the development of diabetic kidney disease. Since then, figuring out the mechanisms promoting glomerulosclerosis in diabetic nephropathy has been a crucial task for researchers.

5.4.1. Classical View of Diabetic Glomerulosclerosis

A broad consensus regarding the primary signaling pathways that drive mesangial cell synthesis of extracellular matrix (ECM) proteins developed during the 1990s. According to the general consensus, elevated extracellular glucose causes the facilitative glucose transporter GLUT1 to express more, which in turn increases glucose uptake. The consequent increase in glucose metabolic flux triggers several metabolic pathways that intensify the production of oxidative stress and advanced glycation end product. These, in turn, trigger several signaling pathways that lead to increased production of extracellular matrix (ECM) through protein kinase β stimulation of AP-1 transcriptional activation, extracellular signal–related kinase (ERK) pathways, and, most importantly, transforming growth factor (TGF)–β1 synthesis, which stimulates its signaling pathways in an autocrine and paracrine manner, thereby inducing ECM protein synthesis. TGF-β1-induced responses seem to be the last common pathway leading to nephrosclerosis. The role of TGF-β and its signaling mechanisms, though crucial in the development of nephrosclerosis in diabetes and most fibrotic kidney diseases, has been the focus of several recent reviews on diabetic nephropathy (Figure 5.3).

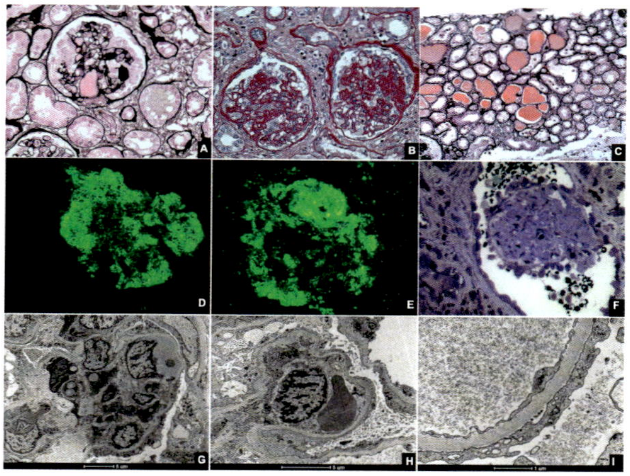

Figure 5.3. *Histopathology of collapsing glomerulopathy. (A, B) Periodic Acid Schiff (PAS) and Jones Methenamine Silver (JMS) (40×), respectively show intense podocyte hyperplasia and glomerular tuft collapse. (C) JMS (20×) exhibits microcytic transformation of distal convoluted tubules with accumulations of hyaline material inside of those. (D, E) Fluorescence microscopy (40×) shows, respectively, IgM and C3 trapping in areas of collapse/sclerosis. (F) Semi-fine stained in Toluidine Blue (63×) with collapse of the entire glomerular tuft and hyperplasia of podocytes and dilated Bowman's space. (G, H) Transmission electron microscopy contrasted with Osmium Tetroxide, Lead Citrate and Uranyl in block shows capillary loop collapse with hyalinosis in addition to diffuse fusion and flattening of the pedicels associated with microvillous transformation. (I) Electron microscopy tubes contrasted with osmium tetroxide, lead citrate, and uranyl in block with detail of disorganization of the cytoskeleton in the podocyte cytoplasm, with extensive effacement of the pedicels.*

Source: By Cutrim ÉMM, Neves PDMM, Campos MAG, Wanderley DC, Teixeira-Júnior AAL, Muniz MPR - Cutrim ÉMM, Neves PDMM, Campos MAG, Wanderley DC, Teixeira-Júnior AAL, Muniz MPR (2022). "Collapsing Glomerulopathy: A Review by the Collapsing Brazilian Consortium." Front Med (Lausanne) 9: 846173. DOI:10.3389/fmed.2022.846173. PMID 35308512. PMC: 8927620.- CC-BY 4.0 license, CC BY 4.0, https://commons.wikimedia.org/w/index.php?curid=139097839.

The majority of the factors have been demonstrated to be predominant in the mesangial cell in vitro, animal models, and, to the extent that human studies can corroborate, in human trials. The idea that enhanced glucose uptake and metabolic flux in mesangial cells can either directly or indirectly result in the activation of the entire program is implied in this pathogenesis schema. This is most likely untrue in living organisms and is undoubtedly untrue even in systems of cultured cells. Weigert et al. did a good job of illustrating how enhanced glucose uptake and metabolism cannot fully explain all downstream changes. who discovered that mesangial cells exposed to high extracellular glucose did not induce the same biochemical pathways as mesangial cells exposed to physiologically occurring glucose concentrations when GLUT1 was overexpressed. Therefore, to activate these crucial (and possibly additional) glomerulosclerosis mechanisms, an increase in extracellular glucose levels needs to cause responses in mesangial cells that are independent of glucose uptake and glucose metabolic flux. Moreover, and perhaps even more crucially, a variety of exogenous factors that do not originate from mesangial cells can induce glomerulosclerosis apart from hyperglycemia itself.

It is essential to understand the impact of various extraglomerular and systemic factors that can cause fibrotic responses in the glomerular tuft in diabetes. Although these factors are too intricate to fully cover in a brief review, glomerular and systemic hypertension, as well as activation of the renin-angiotensin-aldosterone system, are believed to be particularly significant. Some studies indicate that glomerular hypertension and the resulting stretching of mesangial cells can increase the expression of the GLUT1 glucose transporter, leading to a series of intracellular reactions that can ultimately result in glomerulosclerosis.

5.4.2. All Glomerular Cell Types Are Involved in Diabetic Glomerulosclerosis

Although the mesangial cell has traditionally been considered the main player in mediating mesangial sclerosis in diabetic nephropathy, recent studies suggest that podocytes and endothelial cells also play significant roles. The interaction between all three glomerular cell types is crucial in understanding the development of diabetic glomerulosclerosis. While most research has focused on regulating mesangial cell ECM production, it is clear that podocytes also play a key role in the progression of the disease. Podocyte damage and loss have been shown to be early events in diabetic nephropathy and can accurately predict progressive nephropathy in individuals with type 2 diabetes. Additionally, endothelial cell dysfunction has been linked to diabetic glomerulosclerosis, indicating a strong connection between endothelial and mesangial cells. Furthermore, extraglomerular cells, such as bone marrow–derived mesangial cell progenitors and macrophages, may also have a significant impact on the development of glomerulosclerosis in diabetic nephropathy.

Given the evidence supporting the involvement of extraglomerular cells and all three glomerular cell types in the progressive build-up of extracellular matrix proteins in diabetic nephropathy, the pathogenesis of this lesion must be intricate and multifaceted.

5.4.3. Newer Observations on Mechanisms of Diabetic Glomerulosclerosis

While the classic understanding of how diabetic nephropathy develops is still mostly accurate, there have been some new discoveries regarding the mechanisms of diabetic glomerulosclerosis since 2000 that have deepened our knowledge of this complex process. It is important to note that many of these findings come from studies on animals and cell signaling, and have not yet been confirmed in humans. We will highlight any data available on human glomerulosclerosis, but until then, these new mechanisms should be considered potential factors in diabetic injury until proven otherwise in human studies. It is crucial to remember that traditional animal models may not perfectly mimic the disease in humans and have not consistently shown the same level of glomerulosclerosis as seen in human diabetic glomerulopathy.

5.4.3.1. Systemic and Paracrine: Inflammation

Inflammatory pathways have been identified as significant pathogenic factors in diabetic microvascular complications, such as diabetic glomerulosclerosis, by a number of clinical and animal model investigations. While the majority of research on the relationship between inflammation and diabetic nephropathy focuses on the progressive tubulointerstitial injury it causes, several studies also link inflammatory mechanisms to the glomerulosclerosis pathogenesis. Both type 1 and type 2 diabetic patients have elevated levels of circulating markers of inflammation. Several of these markers, including fibrinogen, C-reactive protein, serum amyloid A protein, and interleukin-6, are correlated with an increased risk of end-stage kidney disease progression as well as albuminuria and glomerular ECM protein deposition. Tumor necrosis factor-α and other mediators are examples of inflammatory cytokines that can induce glomerular cells to produce more ECM proteins or slow down their degradation. It has recently come to light that macrophages play a role in the development of glomerulosclerosis. For instance, six months after the onset of diabetes, selective deletion of the macrophage scavenger receptor-A improved a number of the glomerular abnormalities associated with experimental diabetic nephropathy in mice, such as albuminuria, glomerular hypertrophy, mesangial matrix expansion, and TGF-β overexpression. In addition, proinflammatory genes were downregulated, macrophage infiltration was diminished, and monocyte attachment to type IV collagen was diminished in this model. Recent research indicates that interventions aimed at preventing inflammation-induced damage can potentially improve diabetic glomerulosclerosis by linking inflammatory mechanisms to podocyte injury in diabetic models. The fact that many medications that stop or slow the progression of diabetic glomerular disease in humans also have strong anti-inflammatory properties highlights the significance of inflammatory mechanisms in diabetic glomerulosclerosis.

Furthermore, oxidant stress and advanced glycation end products, which are important variables in the development of diabetic nephropathy, both enhance and are enhanced by inflammatory mechanisms of renal injury. Lastly, it should be emphasized that glomerular cells in a diabetic milieu produce a wide range of inflammatory mediators that can exacerbate inflammatory damage and even have systemic effects, particularly as glomerular injury advances.

5.4.3.2. Systemic and Mesangial Cell: Bradykinin 2 Receptor Blockade

Several groups have reported an association between the D-allele of the ACE gene and the onset and progression of type 1 diabetic nephropathy in humans. Furthermore, the cornerstones of renal protection in diabetic nephropathy in humans are ACE inhibitors and angiotensin receptor blockers. However, Smithies and colleagues discovered that significant changes in ACE gene dose led to only modest increases in ACE with minimal effects on blood pressure and angiotensin II levels. Interestingly, however, led to substantial decreases in bradykinin, suggesting that perhaps bradykinin rather than angiotensin II was more important in renal responses in diabetes. These findings were made using knockout and knockin mice as well as computer modeling. Thus, using Akita mice with a C57BL/6 background, this group investigated the role of targeted deletion of the bradykinin 2 receptor in the development of diabetic nephropathy. This model involved the development of profound mesangial sclerosis in diabetic homozygote bradykinin 2 receptor knockout mice, which resembled the glomerular alterations seen in diabetic glomerulosclerosis in humans. Podocytes and glomerular endothelial cells were unaltered. Bradykinin 2 receptors are normally highly expressed in mesangial cells; knocking these receptors down was linked to increased renal expression of several genes involved in progressive glomerulosclerosis, such as TGF-β1, connective tissue growth factor (a TGF-β effector), and p53. The mechanism underlying this increased glomerulosclerosis phenotype is still unknown. Bradykinin 1 receptor levels in these mice are significantly higher than in others, but this did not protect them from the consequences of bradykinin 2 receptor gene deletion. When a particular nonpeptidic bradykinin 2 receptor antagonist was administered to diabetic rats, similar outcomes to bradykinin 2 receptor knockout were observed. Nearly all of the beneficial effects of ACE inhibitors on albuminuria, glomerular TGF-β, ERK, and signaling pathways, as well as glomerular gene expression alterations, were reversed by this agent. In the glomeruli of treated diabetic rats, it also increased oxidative stress. Therefore, bradykinin 2 receptor activation in the kidney, most likely in mesangial cells, is protective and needs to, via an unidentified mechanism or mechanisms, reduce activation of ERK- and TGF-β-dependent prosclerotic pathways.

5.4.3.3. Paracrine and Mesangial Cell: Lipids and Lipid Mediators

Although it is still unknown how elevated circulating lipids might contribute to diabetic glomerulosclerosis, increased glomerular lipid synthesis and elevated circulating lipids have been definitively linked to the disease. Furthermore, increased kidney synthesis of cholesterol and triglycerides has been shown in several studies by Levi and colleagues as well as others. Numerous factors, including increased renal expression of the transcription factor sterol regulatory element–binding protein-1, which, when overexpressed in mice, causes lipid accumulation and induces expression of TGF-β, plasminogen activator inhibitor-1, and vascular endothelial growth factor (VEGF), appear to be responsible for this increased local lipid synthesis in diabetes. Diabetes may cause renal glomerular synthesis of triglycerides and cholesterol, which in turn promotes glomerulosclerosis because this endogenous kidney lipid synthesis pathway appears to directly lead to enhanced accumulation of ECM proteins, mesangial expansion, and glomerulosclerosis. Triglyceride and cholesterol production locally is essentially similar to the synthesis of other lipid mediators locally. These mediators are produced in renal and glomerular vascular cells and have a significant impact on the progression of glomerulosclerosis.

These later mediators, which are referred to as eicosanoids collectively (prostanoids, leukotrienes, hydroxyeicosatetrenoic acids, and epoxyeicosatrienoic acids), have a variety of intricate effects on renal glomeruli. Each eicosanoid has a different effect on different cells depending on gene transcription and other mechanisms. Numerous effects, nevertheless, seem to encourage diabetic glomerulosclerosis. For example, in rats with streptozotocin diabetes and hypertension, selective COX2 inhibition prevents the development of glomerular sclerosis. Further research is necessary to fully understand the role that COX-derived prostanoids play in the pathogenesis of diabetic glomerulosclerosis. Lastly, it is at best artificial to isolate lipid mediators from inflammation as a factor in glomerulosclerosis, given the critical role that many of these lipid mediators play in inflammatory responses.

5.4.3.4. Mesangial Cell: microRNA Regulation of TGF-β Signaling

It has been demonstrated that 22 nucleotide short noncoding RNAs, or microRNAs, are significant players in the expression of mammalian genes. They can play key roles in gene regulation in both physiologic and pathophysiologic conditions in a variety of disease states because they induce posttranscriptional gene regulation by either inducing miRNA degradation or blocking protein translation (by binding to the 3′ untranslated region of their target genes). It is estimated that up to 30% of human protein-coding genes may be regulated by miRNAs, of which more than 500 have been identified. It has been discovered recently that TGF-β treatment of cultured mesangial cells and glomeruli from mice with type 1 and type 2 diabetes both increase the expression of miRNA-192. These researchers discovered that by downregulating the expression of two E-box repressors of collagen-1α2 gene activation, TGF-β–induced miRNA-192 mediates an increase in collagen-1α2 expression. The authors reasoned that hyperglycemia might be a common factor in inducing miRNA-192 expression because miRNA-192 was upregulated in the tissues of both type 1 and type 2 diabetic mice. However, the mechanisms underlying this regulation are still unknown. This seems to be the first instance of an miRNA's functional involvement in kidney disease of any kind. Since miRNA-192 stimulates extracellular matrix synthesis after TGF-β, targeting it for therapy makes more sense because it may have fewer side effects than blocking TGF-β signaling altogether.

5.4.3.5. Mesangial Cell: Janus Kinase/Signal Transducer and Activation of Transcription Pathway Activation

The glomerular response to diabetes may be influenced by the Janus kinase (JAK)/signal transducers and activation of transcription (STAT) signaling pathways, which are activated by a variety of growth factors and agonists, including angiotenisin II. Marerro and colleagues have discovered that in rat kidney glomeruli, high glucose increases the angiotensin II-induced activation of the JAK/STAT pathway, and that in mesangial cells, JAK/STAT signaling is activated to promote the production of TGF-β, collagen IV, and fibronectin. These effects seem to be directly related to hyperglycemia, possibly through increased production of reactive oxygen species. This is because high glucose causes enhanced phosphorylation in cultured mesangial cells, which activates JAK2 and its downstream substrates, STAT1, STAT3, and STAT5A/B. Furthermore, diabetic proteinuria was avoided by blocking JAK2 with AG-490; however, the effects of this inhibitor on diabetic glomerulosclerosis in general have not yet been reported.

5.4.3.6. Endothelial Cell/Podocyte: Reduction in Endothelial Nitric Oxide Synthase and Vascular endothelial Growth Factor

As previously mentioned, there has been a growing focus on the part endothelial cells play in the pathophysiology of diabetic nephrosclerosis. The regulation of endothelial nitric oxide (NO) production is one endothelial abnormality associated with diabetes. Most reports indicate higher NO production early in diabetes but lower levels in progressive diabetic nephropathy, though there is some disagreement on this point. Advanced diabetic nephropathy is linked to eNOS gene polymorphisms that cause a decrease in endothelial NO synthase (eNOS) expression. Endothelial responses play a critical role in diabetic glomerular pathology in animal models, as highlighted by three reports examining the effects of diabetes in mice with targeted deletion of the eNOS gene. Significant mesangial expansion, glomerulosclerosis, including nodular sclerosis, and other indications of advanced diabetic nephropathy, such as a decrease in glomerular filtration rate, were observed in diabetic eNOS knockout mice. It is unclear how decreased NO production leads to glomerular pathology and through what mechanisms. Although paracrine interactions between endothelial cells, podocytes, and mesangial cells appear to be primarily responsible for the remarkable pathology resulting from altered endothelial NO production, subsequent hemodynamic effects may also be important.

VEGF may be involved in the regulation of eNOS in diabetic nephropathy. Diabetic nephropathy has been linked to changes in endothelium and podocytes, which have been linked to VEGF. Through stimulating eNOS activity in the glomerulus, VEGF may partially explain its protective effects. VEGF levels are low in many chronic kidney diseases and are linked to reduced angiogenesis and capillary loss. On the other hand, VEGF levels are raised in the majority of animal models of diabetic nephropathy, indicating a disconnection of the VEGF-NO axis. While such an uncoupling might be relevant in rodent models, the finding that human biopsy samples with progressive diabetic nephropathy actually exhibit decreased VEGF gene expression raises the possibility that lower VEGF levels could inhibit eNOS activity and cause glomerular pathology akin to that observed in eNOS knockout mice with diabetic glomerulosclerosis. Via pathways that may be NO-dependent or -independent, glomerular endothelium can be negatively impacted by both low and high levels of VEGF. Thus, a deeper understanding of the podocyte-endothelial crosstalk in diabetic glomerulosclerosis will require improved characterization of the VEGF and eNOS pathways.

5.4.3.7. Endothelial Cell/Podocyte and Paracrine: Reduction of Activated Protein C

The impact of the thrombomodulin/activated protein C (APC) pathway on glomerular endothelial cells in diabetes was clearly explained in a relatively recent study, providing additional evidence of the critical role endothelial cell responses play in the development of diabetic glomerulosclerosis. The endothelial thrombomodulin–protein C system is dysfunctional in diabetic patients, and glomerular endothelial thrombomodulin A expression and protein C activation are significantly decreased in diabetic mice. In vitro, APC inhibited the apoptosis of glomerular endothelial cells and podocytes caused by high glucose, but not mesangial cells. Using two mouse models—one with impaired protein C activation and the other expressing a hyperactivatable protein C mutation—the role of APC in glomerular injury in diabetes was further investigated. In diabetic mice with impaired protein C activation, mesangial extracellular matrix expansion was enhanced; in mice with the hyperactivatable protein C mutation, it was completely prevented. In addition, mice with reduced protein C activation showed increased podocyte and endothelial apoptosis, while mice with hyperactivatable protein C showed a reduction in apoptotic cells. In a fascinating study, the researchers demonstrated how to use minocycline, a generalized apoptosis inhibitor, to prevent glomerular mesangial growth. It was demonstrated that none of these effects were influenced by variations in coagulation brought on by changed protein C activation. In conclusion, a single thorough investigation demonstrated that in experimental diabetes, a decrease in protein C activation stimulates glomerular capillary dysfunction and endothelial and podocyte apoptosis. Furthermore, to control nephropathy, APC appears to be a remarkable mediator of crosstalk between podocytes, endothelial cells, and the mesangium. New treatment avenues may become available if these intriguing findings are verified through additional analysis and validated in individuals suffering from diabetic nephropathy (Chen et al., 2003; Mason and Wahab, 2003).

5.5. Amyloid Nephropathy

A group of illnesses known as amyloidosis are characterized by the extracellular accumulation of protein fibrils that have the distinctive β-pleated sheet structure. One common symptom and a significant cause of morbidity in these patients is kidney disease. The term "amyloid" was first used by Rudolph Virchow in 1854, and the first amyloid protein to be chemically characterized was the monoclonal light chain, which was discovered in 1971. The ability to identify and classify amyloid has significantly improved thanks to mass spectrometry-based proteomics, and up to 30 amyloidogenic proteins have been found thus far. Amyloid fibrils all have similar chemical and ultrastructural characteristics, such as organizing into insoluble beta-pleated sheets that can be detected by X-ray crystallography, despite the fact that numerous proteins have been linked to amyloidosis.

5.5.1. Histologic Diagnosis and Identification of Amyloid

Regardless of its composition, amyloid has the same histologic characteristics. Amyloid is recognized on tissue sections stained with HandE as extracellular amorphous material that exhibits a mild eosinophilia. These deposits typically show a blue-to-gray hue on the trichrome stain, stain weakly for periodic acid Schiff (PAS), and test negative for Jones methenamine silver (JMS). These tinctorial characteristics are in stark contrast to the collagen histologic appearance, which shows strong positivity for PAS and JMS and is a major component of basement membranes, mesangial matrix, and areas of sclerosis. Every kind of amyloid has a preference for Congo red dye, which gives them an orange-red appearance under light microscopy and a distinctive apple-green birefringence when they polarize. Tissue sections stained with Congo red stain should be cut thicker (>5 μm) than the 2- to 4-μm sections used for standard light microscopy stains to achieve the best results. Although it is less selective than Congo red, thioflavin T can bind beta-sheet-rich structures as well. According to electron microscopy, amyloid deposits are made up of randomly oriented, non-branching fibrils with a diameter of seven to ten nm.

Any of the parenchymal compartments in the kidney, such as the glomeruli, tubules, interstitium, and/or vessels, may contain amyloid deposits. The most frequently affected organs are the glomeruli; a study found that glomerular deposition was present in 97% of cases. Amyloid buildup typically affects the mesangium before the capillary walls. Early on in the process, the involvement of only a few mesangial regions can make it subtle, making routine histologic evaluation easily overlooked. Greater involvement causes the mesangium to enlarge significantly. This mesangium can resemble mesangial sclerotic processes like diabetic glomerulosclerosis and may even develop a nodular appearance. The frequently negative staining with JMS and PAS, however, is more indicative of amyloid. Widely spaced subepithelial spikes, also known as amyloid spicules, can occasionally be seen in subepithelial or intramembranous deposits of amyloid, which are made up of fibrils arranged perpendicular to the glomerular basement membrane. Silver-positive, these spicules are typically longer and more focal than the "spikes" associated with membranous nephropathy. The glomerular architecture eventually completely disappears as amyloid deposition advances. Deposits in the tubulointerstitium and/or renal vessels, especially the interlobular arteries and arterioles, are often seen in conjunction with glomerular involvement. The clinical presentation is influenced by the amyloid's location. Proteinuria frequently predominates in cases with predominantly glomerular involvement, whereas renal insufficiency may be the main symptom when tubulointerstitial or vascular deposits are more prevalent. Large renal medullary deposits can occasionally cause polyuria, nocturia, and abnormalities in urine concentration. Amyloid deposits can, as they frequently do, be observed in several compartments and present with a variety of clinical symptoms.

While the histologic and chemical characteristics of all forms of amyloidosis are similar, the pathogenesis and approach to treatment can differ greatly based on the precursor protein. In the more common forms of amyloidosis, typing is frequently accomplished by routine immunofluorescence or immunohistochemical stains. Kidney biopsy specimens are frequently stained for immunoglobulins (Igs) and light chains using immunofluorescence staining, which can typically detect monotypic light chains. In some light chain amyloidosis (AL) cases, staining may be negative or equivocal. Regular kappa and lambda light chain immunofluorescence antibodies can target domains that are potentially changed or eliminated in amyloidogenic forms. Up to 36% of AL in the kidney do not exhibit light chain staining, according to studies.

The utilization of mass spectrometry-based proteomic analysis coupled with laser microdissection (LMD/MS) has shown to be a reliable and practical method for amyloid typing. Said along with others. published the largest series of renal amyloidosis to date, and with the help of LMD/MS, the cause of the amyloid was identified in over 97% of cases. In situations where standard immunofluorescence and/or immunohistochemical testing are unable to conclusively classify the amyloid deposits, proteomics-based amyloid identification is advised.

5.5.2. The Renal Amyloidoses

Kidney disease is a potential consequence of many amyloidogenic proteins. These cases involve a variety of mechanisms of amyloidogenesis, such as aberrant production of proteins, increased or decreased excretion of proteins of the wild-type, and genetic mutation. Renal amyloidosis is most commonly caused by components of Igs and is linked to plasma cell dyscrasias. They are mostly made of monoclonal light chain (AL), but they can also occasionally be made of Ig heavy chain (AH) or Ig heavy and light chain combined (AHL). The second most common type of amyloid, after AL, is serum amyloid A (SAA)-induced amyloidosis, which usually develops in the context of persistent inflammatory diseases. Two large series have reported amyloidogenic leukocyte chemotactic factor 2 (ALECT2) as the third most common form of renal amyloid; however, given its higher prevalence in patients of Mexican descent, this finding is likely location-dependent. Additional types of amyloid in the kidney include fibrinogen Aα chain (AFib), lysozyme (ALys), transthyretin (ATTR), apolipoproteins AI (AApo AI), AII (AApo AII), AIV (AApo AIV), and gelsolin (AGel). (Table 5.1)

Table 5.1. Renal Amyloidosis

Amyloidogenic Protein	Sporadic (S) or Hereditary (H)/ Local (L) or Systemic (S)	Overall Incidence/ Prevalence of Kidney Impairment, %	Extrarenal Manifestation (Other Organ Tropism)
Ig light chains	S/S	59/53–86	Different organs
Serum amyloid A protein	S/S	2.9/7–40	Different organs
Leukocyte cell-derived chemotaxin-2	S/S	3.1/2.5–19.1	Liver, lungs, spleen, adrenal glands, prostate, gastrointestinal tract, gall bladder
Ig heavy chains	S/S	2.3/0.3–4.6	Different organs
Ig light and heavy chains	S/S	not assessed/3.6	Different organs
Fibrinogen α chain	H/S	0.44/1.3–3.5	Liver, spleen, gastrointestinal tract, fat
Transthyretin	S/S; H/S	28/0.9–1.4	Different organs with heart and peripheral nervous system predominance
Apolipoprotein A–IV	H/S	0.35/0.1–1.06	Heart, gastrointestinal tract, skin, lungs
Gelsolin	H/S	0.18/0.8	Cranial nerves, cornea, liver, gastrointestinal tract, skin, heart, breast, pituitary gland
Apolipoprotein C–II	H/L	<0.1/0.6	-
Apolipoprotein A–I	H/S	0.35/0.1–0.5	Liver, heart, skin, larynx, gastrointestinal tract, muscles, peripheral nervous system
Lysozyme	H/S	<0.1/0.16	Lymphatic nodes, liver, gastrointestinal tract, lungs, fat, heart
Apolipoprotein A–II	H/L	<0.1/<0.1 (extremely rare)	-
Apolipoprotein C–III	H/S	<0.1/<0.1 (extremely rare)	Liver, heart, spleen
Calcitonin	S/S	<0.1/<0.1 (extremely rare)	Thyroid gland, fat

Source: Fedotov SA, Khrabrova MS, Anpilova AO, Dobronravov VA, Rubel AA. Noninvasive Diagnostics of Renal Amyloidosis: Current State and Perspectives. International Journal of Molecular Sciences. 2022; 23(20):12662. https://doi.org/10.3390/ijms232012662

5.5.2.1. AL, AH and AHL

The most prevalent type of amyloid in developed nations is AL. Two studies from the USA and Italy found that 81 and 68% of cases of renal amyloidosis, respectively, were caused by AL. Under the umbrella of Ig-related amyloidosis, AH and AHL are rare types of the disease. Seldom is Ig-related amyloidosis observed in conjunction with other lymphoproliferative disorders; it is linked to plasma cell dyscrasias. Forty patients (21%) out of 190 patients with multiple myeloma undergoing kidney biopsy showed signs of amyloidosis, of which 88% were AL. By a ratio of 3:1, lambda light chain is more frequently the amyloidogenic protein than kappa light chain.

Either the whole light chain (consisting of the constant and variable domains) or just the variable domain makes up AL amyloid fibrils. Increased amyloidogenic properties may arise from mutations in the V λ VI subgroup and the N-terminus, which are both located within the variable domain. Amyloid deposition might also be influenced by proteolysis and modifications to post-translational proteins. Although the pathophysiology of AHL and AH is less known, related mechanisms have been proposed.

The most prevalent presenting symptom of systemic Ig-related amyloidosis, which affects up to 50% of patients, is kidney disease. The male-to-female ratio is approximately 2:1, and numerous studies have shown a slight male predominance. The average age at diagnosis is 65 years old. Renal insufficiency is common when the kidney is involved; in one study, it accounted for 47% of cases. Up to 73% of patients with Ig-related renal amyloid have been reported to have proteinuria, and 25–68% of these patients have full nephrotic syndrome. Compared to patients without AL-λ, those with AL-λ typically exhibit higher levels of proteinuria and lower serum creatinine levels. While there is no discernible difference in serum creatinine, estimated glomerular filtration rate (eGFR), 24-hour urine protein, or the proportion of patients with nephrotic syndrome, AH and AHL amyloid are more commonly linked to hematuria than AL amyloid. Patients with AH and AHL are more likely than those with AL to have overt multiple myeloma, and they are linked to less frequent cardiac involvement outside of the kidney.

All renal parenchymal compartments may be histologically affected by AL/AH/AHL, with the glomerulus being the most frequently impacted. Nasr et al. discovered that there were no appreciable variations in the parenchymal distribution between AH/AHL and AL. A few histologic variations were found, including four cases (or 25%) of AH/AHL with amyloid deposits that were positive for PAS. Unusual findings suggest that AL deposits may be restricted to the vasculature, which was linked to lower proteinuria and a higher serum creatinine level at presentation compared to diffuse AL. There has also been a report of an uncommon case of intratubular AL-λ amyloidosis without glomerular, interstitial, or vascular involvement that manifests as acute kidney injury. Light chain cast nephropathy and light chain deposition disease are two additional monoclonal Ig-associated diseases that amyloidosis can occasionally co-occur with.

The underlying plasma cell dyscrasia is usually the focus of treatment for Ig-related amyloidosis. The median survival time for untreated AL patients is 12 months following diagnosis, and it is less than 5 months for patients with cardiac involvement. The prognosis has improved with developments in stem cell transplantation and anti-plasma cell therapy. Skinner and associates. showed that 312 patients treated with high-dose melphalan followed by an autologous stem cell transplant (ASCT) had a prolonged median survival of 4.6 years. An investigation by Leung et al., renal response was observed in 43% of patients with

AL after receiving high-dose melphalan and ASCT, and it was correlated with the degree of baseline proteinuria. Rarely, kidney transplants have been given to AL patients. Pinney and associates. described a series of kidney transplant recipients who were 25 patients with AL. With 5- and 10-year graft survival rates of 74% and 25%, respectively, the median graft survival was 5 points 8 years. Recurrent renal amyloid was seen in 28% of grafts; amyloid nephropathy was not the cause of graft loss, though. Those without at least a partial clonal response to treatment had a much lower graft survival rate at the time of transplant.

5.5.2.2. AA

The second most prevalent type of systemic amyloidosis is amyloid A amyloidosis. In two US studies, AA was present in 7 and 12.5% of renal biopsies that had amyloidosis. In Europe, where it has been documented in as many as 30–40% of patients with renal amyloid deposition, AA is more common. The SAA protein, an acute-phase reactant and an apolipoprotein component of high-density lipoprotein (HDL), is the source of the amyloid fibrils found in AA. Hepatocytes produce SAA, which is controlled by pro-inflammatory cytokines through transcription. A small percentage of patients may experience protein misfolding and subsequent amyloid deposition if they have a prolonged inflammatory stimulus and SAA overproduction. Chronic inflammatory arthritis, infection, recurrent fever syndromes (like familial Mediterranean fever), inflammatory bowel disease, neoplasia, and Castleman's disease are some of the underlying inflammatory stimuli linked to AA.

The short arm of chromosome 11 contains the three expressed gene products that make up the SAA gene family. The two main isotypes deposited in AA are SAA1 and SAA2, which are primarily expressed during the acute-phase response. Instead of being an acute-phase reactant, SAA4 expression is constitutively active. There has been a report of an AA case caused by a SAA4 mutation without any ongoing inflammation.

Approximately ten years is the average age of AA patients, which is younger than that of AL patients. AA is the most prevalent type of amyloidosis in children. The most common clinical manifestation of AA is kidney disease; in one study, up to 97% of patients had a serum creatinine of >132.6 μmol/L (1.5 mg/dL) or >500 mg of proteinuria per day. There have been reports of elevated serum creatinine in 75–81% of patients and full nephrotic syndrome in 54–63% of patients.

5.5.2.3. ALECT2

One of the newest proteins to be added to the expanding list of amyloidogenic proteins is leukocyte chemotactic factor 2 (LECT2). Hepatocytes produce LECT2, which mainly functions as a neutrophil chemotactic factor and may also be involved in tissue growth and repair after injury. Three percent of cases of renal amyloidosis were found to be ALECT2 cases, making it the third most common form of the disease according to two recent studies conducted in the USA. Although the exact mechanism of amyloidogenesis is unknown, there has been speculation regarding a potential genetic component. Murphy along with others. Four ALECT2 patients had their genes sequenced, and it was discovered that they were all homozygous for the G allele, which is the result of an amino acid substitution (Ile40Val). The majority of cases that have been reported have been found in patients who are Mexican-American, which further supports a genetic component. The majority of ALECT2-related clinical illnesses have been found in the kidney; however, one report showed that ALECT2 deposits were unintentionally found in the adrenal, splenic, colonic, and liver tissues. There have also been reports of ALECT2 deposition in the kidney and lung, which manifests as pulmonary-renal syndrome. Renal insufficiency is the more common presentation of renal ALECT2 than is heavy proteinuria. Said along with others. revealed 13 cases of ALECT2 and discovered that 92% of the cases had renal insufficiency and 17% had nephrotic syndrome. The histologic distribution of amyloid deposits is correlated with this clinical manifestation. All renal compartments exhibit ALECT2 deposition; however, interstitial deposits frequently predominate. The most effective method for identifying ALECT2 is LMD/MS, but when carried out by a skilled laboratory, immunohistochemical characterization is also a helpful technique (Chen et al., 2003; Mason and Wahab, 2003).

5.6. Renal Tubular Disorders

The main method by which the body reabsorbs small molecules is through the renal tubules. Renal tubular dysfunction disorders are classified according to the tubule segment affected and the substrates whose transport is impacted. Reabsorbing mechanisms for molecules are saturable and specific. The majority of the transport proteins connected to particular transport systems have been located and characterized. The majority of transport disorders are caused by proximal tubule abnormalities. Employing energy-dependent mechanisms, the renal tubules reabsorb between 80 and 98% of the filtered small molecules. Primary or secondary disorders that disrupt these mechanisms can result in the loss of various organic acids, sugars, amino acids, bicarbonate, phosphorus, and other cations in the urine. Certain transport systems are regulated by genetics. As a result, inherited diseases may impact the reabsorption of a single or limited set of substances. A more widespread loss of renal tubular mechanisms may result from abnormalities that modify energy metabolism. With the notable exception of phosphorus and bicarbonate, these disorders do not typically result in systemic disease unless an intestinal defect is also present. However, there is emerging evidence that they may be significant in older adults. Problems with cysteine transport deficiency are mainly caused by the compound's low solubility. However, these conditions must be identified because they can be mistaken for metabolic defects, in which elevated serum concentrations of a substance lead to a filtered load that is greater than the tubules' ability to reabsorb it.

5.6.1. The Proximal Tubule

The majority of the solutes found in the glomerular filtrate are primarily transported and reabsorbable by the proximal convoluted tubule (PCT), as well as the location of the production of the key urinary buffer ammonium (NH_4^+):

- In the early part of the PCT (S1), reabsorbed solutes include glucose, amino acids, phosphate, bicarbonate and various filtered low molecular weight proteins.
- In the later part of the PCT (S2) urate is reabsorbed and secreted, and citrate is also reabsorbed.
- Still further along is the proximal straight tubule (S3) where many drugs and their metabolites are secreted (e.g., loop and thiazide diuretics).

The "sodium pump" (Na^+K^+-ATPase) on the basolateral side of the proximal tubular cell (PTC) is necessary for all of this active transport. Due to their high reliance on aerobic respiration and need for energy, PTCs are full of mitochondria and sensitive to hypoxia. This makes them especially vulnerable to damage or necrosis from drug nephrotoxicity and renal ischemia.

5.6.1.1. Disturbance of Active Transport Processes

Reduced reabsorption of the previously mentioned solutes occurs when these active transport processes in the PTCs fail, and this reduced solute content may then show up in the final urine.

- **Glucose:** Many genetic defects impact the transport of amino acids (aminoacidurias) and glucose (isolated renal glycosuria). One of the most prevalent and clinically significant inherited defects of amino acid transport that causes stones in humans is cystinuria, which is caused by the mutation of cystine (dimeric cysteine). It is important to distinguish cystinosis, a lysosomal storage disease that affects the PCT and is caused by an intracellular buildup of cystine, from cystinuria.
- **Bicarbonate:** The clinical manifestation of proximal renal tubular acidosis (pRTA or type 2 RTA) is the disturbance of bicarbonate reabsorption. An acidosis will initially be caused by an alkaline urine pH and a decrease in systemic bicarbonate concentration. Any bicarbonate that is not reabsorbed by the PCT is reabsorbed by the thick ascending limb of the loop of Henle and the collecting duct, which together are sometimes referred to as the "distal nephron," when the threshold for bicarbonate reabsorption is exceeded (typically at a plasma or serum concentration of approximately 16 mmol/l). This prevents additional bicarbonate loss and raises the pH of the urine, in contrast to distal RTA – more on that later. In addition to being brought on by carbonic anhydrase inhibitors (like acetazolamide) and their derivative medications, like the anticonvulsant topiramate, this form of RTA can also manifest in an isolated monogenic form.
- **Renal Fanconi syndrome:** On the other hand, renal Fanconi syndrome, which includes uricosuria, glycosuria, phosphaturia, aminoaciduria, and low molecular weight proteinuria, is typically linked to pRTA. This syndrome can arise from a variety of acquired diseases, including Wilson disease and myeloma, as well as from mitochondrial disease, which can be inherited or related to medication, and as a side effect of certain medications, including ifosfamide, tenofovir, and aminoglycoside antibiotics.

Dent disease is a recessive X-linked condition caused by a mutation in a PCT intracellular chloride transporter CLC-5 or in the intracellular phosphatase enzyme OCRL1, which results in a Dent-like syndrome known as Dent-2. This genetic form of the renal Fanconi syndrome associated with nephrocalcinosis and nephrolithiasis occurs in Dent disease. Lowe syndrome, an inherited renal Fanconi syndrome linked to congenital cataracts and mental retardation (oculocerebrorenal syndrome), is also brought on by OCRLA1 mutations.

5.6.2. The Loop of Henle

The counter-current multiplier located in the loop of Henle is responsible for producing the corticomedullary osmotic gradient, which in turn enables the kidneys to concentrate and dilute the final urine product. Reabsorption of sodium (Na^+) and chloride (Cl^-) along the water impermeable thick ascending limb (TAL) of the loop of Henle, also referred to as the "diluting segment," is necessary for this ability.

5.6.2.1. Bartter Syndrome

Failure of Na+ and Cl-reabsorption in the TAL leads to a lack of urine concentration, which is the cause of Bartter syndrome. This leads to volume depletion, polyuria, and salt waste (often with hypotension). Increased potassium (K+) and hydrogen (H^+) ion excretion in the urine as a result of secondary hyperaldosteronism and increased Na^+ delivery to the downstream collecting duct causes hypokalaemia and metabolic alkalosis. Additionally, normal NaCl reabsorption is necessary for the major sites of calcium (Ca^{2+}) and magnesium (Mg^{2+}) reabsorption, which are located in the TAL. As a result, Bartter syndrome is associated with increased urinary Ca^{2+} and Mg^{2+} losses, and hypomagnesaemia is common in types 1 and 2.

In order for NaCl reabsorption to occur in the TAL, several transporters must cooperate. Na+, K+, and 2Cl− are all transported into the cell by the furosemide-sensitive apical transporter NKCC2, which is triggered by the low intracellular Na^+ concentration that is upheld by the basolateral Na^+–K^+–ATPase. Nonetheless, the concentration of K+ in tubular fluid is significantly lower than that of Na+ and Cl^-. If the apical K+ channel, ROMK, didn't recycle K+ back across the apical membrane into the lumen, this would be limiting. A lumen positive potential difference produced by this K^+ recycling forces the paracellular reabsorption of Ca^{2+}, Mg^{2+}, and some Na+ between the TAL cells. In the meantime, Cl^- is eliminated basolaterally from the TAL cell through the Cl− channels ClC-Kb and ClC-Ka, both of which are controlled by the accessory protein barttin. Bartter syndrome is caused by genetic mutations in any of these transport and regulatory proteins, which reduce NaCl transport along the TAL and have local and downstream effects on the excretion of Ca^{2+}, Mg^{2+}, K+, and H^+.

- Types of Bartter syndrome:

Types 1–4 of Bartter syndrome are autosomal recessive.

- o Types 1 and 2 are linked to nephrocalcinosis and result from mutations in the NKCC2 and ROMK genes, respectively.
- o ClC-Kb mutations cause type 3, which has a milder phenotype, most likely because Cl− channel function is somewhat redundant.
- o Since this protein is also found in the inner ear, a barttin mutation causes a more severe form known as type 4, which is linked to sensorineural deafness.
- o Mutations in the calcium sensing receptor (CaSR) on the basolateral membrane of TAL cells activate type 5, an autosomal dominant form. CaSR activation explains the renal effects of hypercalcemia by inhibiting NaCl reabsorption. Nephrocalcinosis, stones, and hypocalcemia from parathyroid hormone suppression (caused by the expression of the CaSR in the parathyroid gland) are other symptoms experienced by affected patients.

5.6.2.2. Familial Hypomagnesemia with Hypercalciuria

Familial hypomagnesemia with hypercalciuria is another hereditary tubular disease that affects this segment of the nephron. This is caused by a malfunction in the paracellular pathway (discussed above) for the absorption of Ca^{2+} and Mg^{2+}, which is dependent on the claudins, which are cell junction proteins that have selective permeability. This autosomal recessive syndrome, characterized by nephrocalcinosis and poorly understood recurrent urinary tract infections, is caused by mutations in either claudin 16 or 19. It always goes on to become renal failure.

5.6.3. The Distal Convoluted Tubule

The primary functions of the distal convoluted tubule (DCT) include the transport of Na+ and Cl-, along with a minor amount of Ca^{2+} and Mg^{2+} reabsorption. However, in this case, the transport occurs across (transcellular) rather than between (paracellular) DCT cells. Na^+ and Cl^- transport is carried out by an apical NaCl co-transporter (NCC) that is sensitive to thiazides.

- **Gitelman Syndrome:** Loss-of-function mutations of NCC cause Gitelman syndrome,[8] characterized by:
    - o milder renal salt losses and volume contraction than in Bartter syndrome
    - o hypokalaemia and metabolic alkalosis, but with
    - o hypocalciuria, similar to the effect of thiazide diuretic administration rather than the hypercalciuria of Bartter syndrome.

Gitelman syndrome is typically asymptomatic and is frequently discovered by chance in adulthood or late in childhood.

- **Gordon Syndrome:** Gordon syndrome, also known as familial hyperkalaemic hypertension, pseudohypoaldosteronism type 2, or autosomal dominant syndrome, is the mirror image of Gitelman syndrome. This results from mutations in the upstream regulators of NCC, WNK (With No Lysine (K)) kinases 1 and 4, which cause NCC overactivity. Hypertension, hyperkalaemia, metabolic acidosis, and hypercalciuria are the outcomes. Most of the clinical features of Gordon syndrome can be corrected with thiazide diuretics, which are especially sensitive to patients with this syndrome.

5.6.4. The Collecting Duct

The collecting duct comprises two main cell types:

- Na^+ and water reabsorbing, and K^+ secreting, principal cells, and
- acid or bicarbonate secreting intercalated cells.
- **Principal Cells:** Principal cells are the predominant type of cells found in the kidney, containing the Na^+ channel ENaC and the K^+ channel ROMK on their apical side. They also have the Na^+-K^+-ATPase on their basolateral side, which is a common feature in all polarized renal epithelial cells. The activity of ENaC is regulated by aldosterone, which increases the number of open ENaCs, the activity of Na^+-K^+-ATPase, and the number of ROMK channels. This results in increased reabsorption of Na+ and secretion/excretion of K^+.
- **Liddle Syndrome:** Additionally, water reabsorption happens between the main cells through

the apical water channel aquaporin 2, which is regulated by the antidiuretic hormone vasopressin. Liddle syndrome, an autosomal dominant form of hypertension, is brought on by mutations in ENaC that keep the protein from being removed from the apical membrane, thereby preserving elevated ENaC activity. Metabolic alkalosis and hypokalaemia coexist with hypertension. It should come as no surprise that amiloride works wonders for Liddle syndrome patients while spironolactone has no effect.

- **Apparent Mineralocorticoid Excess Syndrome:** A related syndrome called apparent mineralocorticoid excess is caused by mutations in the enzyme 11-hydroxysteroid dehydrogenase-2 (11HSD2) that cause a loss of function. This syndrome is autosomal recessive. The intracellular enzyme 11HSD2 normally metabolizes cortisol, preventing it from activating the mineralocorticoid receptor (MR) in place of aldosterone. Cortisol is present in much higher concentrations than aldosterone, but the MR in the collecting duct can bind it as well. This enzyme, which can lead to hypertension, is inhibited by licorice.
- **Pseudohypoaldosteronism Type 1 (PHA1):** Pseudohypoaldosteronism type 1 is a condition that closely resembles Liddle syndrome, with symptoms similar to Addison's disease. Common traits include salt wasting, low blood pressure, acidosis, and high levels of potassium in the blood.

The syndrome has two forms due to:

- o Autosomal recessive loss-of-function ENaC mutations unresponsive to aldosterone (type 1a). There is a wide distribution of ENaC in the lung, kidney, skin and gastrointestinal tract, so the phenotype is often more severe.
- o Autosomal dominant mutations of the MR that cannot bind aldosterone (type 1b). In this form the phenotype is milder and is confined to the kidney.

- **Hereditary Nephrogenic Diabetes:** Hereditary nephrogenic diabetes insipidus (NDI) is a condition of resistance to the action of vasopressin caused either by:
- o recessive loss-of-function mutations in the V2 vasopressin receptor gene (*AVRP2*) on the X chromosome (>90%), or
- o recessive and autosomal dominant mutations in the water channel aquaporin 2 gene (*AQP2*).

The main symptoms, which are usually connected to mild hypernatraemia, are polyuria, nocturia, and polydipsia, with elevated vasopressin levels. Urine osmolality is low and plasma or serum osmolality is elevated due to the loss of urine concentrating ability. Since thirst is typical, severe hypernatraemia is rare. Because lithium enters the main cells through ENaC, it can result in an acquired form of NDI, a side effect of long-term use. Lithium also interferes with vasopressin signaling through cyclic AMP. Amiloride can either block or lessen this effect.

- **Hereditary Central Diabetes Insipidus:** Autosomal dominant mutations in the AVP-neurophysin II gene (AVP-NPII) cause hereditary central diabetes insipidus, which is characterized by low circulating vasopressin levels and loss of vasopressin secretion (unlike NDI, which is typically progressive rather than obvious at birth).
- **Hereditary Syndrome of Antidiuretic Hormone Secretion (SIADH) and Hyponatremia:** SIADH, as opposed to X-linked NDI, may result from a gain-of-function mutation in the V2 vasopressin receptor and AVRP2 gene. Hyponatraemia and SIADH have also been connected to a loss-of-function polymorphism of the TRPV4 cation channel, suggesting that the hypothalamus uses this ion channel for osmosensing. A lower-than-normal plasma osmolality can be controlled by those affected, who also exhibit a blunted response to hypotonicity and behave as though they have a reset osmostat. This polymorphism affects the normal wild-type allele in a dominant-negative manner.
- **Alpha Intercalated Cells:** By producing H^+ through the intracellular conversion of CO_2 and water to carbonic acid, followed by its breakdown into bicarbonate and H^+ catalyzed by carbonic anhydrase 2 (CA2), alpha intercalated cells excrete acid into the urine. The electrogenic H^+ vH-ATPase secretes H^+ into the tubular lumen, while the Cl^-/bicarbonate anion exchanger AE1 (SLC4A1) transports bicarbonate to the blood.
- **Hereditary Distal renal Tubular Acidosis:** Type 1 RTA, also known as dRTA, is a hereditary distal renal tubular acidosis that can be brought on by loss-of-function mutations in AE1 or the vH-ATPase subunits B1 or a4. Metabolic acidosis, which is exacerbated by rickets, osteomalacia or low bone mineral density, nephrocalcinosis, and stones, can be brought on by a decreased capacity to excrete acid in the urine. Hypokalaemia is also caused by increased excretion of potassium in the urine, though this is harder to explain. In acidotic patients (so-called "complete" dRTA), the propensity to develop calcium phosphate stones is due to hypercalciuria and alkaline urine; urine pH is always higher than 5 points 3 when systemic acidosis is present. Patients may still have "incomplete" dRTA (acidification defect but not acidosis). Urinary acidification testing is required if this is suspected (in the case of nephrocalcinosis or in the event of a family history of stones) (Couser and Johnson, 2014; O'Shaughnessy et al., 2017; Khalighi et al., 2018; Mariani et al., 2019; Satoskar et al., 2020).

A Closer Look

Proteinuria

One indicator of kidney disease is proteinuria. Therefore, measuring the protein content of urine plays a crucial role in any diagnostic work-up for kidney infection. Since glomerular illness is known to be associated with undeniable degrees of proteinuria (nephrotic proteinuria), most proteinuria investigation focuses on estimating the absolute protein content. However, proteinuria may also be physiological or the result of impaired cylinder protein reabsorption.

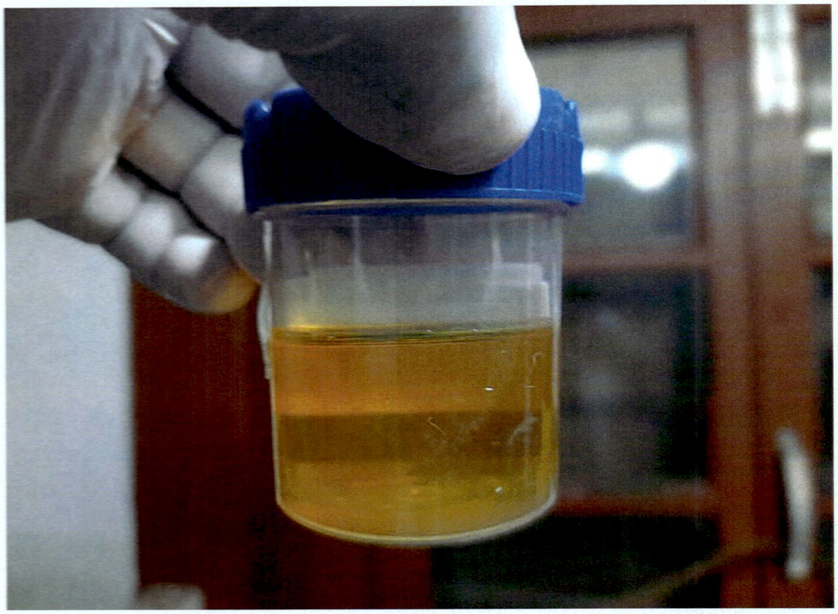

Source: By Ajay Kumar Chaurasiya - Own work, CC BY-SA 4.0, https://commons.wikimedia.org/w/index.php?curid=113879411.

In addition to serum creatinine, blood pressure, and urinalysis, the measurement of urine protein output plays a crucial role in the identification and categorization of renal illness. In fact, as the KIDGO guidelines indicate, even small amounts of proteinuria, or microalbuminuria, are associated with dire outcomes and are therefore remembered for the coordination of chronic kidney disease. This is especially true for proteinuria in the nephrotic range. Proteinuria is an indicator of glomerular illness because large proteins are essentially impermeable to the unimpaired glomerular channel.

Urine is essentially free of protein under normal circumstances (i.e., proteinuria < 4 mg/m2/h or a protein-creatinine ratio of < 180 mg/g (20 mg/mmol)). All things considered, orthostatic proteinuria, febrile proteinuria, and practice proteinuria are the three conditions in which proteinuria may be physiological. Given these conditions, proteinuria is temporary and should be excluded from the first morning urine test collected directly after waking up, following recovery from the fever, or following recovery from strenuous activity, respectively.

The glomerular channel allows water and small solutes up to inulin's (5 kDa) size to pass through without restriction. Porousness is, on the other hand, associated with subatomic size for larger particles. Consequently, a large number of various macromolecules, such as chemicals and cytokines, as well as LMW proteins with an atomic mass between 10 and 20 kDa, such as α1-microglobulin, β-2 microglobulin, cystatin C, and retinol-restricting protein (RBP), also cross the glomerular channel.

Taking everything into account, the final urine has negligible amounts of LMW proteins. This is due to the extensive reabsorption of proteins, such as megalin and cubulin, in the proximal tubule through receptor-interceded multi-ligand endocytosis. Reabsorbed LMW proteins don't always enter the dissemination process because they are broken down at a low pH in proximal tubule lysosomes.

Two head systems (or a combination of the two) can cause obsessive proteinuria: (i) the glomerular boundary's extreme protein porosity, or (ii) the impaired ability of the proximal tubule to reabsorb protein. Although glomerular illness and nephrotic range proteinuria are related, non-glomerular illnesses also have a substantial impact and can result in severe albuminuria and proteinuria.

Summary

- Renal disease, also known as kidney disease, refers to any condition that affects the structure or function of the kidneys. The kidneys play a vital role in filtering waste products and excess fluids from the blood, regulating electrolyte balance, and producing hormones that control blood pressure and stimulate red blood cell production.
- Glomerular disease reduces the kidneys' ability to maintain a balance of certain substances in the bloodstream.
- Symptoms of glomerular disease vary and are related to the type of damage to your glomeruli. Some people with less damage may have few or no symptoms, whereas people with more severe damage may have more noticeable symptoms.
- Glomerular diseases are considered to be the result of inherited or acquired disorders and may manifest in a variety of clinical syndromes, including numerous pictures in terms of severity.
- Post-streptococcal glomerulonephritis is the best-known example of endocapillary glomerulonephritis, the most common form of acute glomerulonephritis seen after some bacterial, viral, fungal, and parasitic infections.
- The rapidly progressive glomerulonephritides are the most serious of all glomerulonephritides with the potential to destroy renal function within days.
- Systemic lupus erythematosus (SLE) is an autoimmune disorder affecting multiple organ systems including kidney, skin, lung, heart, the hematopoietic system and brain.
- The progression of diabetic nephropathy to end-stage kidney disease is mediated by a host of processes, but none is as important as the gradual, inexorable scarring of the renal glomerulus, known as glomerulosclerosis.
- Amyloidosis represents a family of disorders defined by the extracellular deposition of protein fibrils with a characteristic β-pleated sheet conformation.

References

1. Alsaad, K. O., & Herzenberg, A. M. (2007). Distinguishing diabetic nephropathy from other causes of glomerulosclerosis: An update. *Journal of Clinical Pathology, 60*, 18–26.
2. Chen, S., Jim, B., & Ziyadeh, F. N. (2003). Diabetic nephropathy and transforming growth factor-beta: Transforming our view of glomerulosclerosis and fibrosis build-up. *Seminars in Nephrology, 23*, 532–543.
3. Couser, W. G., & Johnson, R. J. (2014). The etiology of glomerulonephritis: Roles of infection and autoimmunity. *Kidney International, 86*(5), 905–914.
4. D'Agord Schaan, B., Lacchini, S., Bertoluci, M. C., Irigoyen, M. C., Machado, U. F., & Schmid, H. (2001). Increased renal GLUT1 abundance and urinary TGF-beta 1 in streptozotocin-induced diabetic rats: Implications for the development of nephropathy complicating diabetes. *Hormone and Metabolic Research, 33*, 664–669.
5. Glenner, G. G., Terry, W., Harada, M., et al. (1971). Amyloid fibril proteins: Proof of homology with immunoglobulin light chains by sequence analyses. *Science, 172*, 1150–1151.

6. Heilig, C. W., Liu, Y., England, R. L., Freytag, S. O., Gilbert, J. D., Heilig, K. O., Zhu, M., Concepcion, L. A., & Brosius, F. C. (1997). D-glucose stimulates mesangial cell GLUT1 expression and basal and IGF-I–sensitive glucose uptake in rat mesangial cells: Implications for diabetic nephropathy. *Diabetes, 46*, 1030–1039.

7. Khalighi, M. A., Al-Rabadi, L., Chalasani, M., Smith, M., Kakani, S., Revelo, M. P., & Meehan, S. M. (2018). Staphylococcal infection-related glomerulonephritis with cryoglobulinemic features. *Kidney International Reports, 3*(5), 1128–1134.

8. Mariani, L. H., Bomback, A. S., Canetta, P. A., et al. (2019). CureGN Study rationale, design, and methods: Establishing a large prospective observational study of glomerular disease. *American Journal of Kidney Diseases, 73*(2), 218–229.

9. Mason, R. M., & Wahab, N. A. (2003). Extracellular matrix metabolism in diabetic nephropathy. *Journal of the American Society of Nephrology, 14*, 1358–1373.

10. O'Shaughnessy, M. M., Hogan, S. L., Poulton, C. J., et al. (2017). Temporal and demographic trends in glomerular disease epidemiology in the southeastern United States, 1986–2015. *Clinical Journal of the American Society of Nephrology, 12*(4), 614–623.

11. O'Shaughnessy, M. M., Hogan, S. L., Thompson, B. D., Coppo, R., Fogo, A. B., & Jennette, J. C. (2018). Glomerular disease frequencies by race, sex, and region: Results from the International Kidney Biopsy Survey. *Nephrology, Dialysis, Transplantation, 33*(4), 661–669.

12. Satoskar, A. A., Parikh, S. V., & Nadasdy, T. (2020). Epidemiology, pathogenesis, treatment and outcomes of infection-associated glomerulonephritis. *Nature Reviews Nephrology, 16*(1), 32–50.

13. Wang, S. Y., Bu, R., Zhang, Q., Liang, S., Wu, J., Liu, X. Z. S., Cai, G. Y., & Chen, X. M. (2016). Clinical, pathological, and prognostic characteristics of glomerulonephritis related to Staphylococcal infection. *Medicine (Baltimore), 95*(15), e3386.

14. Weigert, C., Brodbeck, K., Brosius, F. C., Huber, M., Lehmann, R., Friess, U., Facchin, S., Aulwurm, S., Haring, H. U., Schleicher, E. D., & Heilig, C. W. (2003). Evidence for a novel TGF-β1–independent mechanism of fibronectin production in mesangial cells overexpressing glucose transporters. *Diabetes, 52*, 527–535.

15. Wen, Y. K., & Chen, M. L. (2010). The significance of atypical morphology in the changes of spectrum of postinfectious glomerulonephritis. *Clinical Nephrology, 73*(3), 173–179.

Chapter

CEREBROSPINAL FLUID ANALYSIS

6

Contents

Introduction

The clear and colorless liquid known as cerebrospinal fluid (CSF) surrounds and fills the brain and spinal cord, acting as a mechanical barrier against impacts. CSF, primarily formed in the brain's ventricles, lubricates and supports the brain and spinal cord, acting as a cushion in case of head injury, distributing force and reducing impact. It helps maintain a constant pressure inside the skull, decreasing in proportion to an increase in blood volume or brain tissue. Conversely, CSF volume increases in response to a decrease in cranial matter volume, such as in cases of brain atrophy. Additionally, CSF transports pathological disease products, chemicals, antibodies, and metabolic waste products from the brain and spinal cord to the bloodstream. Composed mainly of water, CSF has a slightly alkaline pH, with the average adult human body containing between 100 and 150 milliliters of CSF.

The precise process by which the CSF is formed is unknown. It most likely passes via the membranes of the nervous system (ependyma) after starting in the brain's ventricles. Every six to eight hours, the entire supply of CSF is replenished, and it is produced continuously. The fluid exits the cerebrospinal spaces in several places, including the areas surrounding the cranial nerves and the spinal roots, before eventually being absorbed into the veins. Gravity's pull downward, the ongoing processes of secretion and absorption, blood pulsations in contingent tissue, breathing, vein pressure, and head and body movements all have an impact on the CSF's movement. Numerous diseases can be diagnosed by CSF examination. A lumbar puncture, also known as a spinal tap, is a procedure used to obtain a fluid sample by inserting a needle into the lumbar region of the lower back below the spinal cord's termination. Meningitis, or inflammation of the lining of the central nervous system, may be present if the CSF is hazy. A hemorrhage in or near the brain could be indicated by blood in the fluid.

Orientation and Directional Terms

Term	Definition	Illustration
Lumbar puncture	A lumbar puncture (spinal tap) is a test used to diagnose certain health conditions. It's performed in your lower back, in the lumbar region.	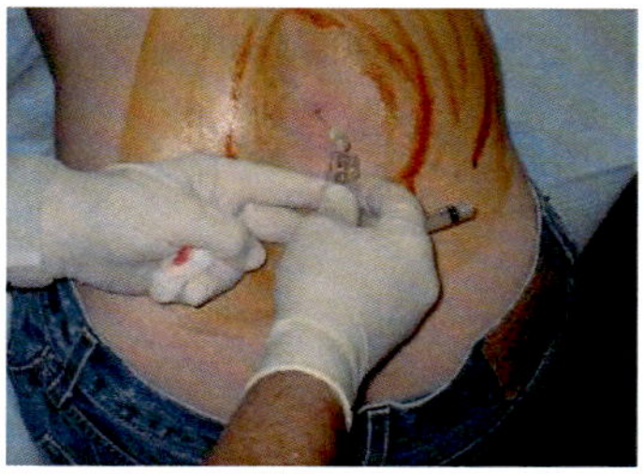
Hemorrhage	A hemorrhage is a loss of blood from a damaged blood vessel. It can be minor or major and internal or external.	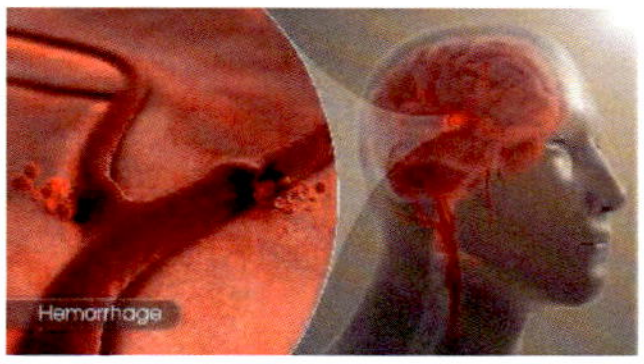
Leukemia	Leukemia is a broad term for cancers of the blood cells. The type of leukemia depends on the type of blood cell that becomes cancer and whether it grows quickly or slowly. Leukemia occurs most often in adults older than 55, but it is also the most common cancer in children younger than 15.	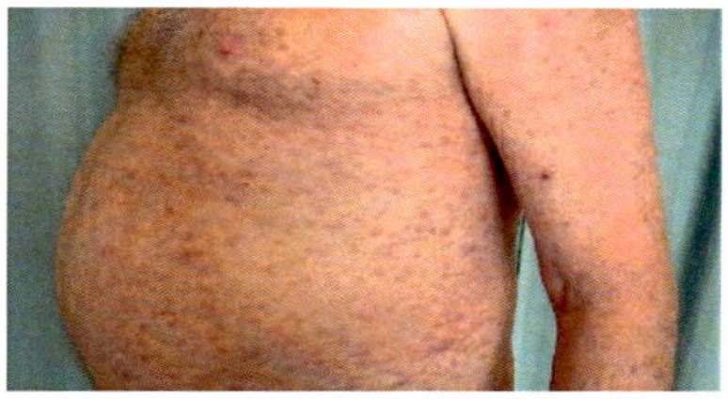
Erythrophagocytosis	Erythrophagocytosis primarily occurs in the spleen and liver and allows for the removal of senescent erythrocytes and recycling of iron, often evident as cytoplasmic accumulations of pigments.	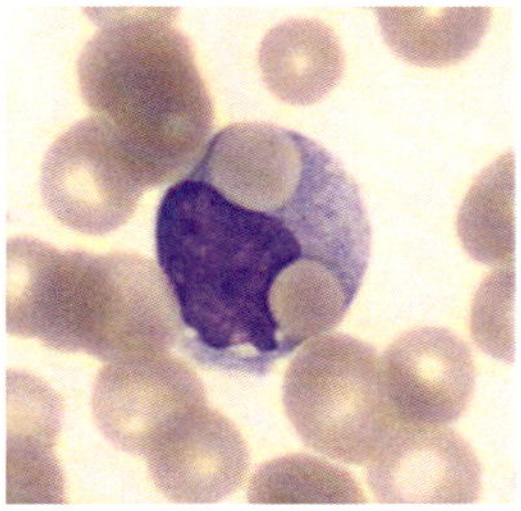
Plasma	Plasma is the liquid portion of your blood that is essential for the components of your blood to circulate throughout your body.	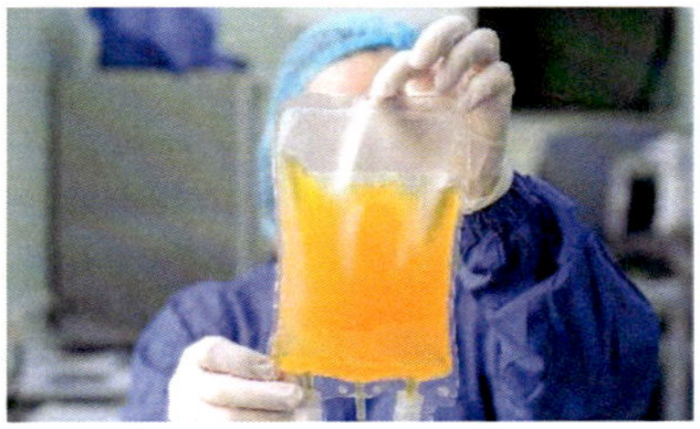

6.1. Structure and Function of Cerebrospinal Fluid (CSF)

All vertebrates have cerebrospinal fluid (CSF), a clear, colorless bodily fluid that is contained in the tissue that envelops the brain and spinal cord. In the choroid plexus of the brain's ventricles, specialized ependymal cells produce CSF, which is then absorbed by arachnoid granulations. About 125 mL of CSF can be found in humans at any given time, and 500 mL can be produced daily. CSF serves as a buffer, cushion, or shock absorber, giving the brain inside the skull fundamental mechanical and immunological protection. The cerebral autoregulation of cerebral blood flow is another essential function of CSF. CSF surrounds and resides inside the brain and spinal cord in the ventricular system as well as the subarachnoid space, which is located between the arachnoid mater and the pia mater. It fills the spinal cord's central canal, the brain's ventricles, cisterns, and sulci. Additionally, the perilymphatic duct, which connects the subarachnoid space to the inner ear's bony labyrinth, is where the perilymph and cerebrospinal fluid meet. Multiple motile cilia on the apical surfaces of the ependymal cells in the choroid plexus beat to force the CSF through the ventricles (Figure 6.1) (Hajdu and Steven, 2003; Brown, 2004; Algotsson and Winblad, 2007; Dr Cal Shipley; Adigun and Al-Dhahir).

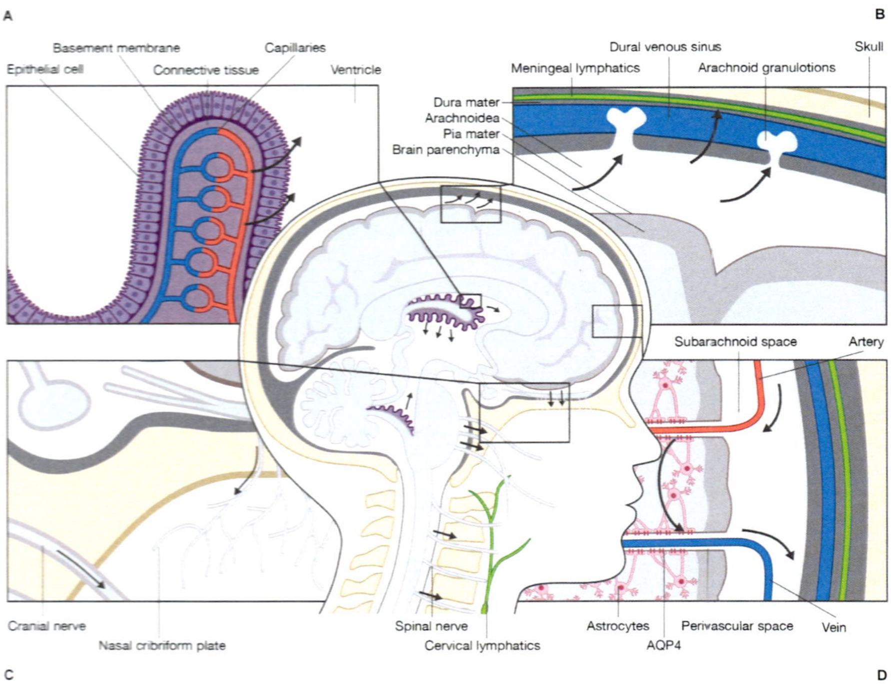

Figure 6.1. *Schematic overview of the cerebrospinal fluid system.*

Source: Thea Overgaard Wichmann, Helle Hasager Damkier, and Michael Pedersen, "A Brief Overview of the Cerebrospinal Fluid System and Its Implications for Brain and Spinal Cord Diseases," Front. Hum. Neurosci., 21 January 2022, Sec. Brain Health and Clinical Neuroscience, Volume 15 - 2021 | https://doi.org/10.3389/fnhum.2021.737217.

The primary site of cerebrospinal fluid (CSF) production is the choroid Plexi located within the lateral, third, and fourth ventricles of the brain. (A) The choroid Plexi consist of leaky epithelial cells, a basement membrane, connective tissue, and fenestrated capillaries. The CSF production is mediated by ionic transport that generates osmotic gradients and water transport from the blood system to the ventricular system. (B) Several anatomical sites are responsible for CSF absorption e.g., arachnoid granulations, meningeal lymphatics, and (C) cranial nerve sheaths and nasal cribriform plate to the cervical lymphatics. (D) One essential function of CSF is the delivery of nutrients and the removal of waste products. The most recently proposed mechanism for removal of waste is the glymphatic system. The CSF enters from the perivascular spaces surrounding arteries into the brain parenchyma via mechanisms that include AQP4 water channels located at the astrocytic end-feet. Within the brain parenchyma, CSF disperses and intermixes with the interstitial fluid (ISF) and waste products. The mixture of CSF, ISF, and waste products enters the perivascular spaces surrounding veins by unknown mechanisms, e.g., AQP4 water channels. From the perivascular spaces, the mixture leaves the brain parenchyma.

6.1.1. Structure

- **Circulation:** The CSF contains between 125 and 150 mL at any given time. The brain's ventricular system is where this CSF circulates. The ventricles are a group of CSF-filled cavities. The two lateral ventricles generate the majority of the CSF. The CSF then travels to the third ventricle via the interventricular foramina and to the fourth ventricle via the cerebral aqueduct. The spinal cord-central canal, the median aperture, and the two lateral apertures are the four openings through which fluid exits the fourth ventricle and enters the subarachnoid space. The subarachnoid space, which surrounds the brain and spinal cord and extends to the sacrum below the end of the spinal cord, contains CSF. In 93% of cases, there is a continuous flow of cerebrospinal fluid and perilymph due to a connection between the subarachnoid space and the inner ear's bony labyrinth.

  While moving in multiple directions in the subarachnoid space, CSF only moves in one direction outward from the ventricles. The pulsating movement of the fluid reflects the pressure waves that the heartbeat produces in the blood vessels. Contrary to what some authors claim, there is bidirectional systolic-diastolic CSF movements to and from the craniospinal circulation that are dependent on the cardiac cycle rather than unidirectional CSF circulation.
- **Contents:** Though it differs slightly in terms of electrolyte levels and is almost entirely protein-free, CSF is derived from blood plasma and is essentially identical to it. Because of its production process, CSF has a higher sodium content and less chloride than plasma. Depending on the sampling location, CSF contains between 15 and 40 mg/dL, or 0.59% plasma proteins. Generally speaking, ventricular CSF has lower concentrations of albumin and globular proteins than lumbar or cisternal fluid. This constant flow into the veins dilutes the concentration of bigger molecules that enter the CSF and brain that are lipid-insoluble. Red blood cells are typically absent from CSF, and fewer than 5 white blood cells per milliliter (mm^3) are present at most (a higher count of white blood cells

is referred to as pleocytosis, which may be an indication of infection or inflammation).

6.1.2. Development

The embryo is a three-layered disc covered in ectoderm, mesoderm, and endoderm at about the fifth week of development. In the midline, a structure known as the notochord—a tube-like structure—develops. The release of extracellular molecules by the notochord influences the conversion of the ectoderm that covers it into nervous tissue. The neural tube, which develops from the ectoderm, has CSF in it before the choroid plexuses do. After the first month of development, the neural tube's open neuropores close, and the CSF pressure progressively rises.

By the fourth week of embryonic development, three swellings have formed inside the embryo around the canal, close to the area where the head will develop, as the brain develops. These enlargements stand in for the prosencephalon (forebrain), mesencephalon (midbrain), and rhombencephalon (hindbrain) as distinct regions of the central nervous system. Around the 32nd day of development, subarachnoid spaces become noticeable close to the rhombencephalon; circulation becomes apparent on the 41st day. The first choroid plexus, which is located in the fourth ventricle, is visible at this point; however, it is unknown when they start secreting CSF.

The neural cord is surrounded by the growing forebrain. The neural cord inside the forebrain develops into a ventricle as it grows, eventually forming the lateral ventricles. The ventricular wall is thin along the inner surface of both ventricles and a choroid plexus forms, generating and secreting CSF. CSF fills the neural canal fast. Arachnoid granulations appear around the 39th week of development, and arachnoid villi begin to form around the 35th week. Arachnoid development continues until the child is 18 months old. To facilitate passage through the cerebral aqueduct, the subcommissural organ secretes SCO-spondin, which forms Reissner's fiber within CSF. It is there in the first stages of intrauterine life but vanishes in the early stages of development (Hajdu and Steven, 2003; Brown, 2004; Algotsson and Winblad, 2007; Dr Cal Shipley; Adigun and Al-Dhahir).

6.1.3. Physiology

6.1.3.1. Function

CSF serves several purposes:

1. **Buoyancy:** The net weight of the human brain suspended in CSF is equal to a mass of 25–50 g, despite the brain's actual mass being approximately 1400–1500 grams. Because of this, the brain is in a state of neutral buoyancy, which prevents it from being negatively impacted by its own weight, which would otherwise cut off blood flow and kill neurons in the lower regions of the brain.
2. **Protection:** CSF provides a fluid cushion that functions as a shock absorber from some types of mechanical injury, protecting the brain tissue from harm when jolted or struck.
3. **Prevention of brain ischemia:** Reducing the volume of CSF in the small area inside the skull helps prevent brain ischemia. This promotes blood perfusion and lowers intracranial pressure overall.
4. **Regulation:** The distribution of substances among brain cells

and neuroendocrine factors, to which minute modifications can result in issues or harm to the nervous system, are homeostatically regulated by CSF. For instance, a high glycine content throws off blood pressure and temperature regulation, while a high CSF pH results in lightheadedness and fainting.

5. **Clearing Waste:** CSF plays a vital role in the brain's lymphatic system, also known as the glymphatic system, which enables waste products to be eliminated from the brain. When CSF is absorbed, metabolic waste products quickly diffuse into it and are eliminated into the bloodstream. When this goes wrong, CSF can become toxic, as in the case of the most prevalent motor neuron disease, amyotrophic lateral sclerosis. (Table 6.1)

6.1.3.2. Production

Cerebrospinal fluid (CSF) is produced by the brain at a rate of about 20 mL per hour, or about 500 mL per day. There is never more than 125–150 mL of this transcellular fluid at any given time due to constant reabsorption.

Table 6.1. Comparison of Serum and Cerebrospinal Fluid

Substance	CSF	Serum
Water content (% wt)	99	93
Protein (mg/dL)	35	7000
Glucose (mg/dL)	60	90
Osmolarity (mOsm/L)	295	295
Sodium (mEq/L)	138	138
Potassium (mEq/L)	2.8	4.5
Calcium (mEq/L)	2.1	4.8
Magnesium (mEq/L)	2.0–2.5	1.7
Chloride (mEq/L)	119	102
pH	7.33	7.41

Source: https://en.wikipedia.org/wiki/Cerebrospinal_fluid.

Children have a larger volume of CSF than adults do, measured in milliliters per kilogram of body weight. The volume of CSF in infants is 4 mL/kg, in children, it is 3 mL/kg, and in adults, it is 1.5–2mL/kg.

Children's CSF volume is greater than adults' on a mL per kg body weight basis. The CSF volume of an infant is 4 mL/kg, that of a child is 3 mL/kg, and that of an adult is 1.5-2 mL/kg. Because of their high CSF volume, infants require a higher mL/kg dose of local anesthetic. Furthermore, the lower incidence of postdural puncture headache in children could be attributed in part to the greater volume of CSF. The choroid plexus produces the majority (roughly two-thirds to 80%) of CSF. Sections of the brain's four ventricles contain a network of blood vessels called the choroid plexus. It is found all over the ventricular system, except the lateral ventricles' frontal and occipital horns and the cerebral aqueduct. The lateral ventricles generate the majority of CSF. In addition, a small amount of CSF is directly produced from the tiny spaces surrounding the blood vessels surrounding the brain, the lining surrounding the subarachnoid space, and the single layer of columnar ependymal cells that line the ventricles.

The choroid plexus produces CSF in a two-step process. Initially, a filtered version of plasma from fenestrated capillaries in the choroid plexus moves into an interstitial space, guided by pressure differences between blood in the capillaries and interstitial fluid. This fluid then must cross epithelial cells lining the choroid plexus into the ventricles, an active process involving the transport of sodium, potassium, and chloride to create osmotic pressure that draws water into CSF. Unlike blood flow into the choroid plexus, the tight junctions between cells in the epithelial lining prevent most substances from freely entering the CSF. Cilia on the ependymal cell apical surfaces help transport the CSF.

The interstitial fluid diffuses into the epithelial cells, bringing with it carbon dioxide and water. The materials are changed into bicarbonate and hydrogen ions inside these cells by carbonic anhydrase. On the surface of the cell facing the interstitium, these are traded for sodium and chloride. Following that, the ventricular lumen actively secretes potassium, sodium, chloride, and bicarbonate. Because of aquaporins, this generates osmotic pressure and pulls water into the CSF. Protein anions are far less prevalent in CSF than in blood plasma. The majority of the anions that make up blood protein are highly negatively charged. As a result, blood plasma contains far fewer chloride anions than sodium cations to maintain electroneutrality. While CSF's concentration of sodium ions is comparable to that of blood plasma, it has a higher concentration of chloride ions due to a smaller imbalance between sodium and chloride caused by fewer protein cations. As a result, the plasma and osmotic pressure differ. Less potassium, calcium, glucose, and protein are present in CSF. Growth factors, iodine, vitamins B_1, B_{12}, C, folate, beta-2 microglobulin, arginine vasopressin, and nitric oxide are also secreted into CSF by choroid plexuses. The surface of the choroid endothelium contains Na/K ATPase and a Na-K-Cl cotransporter, which may be involved in controlling CSF secretion and composition. According to a theory, CSF is not mainly produced by the choroid plexus but rather is continuously produced throughout the entire CSF system as a result of water filtration into the interstitial fluid of the surrounding brain tissue through capillary walls, which is controlled by AQP-4. Although the exact causes of the circadian fluctuations in CSF secretion are unknown, they may be related to variations in the autonomic nervous system's activation throughout the day. The anterior choroidal artery supplies the arterial blood that the choroid plexus of the lateral ventricle uses to produce CSF. The arterial blood from the anterior inferior cerebellar artery (cerebellopontine angle and the surrounding portion of the lateral recess), posterior inferior cerebellar artery (roof and median opening), and superior cerebellar artery is used to create CSF in the fourth ventricle.

6.1.3.3. Reabsorption

Through arachnoid granulations, CSF re-enters the vascular system by entering the dural venous sinuses. These are arachnoid mater outpouchings that have valves to maintain one-way drainage into the venous sinuses surrounding the brain. A pressure differential between the venous sinuses and the arachnoid mater is the cause of this. Additionally, CSF has been observed to drain into lymphatic vessels, especially those that surround the nose, by passing through the cribriform plate and the olfactory nerve. Although the exact route and extent are unknown at this time, it may involve CSF flow along certain cranial nerves and be more noticeable in newborns. Three to four times a day, the CSF is replaced. Additionally, it has been observed that CSF is reabsorbed via the ependyma and the sheaths surrounding the spinal and cranial nerves.

6.1.3.4. Regulation

Hormones, blood pressure, and CSF content all affect the composition and rate of CSF generation. For instance, a higher CSF pressure reduces the pressure differential between the capillary blood in choroid plexuses and the CSF, which slows down the flow of fluids into the plexus and the production of CSF. Choroid plexus CSF secretion is influenced by the autonomic nervous system;

activation of the parasympathetic nervous system increases secretion, and activation of the sympathetic nervous system decreases it. Blood pH fluctuations can impact the activity of carbonic anhydrase, and certain medications (like furosemide, which acts on the Na-K-Cl cotransporter) may have an effect on membrane channels.

6.2. Lumbar Puncture

A spinal tap, sometimes referred to as a lumbar puncture (LP), is a medical procedure in which a needle is inserted into the spinal canal, usually to collect cerebrospinal fluid (CSF) for diagnostic testing. The primary goal of a lumbar puncture is to aid in the diagnosis of disorders affecting the brain and spine, which is the central nervous system. Meningitis and subarachnoid hemorrhage are a couple of these ailments. For some conditions, it can also be used therapeutically. Because of the possibility of compressed brain matter pushing toward the spine, increased intracranial pressure—or pressure inside the skull—must be avoided. There are instances when lumbar punctures cannot be done safely (due to a severe bleeding tendency, for example). Although post-dural puncture headaches are rare, they can occur if a small, atraumatic needle is not used, despite the procedure being thought to be safe. Usually, the process is carried out sterilely while under local anesthesia. To access and collect fluid from the subarachnoid space, a hypodermic needle is used. It is possible to send fluid for cytological, microbiological, and biochemical analysis. Using ultrasonography for landmarking could improve outcomes. Heinrich Quincke, a German doctor, invented the lumbar puncture in 1891.

6.2.1. Medical Uses

As explained below, a lumbar puncture may be performed for diagnostic or therapeutic purposes.

- **Diagnosis:** The primary purpose of lumbar punctures is to obtain cerebrospinal fluid (CSF) for diagnostic purposes. Diseases affecting the central nervous system that are inflammatory, neoplastic, or infectious may be excluded from the analysis of CSF. The most frequent reason is when meningitis is suspected because there isn't another trustworthy method to rule out meningitis, a potentially fatal but highly treatable illness. Lumbar punctures are frequently necessary in young infants as part of the standard workup for fever without a cause. This is because meningitis rates are higher than in the elderly. Additionally, unlike adults, infants do not consistently exhibit the traditional signs of meningeal irritation (meningismus), such as headaches and stiff necks. This test may be used to confirm or rule out subarachnoid hemorrhage, hydrocephalus, benign intracranial hypertension, and many other diagnoses in any age group. Additionally, it can be used to find cancerous cells in the CSF, such as those found in medulloblastoma or carcinomatous meningitis. When evaluating CSF for subarachnoid hemorrhage, for instance, a negative tap is defined as less than 10 red blood cells (RBCs)/mm3. Positive taps have an RBC count of at least $100/mm^3$.
- **Treatment:** Additionally, lumbar punctures can be used to inject drugs intrathecally (into the cerebrospinal fluid), especially for chemotherapy or spinal anesthesia.

For the temporary management of idiopathic intracranial hypertension (IIH), serial lumbar punctures may be helpful. The hallmark of this illness is elevated CSF pressure, which can result in headaches and irreversible vision loss. Medication is the cornerstone of treatment, but occasionally multiple lumbar punctures can alleviate symptoms. It is not advised as a mainstay of care because of the procedure's discomfort and risk as well as its brief duration of effectiveness. Furthermore, some patients with normal pressure hydrocephalus—a condition marked by dementia, altered gait, and incontinence—experience some degree of symptom relief following CSF withdrawal.

6.2.2. Contraindications

The following circumstances should not be handled by lumbar puncture:

- Idiopathic elevated intracranial pressure (ICP; unknown cause).
    - o **Rationale:** Performing a lumbar puncture when intracranial pressure is elevated may result in uncal herniation.
    - o **Exception:** ICP can be lowered therapeutically with lumbar puncture, but only after all other options have been exhausted, such as obstruction in the brain's third ventricle.
    - o **Precaution**
        - CT brain, particularly in the circumstances listed below.
            - Ø Age >65
            - Ø Reduced GCS
            - Ø Recent history of seizure
            - Ø Focal neurological signs
            - Ø Abnormal respiratory pattern
            - Ø Bradycardia, hypertension, and declining consciousness.
        - Ophthalmoscopy for papilledema
- Bleeding diathesis (relative)
    - o Coagulopathy
    - o Decreased platelet count (<50 x 10^9/L)
- Infections
    - o Skin infection at the puncture site
- Vertebral malformations (kyphosis or scoliosis) in the care of a medical professional lacking experience.

6.2.3. Adverse Effects

- **Headache:** The most frequent side effect is post-dural puncture headache accompanied by nausea; it frequently goes away with painkillers and fluid infusions. It has long been believed that this complication can be avoided by strictly maintaining a supine position for two hours following the successful puncture; however, recent large-scale studies have not supported this theory. Performing the surgery with the patient at their side may help to lower the risk. An intravenous caffeine injection can frequently effectively stop these headaches in the back. A headache that only happens when sitting up and that lasts for a long-time during bed rest could be a sign of a CSF leak from the lumbar puncture site. Additional bed rest or an epidural blood patch, which involves injecting the patient's own blood back into the leak site to create a clot and stop the leak, are two possible treatments.

When using atraumatic needles, there is a significantly lower chance of headaches and a need for analgesics and blood patches. This has no further impact on the procedure's success rate. While the cost and difficulty are comparable, adoption is still quite low, at about 16%. 2014. The dura mater may have been accidentally punctured, which would explain the headaches.

- **Other:** Paresthesia, or abnormal sensations in the leg caused by contact between the side of the lumbar puncture needle and a spinal nerve root, is a harmless side effect that can be warned about ahead of time to reduce anxiety if it happens.

When a lumbar puncture is done correctly, serious complications are very rare. These comprise spinal or epidural hemorrhage, adhesive arachnoiditis, and injuries to the spinal nerve roots or spinal cord that cause paraplegia, weakness, or loss of feeling. The latter is extremely uncommon because it occurs several vertebral spaces above the appropriate location for a lumbar puncture (L3/L4), where the spinal cord normally ends (the inferior border of L1, though it is slightly lower in infants). Although extremely rare, there have been case reports of lumbar punctures leading to the perforation of aberrant dural arterio-venous malformations and catastrophic epidural hemorrhage.

When there is a risk of infection at the puncture site due to topical infections or dermatological conditions, when there is an epidural infection present or suspected, or in patients who suffer from severe psychosis or neurosis and have back pain, the procedure is not advised. Some experts think that removing fluid when initial pressures are abnormal could cause cerebral herniation or spinal cord compression; others think that these events are just coincidental, happening separately as a result of the same pathology that the lumbar puncture was done to diagnose. In any event, if an intracranial mass is suspected, computed tomography of the brain is frequently carried out before lumbar puncture. A lumbar puncture procedure may cause CSF leaks.

6.2.4. Technique

- **Mechanism:** Below this point in the spine, nerves continue, but they form the cauda equina, a loose bundle of nerve fibers. Because these loose fibers move out of the way of the needle without being damaged, there is less risk involved when inserting a needle into the spine at the cauda equina level.

Up to the S2 vertebra, the lumbar cistern extends into the sacrum.

6.2.5. Procedure

Usually, the person is positioned on their side (left side more frequently than right). The patient hunches over, bends the neck so the chin is near the chest, and brings the knees up to the chest. This is as close to a fetal position as it gets. Patients may also lean their head and shoulders forward while sitting on a stool. An aseptic technique is used to prepare the region surrounding the lower back. Following palpation of the proper location, local anesthetic is injected along the spinal needle's intended path after penetrating the skin. A spinal needle is pushed in until it gives way as it enters the lumbar cistern, which houses the ligamentum flavum, between the lumbar vertebrae L3/L4, L4/L5, or L5/S1. Once more, the needle is pushed until a second "give" occurs, signifying that the dura mater has been passed. The fluid pressure from CSF in the subarachnoid space pushes the arachnoid membrane out towards the dura, causing the arachnoid membrane and dura mater to exist in flush contact with one another in the spine of a living individual. As a result, the needle has passed through the thinner arachnoid membrane after penetrating the dura mater. At that point, the needle is in the subarachnoid space. Following the withdrawal of the spinal needle's stylet, drops of cerebrospinal fluid are collected. Using a straightforward column manometer, the opening pressure of the cerebrospinal fluid can be measured during this collection. With pressure applied to the puncture site, the needle is removed to complete the procedure. The choice of the spinal level was made to prevent spinal injuries. The patient used to be kept under observation for any indications of neurological issues while they remained on their back for at least six hours. There isn't any scientific proof that this is beneficial. With the exception of the fact that spinal anesthesia is typically administered while the patient is seated, the technique described is nearly identical to that of spinal anesthesia (Figure 6.2).

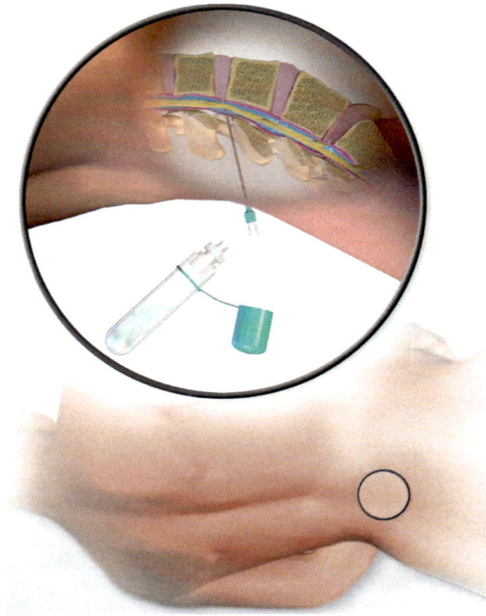

Figure 6.2. *Illustration depicting lumbar puncture (spinal tap).*

Source: By BruceBlaus, Own work, CC BY 3.0, https://commons.wikimedia.org/w/index.php?curid=27796935.

The benefit of sitting up straight is that the spinal anatomy is less distorted, making fluid withdrawal simpler. When performing a lumbar puncture on an obese patient, some medical professionals prefer not to lie on their side because this can result in scoliosis and inaccurate anatomical landmarks. On the other hand, opening pressure measurements made while seated are infamously inaccurate. Therefore, if healthcare professionals need to measure opening pressure, patients should ideally lie on their side.

The frequency of headaches following lumbar puncture may be reduced by re-introducing the stylet (Figure 6.3).

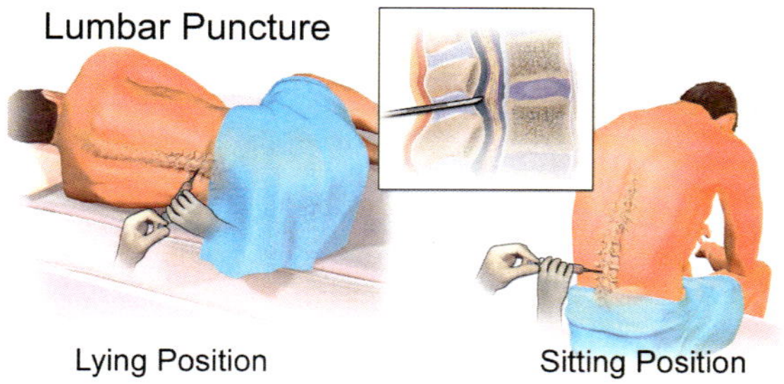

Figure 6.3. *Illustration depicting common positions for lumbar puncture procedure.*

Source: By BruceBlaus, Own work, CC BY 3.0, https://commons.wikimedia.org/w/index.php?curid=29987039.

Ultrasonography is useful for determining the depth of the spine from the skin and for visualizing the interspinous space, though it is not always available in clinical settings. By using ultrasound, fewer needle insertions and redirections are made, and the success rate of lumbar punctures is increased. In cases where the procedure presents difficulties, such as in individuals with scoliosis or other spinal deformities, fluoroscopy (constant X-ray imaging) can also be used.

- **Children:** Sitting flexed was just as effective as lying on the side in obtaining non-traumatic CSF, CSF for culture, and cell count in children. When infants under 12 months old were positioned with their heads bent forward, they had a greater success rate when trying to obtain CSF for the first time.

  An infant's spine is not the same as an adult's spine at birth. In adults, the conus medullaris, or bottom of the spinal cord, ends at level L1, but in term neonates, or newborn babies, it can vary from L1 to L3. It is crucial to place the spinal needle at the L3/L4 or L4/L5 interspinous levels, below the conus medullaris.

  By the time a child is two years old, the conus usually reaches the adult level (L1) due to spinal growth.

Compared to adults, the ligamentum flavum and dura mater are thinner in newborns and young children. Because of this, it can be challenging to determine when the needle enters the subarachnoid space during a pediatric lumbar puncture because the typical pop or give may be weak or nonexistent. Some clinicians employ the Cincinnati technique to reduce the possibility of inserting the spinal needle too far. With this technique, the spinal needle's stylet is removed after the needle has penetrated the dermis. The stylet is removed, and then the needle is inserted until CSF begins to emerge from it. The stylet is then put back in before the needle is taken out after all of the CSF has been collected.

- **Newborn Infants:** When very young babies have lumbar punctures, they are frequently used to diagnose or confirm an infection. If proper pain management (analgesia) is not applied, these procedures can be very painful. For babies having this surgery, pain management is crucial. Topical painkillers (anesthetics like lidocaine) are one method of managing pain. It's unclear which method of pain management works best for newborns who need lumbar punctures.

6.2.6. Interpretation

Counting the number of cells in the cerebrospinal fluid and figuring out its glucose and protein concentrations are standard procedures for analyzing it. The diagnostic suspicion guides the other analytical investigations of cerebrospinal fluid.

- **Pressure Determination:**

Congestive heart failure, cerebral edema, subarachnoid hemorrhage, hypo-osmolality from hemodialysis, meningeal inflammation, purulent meningitis or tuberculous meningitis, hydrocephalus, or pseudotumor cerebri can all be indicated by elevated CSF pressure. A lumbar puncture may be beneficial in the case of raised pressure hydrocephalus, also known as normal pressure hydrocephalus, in which the CSF level is high but the pressure is normal. Reduced CSF pressure may be a sign of circulatory collapse, severe dehydration, hyperosmolality, spinal fluid leakage, or total subarachnoid blockage. Significant pressure changes during the procedure may be a sign of hydrocephalus, tumors, or spinal blockage that results in a large pool of CSF.

- **Cell Count:** Pleocytosis is the term used to describe the presence of white blood cells in cerebrospinal fluid. Granulocytes are always an abnormal finding; monocytes in small numbers can be normal. A high granulocyte count frequently signals the presence of bacterial meningitis. White cells can also be an indication of leukemia, a recent epileptic seizure, a metastatic tumor, central nervous system hemorrhage, reactions to previous injections of medications or dyes, or repeated lumbar punctures. White blood cells and erythrocytes will be present in the withdrawn CSF if peripheral blood contaminates it, which is a common procedural complication. The ratio of white blood cells to erythrocytes will also be the same.

The presence of phagocytosed erythrocytes, or erythrophagocytosis, indicates hemorrhage into the CSF before lumbar puncture. Erythrophagocytosis, therefore, indicates causes other than a traumatic tap when erythrocytes are found in the CSF sample, such as intracranial hemorrhage and hemorrhagic herpetic encephalitis. If so, additional research, including imaging and viral culture, is necessary.

- **Microbiology:** To diagnose infections, CSF can be sent to the microbiology lab for a variety of smears and cultures.
  - Gram staining can reveal gram-positive bacteria in cases of meningitis caused by bacteria.
  - The gold standard for identifying bacterial meningitis is microbiological culture. Different methods can be used to cultivate viruses, fungi, and bacteria.
  - In the diagnosis of certain types of meningitis, such as enterovirus and herpesvirus meningitis, polymerase chain reaction (PCR) has greatly advanced diagnostic techniques. It is quick, requires little amounts of CSF, and has excellent sensitivity and specificity for a wide range of CNS infections. Despite the high cost of testing, cost analyses of PCR testing in newborn patients showed savings through lower hospitalization costs.
  - Measured IgG and total protein levels are used to calculate the IgG synthetic rate, which is higher in immune disorders

like multiple sclerosis, transverse myelitis, and Devic's neuromyelitis Optica. The presence of oligoclonal bands in CSF but not serum suggests intrathecal antibody production. (Table 6.2)

Table 6.2. Diagnostic Measurement

Infection	**Appearance**	**WBCs / mm^3**	**Protein (g/L)**	**Glucose**
Normal	Clear	<5	0.15 to 0.45	> 2/3 of blood glucose
Bacterial	Yellowish, turbid	> 1,000 (mostly PMNs)	> 1	Low
Viral	Clear	< 200 (mostly lymphocytes)	Mild increase	Normal or mildly low
Tuberculosis	Yellowish and viscous	Modest increase	Markedly Increased	Decreased
Fungal	Yellowish and viscous	< 50 (mostly lymphocytes)	Initially normal, then increased	Normal or mildly low

Source: https://en.wikipedia.org/wiki/Lumbar_puncture#Technique.

6.3. Processing and Testing of CSF

One of the most important tools available to medical professionals for the diagnosis of disorders affecting the brain and spinal cord is cerebrospinal fluid (CSF) samples. These regions are surrounded by a clear fluid that serves as a cushion for the central nervous system, protecting it from harm while also supplying the brain with nourishment and eliminating waste from the intricate organ. CSF samples provide insight into the levels and concentrations of various cells, substances, and contaminants in the fluid when things aren't working as they should. A variety of disorders affecting the central nervous system, such as meningitis, encephalitis, tuberculosis, and fungal infections, are diagnosed using the results. CSF analysis is also used to identify immune response abnormalities, brain and spinal tumors, and hemorrhages. When gathering and processing CSF samples, it's imperative to follow best-practice guidelines because there is so much potential for benefit.

6.3.1. CSF Specimen Collection Process

A doctor will typically perform a lumbar puncture in the L3–L4 region to obtain a CSF sample. To lower the chance of infection, sterile technique is always employed. To prevent damage to neural tissue, caution must be used. An adult's spinal fluid can be removed with a syringe in 6 to 15 milliliters. Nevertheless, no more than 2 mL of CSF would be removed if the opening pressure was first measured and found to be elevated by more than 200 mm. Small children and babies lose less fluid. Three to four tubes, each holding two to four milliliters of the CSF sample, are used. Because of the possibility of cell adhesion affecting the cell count or differential, glass tubes should not be used. The order in which the CSF is obtained determines the tube numbers.

6.3.2. Procedure for CSF Collection

- **Item 1: Minimum Withdrawal Volume of 12 Milliliters:** The amount of CSF used can affect the biomarker concentration.
- **Item 2: Vertebral Body Puncture Site: L3–L5:** Usually, a lumbar puncture is used to obtain diagnostic CSF. The site of CSF withdrawal needs to be noted due to the increasing gradient in protein concentration from ventricular to lumbar CSF.
- **Item 3: Removal of Bloody CSF Samples**: In between 14% to 20% of routine lumbar punctures, there is a traumatic tap that results in blood contamination of the CSF. False-positive results can arise from blood contamination for biomarkers with high serum concentrations, like coagulation factors. Furthermore, suppressed matrix-assisted laser desorption/ionization time-of-flight (MALDI-TOF)/MS proteomics patterns in CSF are caused by blood proteins. Nevertheless, once the blood cells are removed by centrifugation prior to initial freezing, this suppression by blood proteins is significantly diminished. To choose CSF samples suitable for these measurements, the erythrocyte count must be recorded. For biomarker studies, CSF samples with an erythrocyte count greater than 500/µL ought not to be utilized.
- **Item 4: Using an Atraumatic Needle (Such as a Whitacre or Sprotte Needle):** There's no proof that the kind of lumbar puncture needle used affects the levels of biomarkers. The risk of post-lumbar puncture headache is lower with atraumatic needles, which patients can tolerate the best. Approximately 12% of patients will experience this type of headache with a needle size of 20–22 gauge, compared to about 70% with a needle size of 16–19 gauge.
- **Item 5: Polypropylene Collection Tubes are Used:** Numerous reports demonstrate that the type of collection tube affects the results of biomarkers, e.g., amyloid-β peptides and total tau proteins. Standardization is crucial as a result. We suggest collecting CSF in polypropylene tubes because of their low potential for protein binding. Use of additives is not advised. Glass tubes should not be used by staff members for safety reasons.
- **Item 6: Time of Day of Withdrawal:** It matters what time of withdrawal biomarkers are affected by circadian rhythms. Since standardizing withdrawal times in routine clinical practice is frequently challenging, documentation is required to choose the right samples and reduce the impact of this variable.
- **Items 7 and 8: DNA, Serum, and Plasma Connected to the CSF Sample:** To evaluate CSF biomarkers, matched serum and/or plasma samples must be obtained because the marker's concentration in blood frequently affects its concentration in CSF. Additionally, serum/plasma pairs are necessary to investigate a biomarker's intrathecal

origin and CNS specificity. Moreover, CNS markers in serum or plasma may help with disease monitoring. Ethylenediaminetetraacetic acid (in dried format) vacuum tubes are preferred over those using citrate (in solution) tubes because the incomplete filling of tubes with a standard volume of citrate dilutes the final biomarker concentration artificially. We advise collecting both serum and plasma, depending on the type of biomarkers and research methods; for some methods, plasma is better than serum, and vice versa. Samples of serum or plasma shouldn't be hemolytic. Finally, obtaining DNA increases the opportunities for researching individual phenotypes and genotypes.

- **Item 9: Holding it at Room Temperature Until it Spins and Separates into Individual Portions: There** is currently insufficient data to support the recommendation to process CSF samples at 4°C or room temperature. This is especially important for serum/plasma.
- **Item 10: Uniform Spinning Parameters:** When fragile cells need to be preserved for RNA isolation, we advise using a standard spinning protocol of 400 g for 10 minutes at room temperature; alternatively, spinning at 2,000 g is recommended. It is suggested to spin the serum for ten minutes at room temperature at 2,000 g. Standardizing the temperature and speed of spinning may have an impact on specific biomarkers, although research on these preanalytical factors for CSF is lacking. The processing temperature of plasma and serum is crucial for certain biomarkers. The supernatant must be separated into aliquots and promptly stored after centrifugation. It is important to document the processing time if this is not done.

6.3.3. Cerebrospinal Fluid (CSF) Testing

The results of CSF testing may more clearly indicate the underlying cause of disorders affecting the central nervous system, even though obtaining a sample of CSF may be more challenging than, say, obtaining a sample of blood or urine.

Testing on cerebrospinal fluid (CSF) can assist in the diagnosis of a broad range of illnesses and disorders affecting the brain and spinal cord (central nervous system). Here are a few instances:

- Testing is used to identify the cause of infections, such as meningitis and encephalitis, and to differentiate them from other medical conditions. Infections can be caused by bacteria, viruses, fungi, or, less frequently, Mycobacterium tuberculosis. Moreover, CSF testing can be used to find infections in or close to the spinal cord.
- Hemorrhaging, or bleeding, in and around the brain.
- Immune conditions that impact the central nervous system, like multiple sclerosis and Guillain-Barré syndrome.
- Primary tumors inside the central nervous system or metastatic cancers, or cancers that spread to the central nervous system.

- Alzheimer disease is a type of dementia that cannot be reversed.

When a CSF analysis is requested, a basic initial set of tests is typically conducted as part of CSF testing.

- CSF color, clarity and pressure during CSF collection
- CSF protein
- CSF glucose
- CSF cell count (total number of cells present)
- CSF differential cell count (the quantity of various cell types present).
- CSF Gram stain, routine culture, and molecular tests that identify the genetic makeup of any present microbes should be performed if an infection is suspected.

Depending on the findings of the initial set of tests or the suspected diagnosis, a wide range of additional tests may be ordered as follow-up. The precise tests that are prescribed are determined by your symptoms and the ailment that your doctor believes could be the Source: Based on the kind of exam that is administered, each of these assessments can be categorized.

6.4. Physical Characteristics of Normal CSF

Examining the fluid surrounding the brain and spinal cord is done through the collection of CSF. CSF serves as a cushion to prevent damage to the spine and brain. Normally, the liquid is clear. Its consistency is the same as that of water. The test is also used to gauge spinal fluid pressure.

6.4.1. Normal Volume and Circulation of the CSF

An average-sized person generates 20–24 ml of CSF per hour, with 125–150 ml of it in their body. This transparent acellular fluid is secreted by the choroid plexus through a combination of active transport and ultrafiltration. Since the concentration of electrolytes in the CSF is tightly regulated and would not happen if the choroid plexus carelessly forced plasma through a filter, ultrafiltration most likely has little effect. The active transport of sodium and chloride, along with water movement through aquaporins and leaky cellular junctions, are essential for the active transport component of CSF production.

The production of CSF is estimated to occur at a rate of 0.4 milliliters per minute. Therefore, if all of the generated CSF issues forth through the EVD instead of circulating around normally, one can anticipate that their EVD output will be 24 ml/hr. This means that a person should produce roughly 576 milliliters of CSF per day, which sounds like a lot.

6.4.2. Biochemical Properties of the CSF

This material is essentially plasma. There is, however, one noteworthy distinction: protein is almost completely absent. This affects the ion concentration in the CSF. After all, in the lack of anionic protein, who will supply all that additional negative charge?

Definitely not the bicarbonate. Because CO_2 diffuses freely into and out of the CSF space and is converted into HCO_{3-}, the pH of the CSF and plasma are very similar. However, since the CSF lacks all those beneficial buffering proteins, there may be a slight difference in the pH of the HCO_{3-} in the CSF compared to the plasma. However, this is off-topic. Dog studies conducted in the early 1960s contrasted plasma electrolytes with CSF electrolytes. The majority of the cation concentrations were essentially the same within the typical measurement error ranges, with the possible exception of slightly less potassium in the CSF. Obviously not the case for the anions. The concentration of chloride in the CSF is roughly 15-20 mmol higher than that of the plasma when albumin is not present to donate anionic charge. According to the dog research, it is roughly 132 mmol/L (Hajdu and Steven, 2003; Brown, 2004; Algotsson and Winblad, 2007; Dr Cal Shipley; Adigun and Al-Dhahir).

6.4.3. Protein Content of the CSF

Protein is almost entirely excluded by the blood-CSF barrier. In fact, the CSF contains 100–200 times less protein than the total serum protein, which means that while the total serum protein may be 80 g/L, the CSF protein will only be 0.4 g/L. An excessive amount of protein in the CSF may be found in certain circumstances, and this is usually an indication of bad things happening.

1. **Elevated CSF Protein in Intracranial Bleeding:** It is conceivable that extra protein in the CSF originated from the plasma due to an unsatisfactory interaction between the CSF and blood. This could be the consequence of a painful tap or a legitimate intracranial hemorrhage. Generally speaking, there should be a negligible additional 0.01g/L of protein for every 1000 RBCs per microlitre.
2. **Elevated CSF Protein in Infectious and Non-infectious Conditions:** Relative to common perception, a slightly elevated CSF protein does not necessarily indicate an infection. There are several possible causes for an increased protein level.

i. Increased CSF Protein due to Exudation of Protein

a. Protein exudes from inflamed meninges in cases of meningitis caused by bacteria or viruses.

b. Viral or bacterial encephalitis

c. Malignancy, damaged blood-brain barriers, and protein seeping into the CSF through immature capillaries.

d. Mycobacterial infection, CNS tuberculosis

ii. **Increased CSF Protein due to Increased Local Synthesis:** IgG is the particular protein that we are discussing here. This is the CSF's main immunoglobulin.

It can be raised under a wide range of circumstances:

a. Multiple sclerosis

b. Neurosyphilis

c. Sarcoidosis

d. Meningitis or encephalitis caused by bacteria or viruses.

iii. **Increased CSF Protein due to Decreased Protein Resorption:** This is usually the case when someone has hydrocephalus, especially if they have communicating hydrocephalus, which arises from a significant subarachnoid hemorrhage. On the other hand, there is a persistently low level of CSF protein in the setting of a chronic CSF leak.

6.4.4. Glucose Content of the CSF

By facilitating transport, glucose enters the CSF and is subsequently drawn out once more by the cistern walls. The cells devour it completely. As a result, the CSF's glucose content is consistently slightly lower than the serum's; the ratio is roughly 0 to 6. As a result, a patient's CSF glucose level should be 6 mmol/L if their BSL is 10 mmol/L.

Many cells, organisms, and chemical reactions metabolize glucose, so there are many possible explanations for the CSF's abnormally low glucose levels.

Causes of low CSF glucose:

- Bacterial meningitis
- viral meningitis, to a far lesser extent
- Intracranial malignancy
- CNS sarcoidosis
- Subarachnoid hemorrhage—in which glucose is also consumed by the RBCs.

Bacterial meningitis would have the lowest glucose concentrations of all of these. Since all those organisms are constantly consuming glucose, the CSF value is usually less than 1.0 mmol/L. In cases of viral meningitis or encephalitis, CSF glucose is typically normal. Typically. There are, of course, always exceptions. A diagnosis would not be made solely based on the CSF protein.

6.4.5. Cellular Content of the CSF

Even though this fluid is described as acellular, some rogue cells may still be present in normal CSF. It is considered normal to have 4-5 RBCs per milliliter; exceeding 3 WCCs is usually considered abnormal. According to conventional wisdom, a neutrophil-dominant WCC of 500 is suggestive of meningitis caused by bacteria, while a monocyte-dominant WCC of 100 is more suggestive of meningitis caused by viruses. There aren't really any set rules, though. If CSF is drawn too soon during bacterial meningitis, the WCC count may be quite normal because the CSF hasn't had time to transform into frank pus.

Causes of raised CSF granulocytes:

- Meningitis caused by bacteria, encephalitis, or burst brain abscess.
- Early phases of meningitis in any form.
- hemorrhagic stroke (as it goes away bit by bit).
- Recently injected intrathecal drugs

Increased CSF monocytes and lymphocytes can be caused by:

- Mycobacterial, fungal or viral meningitis
- Guillain-Barre syndrome
- CNS vasculitis

6.4.6. Other Tests Performed on the CSF

Though none of these are particularly common, it's still important to be aware of them.

- **CSF Lactate:** Any number of conditions, including bacterial meningitis, acute brain injury, and stroke, can cause an increase in CSF lactate. It's not really a particular indicator of anything.
- **CSF LDH:** In the CSF, lactate dehydrogenase increases in reaction to non-specific cell damage. LDH levels in CSF are typically ten times lower than those in serum. Serum LDH levels are reported to be significantly elevated in cases of bacterial meningitis, but only slightly elevated or normal in cases of viral meningitis.
- **CSF CK:** The breakdown of neurons in the brain produces creatine kinase, and there is a correlation between the amount of this enzyme and the degree of brain damage. Naturally, the CSF CK level rises with increased brain tissue compression and subsequent CK leakage.

- **CSF β_2 Transferrin:** Rarely are there any proteins that are unique to the CSF and not present in the plasma. Of these, β_2 transferrin is one. It is the result of regular transferrin that penetrates the CSF and is subsequently processed by CNS neuraminidase.

6.4.7. Changes in CSF in Common Clinical Situations

- **Post Neurosurgical Patients, with EVD in Situ:** These patients suffer from the unusual condition of having a thin silicone rubber tube in their brains in addition to having had their heads cut open. This is acceptable for about three days, after which the risk of infection starts to skyrocket. Unfortunately, it is challenging to diagnose such an infection because the actual presence of such a brain tube tends to irritate the delicate brain parenchyma, causing an increase in CSF WCC and protein. Fever is typically the deciding factor, though the CSF culture is always a possibility.
- **Subarachnoid Hemorrhage:** The SAH patient will exhibit boring old xanthochromia, red blood cells (RBCs), and a drop in CSF glucose due to RBC metabolism.
- **Guillain-Barre Syndrome:** These individuals experience some CSF lymphocytosis later in the game, but the protein is really what matters. An increase in CSF protein is one of the disease's pathognomonic features. Strangely, although not nearly to the same extent as GBS, critical illness polyneuropathy also tends to have an elevated CSF protein.
- **Status Epilepticus:** Somehow, a leaky blood-brain barrier is the outcome of epilepsy. Thus, plasma protein (though not usually cells; occasionally, the CSF WCC is slightly elevated) is enriched in the CSF. It is therefore reasonable to anticipate a small increase in CSF protein following extended seizures.

6.5. Clinical Significance

6.5.1. Pressure

By performing a lumbar puncture, the patient's CSF pressure can be determined by measuring 10–18 cmH_2O (8–15 mmHg or 1.1-2 kPa) when they are lying on their side and 20–30 cmH_2O (16–24 mmHg or 2.1-3 kPa) when they are sitting up. The CSF pressure in newborns is between 8 and 10 cmH_2O, or 0–78–0–98 kPa (4–7–3 mmHg). The majority of variations are brought on by internal compression of the jugular veins in the neck or coughing. When in a supine position, the intracranial pressure and CSF pressure as determined by lumbar puncture are comparable.

An abnormal buildup of CSF in the brain's ventricles is known as hydrocephalus. A blockage of the CSF's passage, such as one brought on by an infection, wound, tumor, or congenital anomaly, can result in hydrocephalus. It is also possible to develop hydrocephalus without obstruction linked to normal CSF pressure. The symptoms may include nausea and vomiting, urinary incontinence, problems with coordination and gait, and gradually worsening cognitive decline. Because the bones in an infant's skull have not yet fused, hydrocephalus can result in an enlarged head, seizures, irritability, and sleepiness. Lumbar puncture can be used to demonstrate and, in certain cases, relieve high intracranial pressure. A CT or MRI scan can show enlargement of one or both lateral ventricles, as well as the mass or lesion causing the increased pressure. A shunt, such as a ventriculo-peritoneal shunt, is typically inserted to treat hydrocephalus by redirecting fluid to a different area of the body.

CSF pressure rises in idiopathic intracranial hypertension, a disorder for which there is no known cause. It is linked to headaches, enlarged optic discs, double vision, and visual problems. It can happen for any reason at all, especially in younger obese women, or it can be related to the use of vitamin A and tetracycline antibiotics. A carbonic anhydrase inhibitor like acetazolamide, repeated lumbar punctures for drainage, or the implantation of a ventriculo-peritoneal shunt are some possible management options.

6.5.2. CSF Leak

CSF may escape from the dura due to various factors, such as physical injury or a lumbar puncture, or for unknown reasons known as a spontaneous cerebrospinal fluid leak. This type of leak is typically linked to intracranial hypotension, resulting in low CSF pressure. Symptoms can include worsening headaches when standing, moving, or coughing, as the brain sags downward due to the low pressure, putting pressure on lower structures. A beta-2 transferrin test can confirm a leak, while imaging tests like CT scans and MRI scans can be used to find a leak that isn't immediately visible. Treatment options may include an epidural blood patch injection, spinal surgery, or fibrin glue, with caffeine often providing relief for symptoms.

6.5.3. Lumbar Puncture

Following a lumbar puncture, headaches affect about one-third of patients, and pain or discomfort at the needle entry site is typical. Less common side effects could be bruises, meningitis, or persistent CSF leakage following a lumbar puncture.

A typical test would look at the fluid's color, gauge the CSF pressure, count and identify the white and red blood cells in it, measure the fluid's protein and glucose levels, and culture it. Elevated white blood cell counts may be a sign of central nervous system infections like meningitis, while the presence of red blood cells and xanthochromia may indicate subarachnoid hemorrhage. The microorganism causing the infection may be obtained through a CSF culture, or PCR may be employed to determine if a virus is to blame. Research on the overall makeup and characteristics of proteins points to certain illnesses, such as paraneoplastic syndromes, systemic lupus erythematosus, cerebral angiitis, multiple sclerosis, and neurosarcoidosis. Tests for particular antibodies, like aquaporin-4, can help identify autoimmune diseases. Certain conditions such as normal pressure hydrocephalus and idiopathic intracranial hypertension may also be treated with a lumbar puncture that drains CSF.

Measurements of intracranial pressure, which may be elevated in specific cases of hydrocephalus, can also be made by lumbar puncture. However, because it can result in a deadly brain herniation, a lumbar puncture should never be carried out if elevated intracranial pressure is suspected as a result of specific circumstances, such as a tumor.

6.5.4. Anesthesia and Chemotherapy

Substances that cannot cross the blood–brain barrier can nevertheless be active throughout the central nervous system because some anesthetics and chemotherapy are injected intrathecally into the subarachnoid space, where they spread around CSF. In regional anesthesia, baricity—a term that describes a substance's density in relation to that of human cerebrospinal fluid—is used to predict how a given drug will distribute within the intrathecal space. Filtering the CSF to remove endogenous or exogenous pathogens is known as liquorpheresis.

6.6. Protein Electrophoretic Patterns of CSF

Proteins are essential components of cells and tissues, serving as the foundation for organs and making up enzymes and hormones that control bodily functions. Protein electrophoresis is a laboratory technique that segregates proteins by size and charge. Analyzing the presence, absence, levels, or changes in proteins in bodily fluids like blood can aid in the diagnosis and management of different illnesses and conditions.

Blood, urine, and cerebrospinal fluid (CSF) are examples of bodily fluids that contain a wide variety of proteins with a variety of functions, including removing toxins, carrying nutrients, and regulating bodily processes.

The two major types of proteins are:

- About 60% of the protein in the blood is made up of albumin, which is produced in the liver.
- Proteins other than albumin are collectively referred to as globulins. The majority of globulins, with the exception of some complement proteins and antibodies (immunoglobulins), are also made in the liver.

A regulated electric current is applied to the different proteins present in bodily fluids, causing them to separate into a characteristic band or peak pattern that can be measured. The proteins are categorized into six groups: albumin, alpha 1, alpha 2, beta, gamma, and prealbumin (rarely detected on serum or urine protein electrophoresis). There are two subgroups within the beta fraction: beta 1 and beta 2.

These protein groups, also known as electrophoresis fractions, are unique and exist in particular concentrations. The diagnostic process can be aided by the patterns frequently observed in specific illnesses and ailments. The table titled Protein Groups lists the major serum proteins and their functions based on their electrophoretic region or fraction (the visible band that they are part of). Protein production and/or loss can be impacted by a number of illnesses and ailments, which can alter the pattern of bands observed on a protein electrophoresis. The emergence of a distinct, monoclonal band in the gamma region is the most significant example. For example, excessive production of a single type of immunoglobulin (monoclonal immunoglobulin) results from the unchecked growth and division of a malignant plasma cell, as observed in multiple myeloma.

When an abnormal protein is discovered during testing, further evaluations are conducted to determine the specific type of protein through a process known as immunotyping. Methods such as immunofixation electrophoresis or immunosubtraction electrophoresis can be used to identify abnormal bands in the gamma region of protein electrophoresis, helping to establish whether there is an overproduction of a specific antibody type (such as IgG, IgA, or IgM). In cases of multiple myeloma, an excess of a single intact immunoglobulin is commonly present, although in some instances there may be an abundance of a section of an immunoglobulin known as a "free light chain." These excess free light chains are released into the bloodstream, filtered by the kidneys, and excreted in the urine, where they are sometimes referred to as Bence Jones proteins.

In blood, urine, or other bodily fluids, protein electrophoresis is used to measure and identify the presence of abnormal proteins, the absence of normal proteins, and/or to find different patterns in the electrophoresis of proteins linked to specific conditions. Although the results of protein electrophoresis typically do not offer a conclusive diagnosis, the data can indicate that a disease or condition is affecting the production or loss of protein. Rather, more tests must be performed to look into the reason and attempt to determine the type of underlying illness.

Serum electrophoresis may be used to:

- Assist in the diagnosis and treatment of monoclonal gammopathies, including multiple myeloma, chronic lymphocytic leukemia, and lymphomas.
- Examine anomalous results from additional lab tests, including those measuring total protein, albumin, calcium, or red or white blood cell counts.
- Examine a person for liver or kidney disease, infection, autoimmune disease, or inflammation.

Urine protein electrophoresis may be used:

- In the multiple myeloma investigation.
- To look into the causes of abnormally high urine protein levels (proteinuria, various forms and causes).

Immunofixation electrophoresis (IFE) or immunosubtraction electrophoresis can be used as follow-up tests to further identify abnormal proteins when an abnormal band on either a serum or a urine electrophoresis pattern suggests the presence of a single type of immunoglobulin (monoclonal).

CSF protein electrophoresis may be used:

- To search for oligoclonal bands, the distinctive banding pattern that multiple sclerosis patients may exhibit.
- To assess a patient exhibiting headaches or other neurologic symptoms and search for proteins that could indicate an infection or inflammation and thus account for the symptoms.

One test that's frequently ordered when you have symptoms that point to a certain condition is protein electrophoresis. Here are a few instances. If you experience any of the following multiple myeloma signs and symptoms, serum and urine protein electrophoresis may be ordered.

- Weakened bones that may cause bone pain, soft spots, fractures, and lesions.
- Carpal tunnel syndrome
- Destruction of bone, which frequently raises blood calcium levels and causes symptoms like fatigue, constipation, nausea, hunger loss, and confusion.
- Anemia
- Frequent infections
- Excessive bleeding and bruising
- Kidney disease: elevated protein levels in the urine brought on by specific types of multiple myeloma (i.e., kidneys and may cause long-term harm (e.g., Bence Jones proteins).
- Hyperviscosity syndrome, a condition where the blood's thickness increases, can occasionally cause headaches, vision issues, seizures, or even coma.

If your urine protein levels are unusually high, you might need to have urine protein electrophoresis. When an aberrant band on a serum or urine electrophoresis is found, suggesting the presence of a monoclonal immunoglobulin, immunofixation or immunosubtraction electrophoresis may be ordered.

CSF protein electrophoresis may be ordered:

- When you exhibit indications and symptoms that point to multiple sclerosis, such as:
  - sensory symptoms include burning, itching, numbness, tingling, pain, facial pain, and blurred vision.
  - Speech difficulties, weakness, tremor, trouble walking, lack of coordination, constipation, and issues controlling urination are examples of motor symptoms.
  - psychological symptoms include mood swings, depression, and cognitive, memory, and learning difficulties.
  - Fatigue
- When experiencing headaches or other neurological symptoms, it is advisable to check for proteins that may indicate infection or inflammation.

Following a diagnosis, electrophoresis may be requested on a regular basis to track the progress or recurrence of a disease as well as the efficacy of treatment.

6.6.1. Serum Protein Electrophoresis

The illnesses or ailments that can be linked to variations in different serum protein levels are listed in the Table 6.3.

Table 6.3. Changes in Serum Proteins for Antibody Deficiency

Age Group	**AUC**	**95% CI**	**p value**	**Gamma Cutoff value (g/L)**[a]	**Sensitivity**	**Specificity**	**Number of patients with IgG**	
							Below reference values	**Normal**
1 to 5 mos (n = 21)	–	–	–	–	–	–	0	21
6 to 11 mos (n = 53)	–	–	–	–	–	–	0	53
1 yo to <4 yo (n = 370)	1	1 - 1	<0,001	3,55	1	0,997	6	364
4 yoto <10 yo (n = 441)	0,997	0,99 - 1	<0,001	5,65	1	0,979	12	429

10 yo to <18 yo (n = 329)	0,995	0,99 - 1	<0,001	6,2	1	0,981	11	318
All (n = 1214)	0,963	0,95 - 0,98	<0,001	6,15	1	0,878	29	1185

Source: Piza CFSdT, Aranda CS, Solé D, Jolles S and Condino-Neto A (2021) Serum Protein Electrophoresis May Be Used as a Screening Tool for Antibody Deficiency in Children and Adolescents. Front. Immunol. 12:712637. doi: 10.3389/fimmu.2021.712637.

6.6.2. CSF Protein Electrophoresis

- Multiple sclerosis (MS) is suggested by the presence of multiple distinct bands in the gamma region (oligoclonal bands) that are present in CSF but absent in serum. The majority of patients with multiple sclerosis and certain other inflammatory brain conditions have these kinds of bands. Because not all individuals whose CSF displays this pattern have MS, oligoclonal bands are not a specific finding for MS. Additional testing and assessments (e.g., CT scan, or MRI) are required to aid in the diagnosis.
- Increased levels of polyclonal immunoglobulins, which are produced by multiple plasma cells, indicate a possible central nervous system infection.

The type of immunoglobulin protein(s) present as monoclonal bands on a protein electrophoresis pattern can be determined using immunofixation electrophoresis or immunosubtraction capillary electrophoresis. Usually, the results of this testing identify the kind and quantity of monoclonal proteins (like IgG kappa).

6.7. Role of CSF Immunologic Tests in the Diagnosis of Diseases

In a number of acute neurological conditions, CSF analysis is especially helpful in making a quick diagnosis and starting treatment. Opening pressure measurement, biochemical analysis, cytology, biomarkers assay, and microbiological evaluation are typically included in CSF analysis. Lumbar puncture and drainage may also be therapeutic measures in certain clinical conditions.

6.7.1. Approach to CSF Analysis in Acute Brain Conditions

6.7.1.1. CSF in Subarachnoid Hemorrhage (SAH)

One acute neurological condition that requires a patient to be admitted to intensive care is subarachnoid hemorrhage (SAH). Intracerebral aneurysm rupture, arteriovenous malformations (AVM), vasculitis, traumatic brain injury, and idiopathic causes are among the possible causes of SAH. Most frequently, patients arrive with a severe headache that starts suddenly, gets worse within an hour, and is frequently described as the worst headache they have ever had. Patients may experience seizures, cranial nerve palsies, loss of consciousness (LOC), and different patterns of motor deficits in severe cases. It's critical to identify the condition right away because rebleeding in the event of an aneurysmal cause can have disastrous consequences. Given that headaches frequently indicate intracranial diseases, a high index of suspicion is required.

LP was the primary diagnostic method for SAH prior to the development of CT scanners. Currently, a simple CT scan is the first line of diagnosis. Occasionally, though, a CT scan may come back negative for SAH even in the face of clinical suspicion. CT is thought to be extremely sensitive for five days following the SAH. In these situations, lumbar puncture is a helpful diagnostic procedure that is typically carried out 12 hours after the onset of symptoms. If there is a high clinical suspicion of SAH but a negative CT scan, LP is recommended. LP is typically finished in a few hours. The diagnosis of SAH is confirmed by the presence of xanthochromia (Level 2 evidence recommendation B) or RBCs (More than 1000 cells/cu mm).

LP can complicate RBC leading to false positive results. To differentiate between traumatic tap and SAH, CSF is collected in three tubes and the red cells in the consecutive tubes are counted. A decrease in red cells typically indicates a traumatic tap. Another method involves centrifuging the CSF to look for xanthochromia in the supernatant fluid. Spectrophotometry is recommended for detecting xanthochromia, which can be seen as early as 12 hours due to RBC lysis and release of pigments like oxyhemoglobin, methemoglobin, and bilirubin. However, for diagnosing rebleeding of SAH, LP is not useful as pigments can be present for up to 3 weeks after the initial SAH.

6.7.2. CSF Analysis in Acute Demyelinating/Autoimmune Diseases

Acute neurological conditions are a possible presentation for patients with demyelinating diseases in the emergency department. CSF analysis can be highly helpful in the diagnosis of some conditions, as well as in tracking the course of the illness and the prognosis after treatment. Acute disseminated encephalomyelitis, multiple sclerosis, and neuromyelitis Optica (NMO) are among the demyelinating diseases. Apart from the conditions mentioned above, different autoimmune disorders such as Guillain-Barrie syndrome, Transverse myelitis, and so on can also result in different degrees of degeneration and demyelination. Because of the severe inflammatory destruction of CNS tissues or complications resulting from it, these conditions may cause acute emergencies.

Table 6.5. Patient Characteristics and Cerebrospinal Fluid Analysis from the Definite Diagnosis of Viral Meningitis and Clinical Diagnosis of Tuberculous Meningitis

	Clinical TBM (14)	**Definite TBM (12)**	**P-value**	**Definite VM (14)**	**P-value**
Patient characteristics					
Age	43.5 (35.5–54.0)	70.5 (57.75–77.0)	0.039	51.5 (40.25–60.75)	0.514
Sex (male), N (%)	12 (85.7)	3 (25.0)	0.004	6 (42.9)	0.046
CSF analysis					
ADA (IU/L)	13.65 (11.57–17.48)	20.20 (13.78–29.30)	0.024	14.00 (10.95–16.07)	0.713
RBC (/mm^3)	7 (2.5–14.25)	30 (11.25–94)	0.054	11 (2.25–69.5)	0.613

WBC (/mm³)	95 (76.25–126.25)	170.0 (72.5–360)	0.425	130.0 (52.25–340)	0.800
PMN (%)	0.5 (0–2.75)	58 (23.5–89.25)	0.001	1 (0–1)	0.751
Lymphocyte (%)	87 (76.50–89.75)	16 (3–51.5)	0.001	77 (70.75–81.5)	0.085
Eosinophil (%)	0 (0–0)	0 (0–0)	0.105	0 (0–0)	0.290
Other types (%)	11 (9.25–13)	9.5 (7.75–17.25)	0.718	22.5 (18–28.5)	<0.001
pH	7.20 (7.20–7.30)	7.20 (7.18–7.30)	0.441	7.25 (7.20–7.30)	0.528
Glucose (mg/dl)	59 (49.25–76)	34.5 (25.25–48)	0.008	59.5 (49–78.75)	0.890
Protein (mg/dl)	113.60 (72.12–131.35)	181.95 (83.58–292.93)	0.160	122.95 (89.45–157.43)	0.603
LDH (U/L) [a]	109.0 (65.0–141.5)	166.0 (108.0–524.5)	0.139	162.5 (116.2–220.0)	0.256

Source: Song J, Kim S-H, Jung Y-R, Choe J, Kang C-I and Min J-H (2022) 10-Year Retrospective Review of the Etiologies for Meningitis With Elevated Adenosine Deaminase in Cerebrospinal Fluid: Etiologies Other Than TB. Front. Cell. Infect. Microbiol. 12:858724. doi: 10.3389/fcimb.2022.858724.

Axonal injury, activation of microglia and astrocytes, and focal collections of lymphocytes and monocytes with variable degrees of demyelination are among the pathological findings in this group of diseases. Vasculitis of the blood vessel can also be observed in addition to complement factors deposition. Usually, a post-infectious, post-vaccination, or systemic inflammatory response precedes the pathology. This results in an inflammatory or autoimmune reaction to brain tissue. Since the majority of these illnesses respond well to therapy, patients benefit more from early diagnosis and treatment. CSF analysis provides important details about the disease's diagnosis, course, or recurrence, as well as the results of treatment (Table 6.5).

6.7.3. Brain and Spinal Cord Neoplasms

Brain neoplasms for which a CSF analysis is useful are typically caused by secondary leptomeningeal deposits or primary CNS lymphomas. Acute presentations of elevated intracranial pressure resulting from cerebral edema, herniations, or mass effect are possible. Making the diagnosis will be aided by radiological examinations. Distinguishing between secondary and primary tutors or infections such as abscesses can pose a challenge occasionally. A CSF study could be beneficial. Centrifuged CSF can be used to check for the presence or absence of cancerous cells and different tumor markers, such as colon, lung, prostate, etc., after the initial CT scan, MRI, or brain scan.

- **CSF Analysis in Spinal Cord Diseases**

Guillain Barre Syndrome (GBS)

- **Albumino-Cytologic Dissociation:** Albuminocytologic dissociation, or elevated CSF protein with normal cell count, is the classic immunologic alteration of CSF. Rarely, pleocytosis may also take place.
- **Neurofilament Light (NFL) Protein Assay:** The NFL level was a strong predictor of long-term disability and correlated with disability during the acute phase of GBS. NFL levels were correlated with albuminocytologic dissociation, a measure of the health of the blood-brain barrier in patients, and were age-dependent

in the control group regardless of gender.

- **Amyotrophic Lateral Sclerosis (ALS):** Since the majority of miR-218 levels are maintained within the surviving motor neurons, the depletion of microRNA (miR), specifically miR-218, in ALS spinal cord tissue is most likely caused by the loss of motor neurons. In both animal and human models of motor neuron loss and disease, miR-218 release is associated with motor neuron dysfunction and death.
- **Spinal Cord Ependymoma:** Tumor-derived cell free DNA (cfDNA) can be found when the tumor is not surrounded by parenchyma or separated by arachnoid membranes. Six out of seven tumor patients had CSF containing cfDNA derived from their tumors.
- **Infectious vs Non-infectious Spine Pathology:** Differentiating infections from non-infectious spinal cord issues is crucial, and CSF analysis can help in making these diagnoses. Various cytokines have been identified as potential aids in distinguishing CNS diseases, with each one playing a specific role in different disease processes. The analysis of certain cytokines, such as MDC/CCL22, GRO/CXCL10, IL-12p70, IP-10/CXCL10, and PDGF-AA, is essential in diagnosing spine pathologies.

In the diagnostic algorithm, determining the IP-10/CXCL10 CSF levels offers a crucial early branch point. The diagnosis of infectious versus non-infectious spinal cord pathology must be made, and CSF analysis will support this process. Increased levels of IP-10/CXCL10 quickly reveal a potential infection. An infectious case can be further subclassified by evaluating the MDC/CCL22 levels. Rather than a viral pathogen, high MDC/CCL22 levels point to a non-viral infectious agent. Within the algorithm's non-infectious arm I. e.g., low IP-10/CXCL10 levels), higher IL-8 and GRO/CXCL1 levels support a diffuse glioma. PDGF-AA can be used to further distinguish between CNS B-cell lymphoma and Autoimmune/Demyelination (DM).

- **CSF Analysis and Biomarkers in Spinal Cord Injury:** A number of biomarkers may be elevated following a spinal cord injury. Among them were cleaved Tau proteins, glial fibrillary proteins, neurofilaments (NF), neuron specific enolase (NSE), microRNA (mRNA), and interleukein (IL6). These stand for various damage components, including vascular injury, glial cells, neurons, axons, and the food-spinal cord barrier. examination of several biomarkers in the CSF of patients who have had spinal cord injuries. can aid in both prognosticating patients and determining the extent of injuries.

A very helpful investigation for patients presenting with acute neurological conditions is CSF analysis. While microbial organism identification is required for acute meningitis, it will also be helpful as a supporting investigation to establish diagnosis, prognosticate, and evaluate the impact of different therapies to treat the patient conditions. Over the years, CSF analysis has changed from basic analysis to the evaluation of different biomarkers to help the physician. Because these tests are expensive and not readily available, it is therefore crucial that the doctor knows when to order them (Venkatesh et al., 2000; Anckarsäter et al., 2005; Luque and Jaffe, 2007; Beer et al., 2008).

A Closer Look

Hydrocephalus

An abnormal rise in the amount of CSF inside the ventricular system is known as hydrocephalus. The increased pressure inside the skull as a result of this volume increase has the potential to permanently harm brain tissue. Hydrocephalus comes in two flavors: non-communicating (obstructive) and communicating (non-obstructive).

An imbalance in the production and absorption of CSF results in non-obstructive hydrocephalus, or communicating hydrocephalus. Either the absorption process fails, or there is a rise in CSF production. Choroid plexus tumors may be the cause of the increased CSF production, although this is an extremely uncommon occurrence. More often than not, communicating hydrocephalus is caused by insufficient CSF reabsorption into the dural venous sinuses due to compromised arachnoid villi function. This may be related to meningitis or subarachnoid hemorrhage, which results in subarachnoid space fibrosis and scarring.

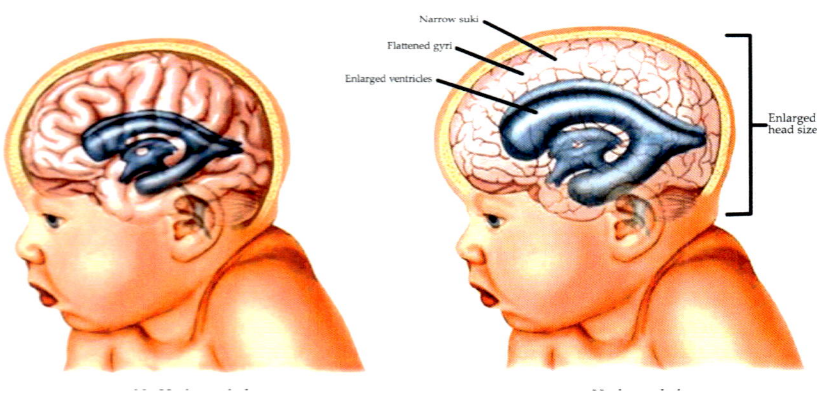

Source: By CDC - http://www.nj.gov/health/fhs/sch/documents/facts_ccns.pdf, Public Domain, https://commons.wikimedia.org/w/index.php?curid=42126065.

CSF outflow obstruction is the cause of non-communicating (obstructive) hydrocephalus. Numerous distinct pathophysiologies, including tumors, vascular malformations, and congenital malformations, can cause these obstructions. These are most likely to happen at constriction sites like the cerebral aqueduct, medial foramen of Magendie, interventricular foramen, or the lateral apertures of the fourth ventricle. The ventricular system dilates proximally to the obstruction as a result of the obstruction.

A ventriculoperitoneal shunt, which connects the ventricles to the abdominal cavity, is used to treat hydrocephalus. Since it's a surgical procedure, infection is a possibility. But it's the only option for long-term care.

Summary

- Cerebrospinal fluid (CSF) is a clear, colorless body fluid found within the tissue that surrounds the brain and spinal cord of all vertebrates. CSF is produced by specialized ependymal cells in the choroid plexus of the ventricles of the brain, and absorbed in the arachnoid granulations.
- In humans, there is about 125–150 mL of CSF at any one time. This CSF circulates within the ventricular system of the brain. The ventricles are a series of cavities filled with CSF. The majority of CSF is produced from within the two lateral ventricles.
- Lumbar puncture (LP), also known as a spinal tap, is a medical procedure in which a needle is inserted into the spinal canal, most commonly to collect cerebrospinal fluid (CSF) for diagnostic testing.
- The chief diagnostic indications of lumbar puncture are for collection of cerebrospinal fluid (CSF). Analysis of CSF may exclude infectious, inflammatory, and neoplastic diseases affecting the central nervous system.
- Analysis of the cerebrospinal fluid generally includes a cell count and determination of the glucose and protein concentrations.
- Cerebrospinal fluid (CSF) samples are one of the most valuable resources doctors can acquire when diagnosing conditions that affect the brain and spinal cord. The clear fluid surrounds these areas and acts as a cushion for the central nervous system, protecting against injury while simultaneously delivering nutrients to the brain and removing waste from the complex organ.
- Cerebrospinal fluid (CSF) is a clear, watery liquid that flows around the brain and spinal cord, surrounding and protecting them. CSF testing is performed to evaluate the level or concentration of different substances and cells in CSF to diagnose conditions affecting the brain and spinal cord (central nervous system).
- Cerebrospinal fluid (CSF) collection is a test to look at the fluid that surrounds the brain and spinal cord. CSF acts as a cushion, protecting the brain and spine from injury. The fluid is normally clear. It has the same consistency as water. The test is also used to measure pressure in the spinal fluid.
- Proteins are important building blocks of all cells and tissues. They form the structural part of most organs and make up enzymes and some hormones that regulate bodily functions. Protein electrophoresis is a lab method that separates proteins based on their size and electrical charge. Knowing which proteins are present, absent, elevated, or decreased in body fluids such as blood can help diagnose and/or monitor various diseases and conditions.
- CSF analysis is particularly useful in various acute neurological conditions and helps in rapid diagnosis of the conditions and initiate therapeutic measures. CSF analysis usually consists of opening pressure measurement, biochemical analysis, cytology, biomarkers assay, and microbiological evaluation.

References

1. Adigun OO, Al-Dhahir MA. Anatomy, Head and Neck: Cerebrospinal Fluid. [Updated 2023 Jul 17]. In: StatPearls [Internet]. Treasure Island (FL): StatPearls Publishing; 2024 Jan-. Available from: https://www.ncbi.nlm.nih.gov/books/NBK459286/
2. Algotsson, A., & Winblad, B. (2007). The integrity of the blood–brain barrier in Alzheimer's disease. *Acta. Neurologica. Scandinavica., 115*(6), 403–408. doi:10.1111/j.1600-0404.2007.00823.x.
3. Anckarsäter, H., Forsman, A., & Blennow, K. (2005). Increased CSF/serum albumin ratio: a recurrent finding in violent offenders. *Acta. Neurologica. Scandinavica., 112*(1), 48–50. doi:10.1111/j.1600-0404.2005.00433.x.
4. Beer, R., Lackner, P., & Pfausler, B. (2008). Nosocomial ventriculitis and meningitis in neurocritical care patients. *Journal of Neurology, 255*(11), 1617–1624.
5. Brown, P. D., et al. (2004). Molecular mechanisms of cerebrospinal fluid production. *Neuroscience, 129*(4), 955–968.
6. Hajdu, S. I. (2003). Discovery of the cerebrospinal fluid. *Annals of Clinical & Laboratory Science, 33*(3), 334–336.
7. Huff T, Tadi P, Weisbrod LJ, et al. Neuroanatomy, Cerebrospinal Fluid. [Updated 2023 Aug 28]. In: StatPearls [Internet]. Treasure Island (FL): StatPearls Publishing; 2024 Jan-. Available from: https://www.ncbi.nlm.nih.gov/books/NBK470578/
8. Luque, F. A., & Jaffe, S. L. (2007). Cerebrospinal fluid analysis in multiple sclerosis. *International Review of Neurobiology, 79*, 341–356. doi:10.1016/S0074-7742(07)79015-3.
9. Matsumae, M., Sato, O., Hirayama, A., Hayashi, N., Takizawa, K., Atsumi, H., & Sorimachi, T. (n.d.). Research into the physiology of cerebrospinal fluid reaches a new horizon: intimate exchange between cerebrospinal fluid and interstitial fluid may contribute to maintenance of homeostasis in the central nervous system, Neurol Med Chir (Tokyo). 2016 Jul 15;56(7):416-41.
10. Telano LN, Baker S. Physiology, Cerebral Spinal Fluid. [Updated 2023 Jul 4]. In: StatPearls [Internet]. Treasure Island (FL): StatPearls Publishing; 2024 Jan-. Available from: https://www.ncbi.nlm.nih.gov/books/NBK519007
11. Venkatesh, B., Scott, P., & Ziegenfuss, M. (2000). Cerebrospinal fluid in critical illness. *Critical Care and Resuscitation, 2*, 42–54.

Chapter

7

PLEURAL, PERICARDIAL, AND PERITONEAL FLUID ANALYSIS

Contents

Introduction

The purpose of these diagnostic procedures is to assess the properties and makeup of fluids located in the pericardial, pleural, and peritoneal cavities, respectively. The serous membranes that surround these body cavities secrete a tiny quantity of fluid to cushion and lubricate the organs within. Effusion, or the abnormal buildup of fluid in these cavities, can, however, be caused by a number of underlying medical conditions, including infections, inflammation, cancer, or malfunctioning organs. Examining fluid extracted from the pleural space between the layers of the pleura, the membrane encircling the lungs, is known as pleural fluid analysis. Common uses for this procedure include the diagnosis of heart failure, lung cancer, pneumonia, and tuberculosis. Comparably, pericardial fluid analysis comprises the analysis of fluid from the heart's outermost membrane, the pericardial sac. Analysis of pericardial effusion can help diagnose myocardial infarction, pericarditis, or autoimmune diseases of the heart. Pericardial effusion can be caused by infections, inflammation, trauma, or cancer. Analyzing peritoneal fluid entails assessing fluid that has accumulated in the area surrounding the abdominal organs, or the peritoneal cavity. Liver cirrhosis, pancreatitis, peritonitis, and internal or ovarian cancers are among the conditions that can cause peritoneal effusion. Usually, multiple components are included in the analysis of these fluids. Assessing the fluid's appearance, volume, and odor during a physical examination can provide preliminary hints about its nature. Microscopic examination entails observing the presence of bacteria or malignant cells in addition to cellular components like red blood cells, white blood cells, and mesothelial cells. Proteins, glucose, lactate dehydrogenase (LDH), and other biochemical markers are measured by biochemical analysis, which helps distinguish between different etiologies. Furthermore, microbiological cultures are carried out to detect any infectious agents in the fluid and to direct the proper course of antimicrobial therapy. Adenosine deaminase (ADA) levels in pleural fluid, for example, can help with the diagnosis of tuberculosis, and cytology can identify cancerous cells that may be a sign of cancerous processes. In addition to providing structural information and identifying underlying causes of effusion, such as tumors or organ abnormalities, imaging studies like computed tomography (CT) scans, ultrasounds, and chest X-rays can also be used in conjunction with fluid analysis.

Orientation and Directional Terms

Term	Definition	Illustration
Lactate dehydrogenase (LDH)	Lactate dehydrogenase (LDH) is an enzyme that's in almost all body tissues. It helps the body turns glucose (sugar) from food into usable energy for our cells.	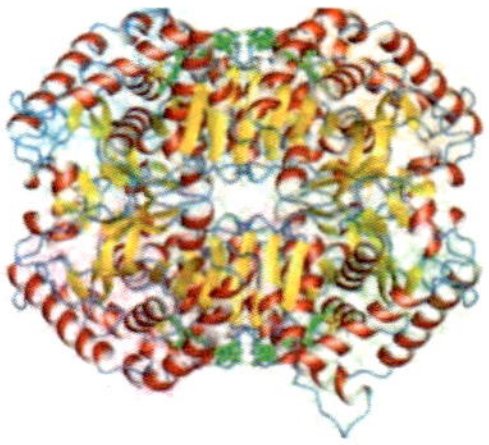
Biochemical Markers	Biochemical markers are molecules produced during the disease process, either at the initiation of the disease or during progression.	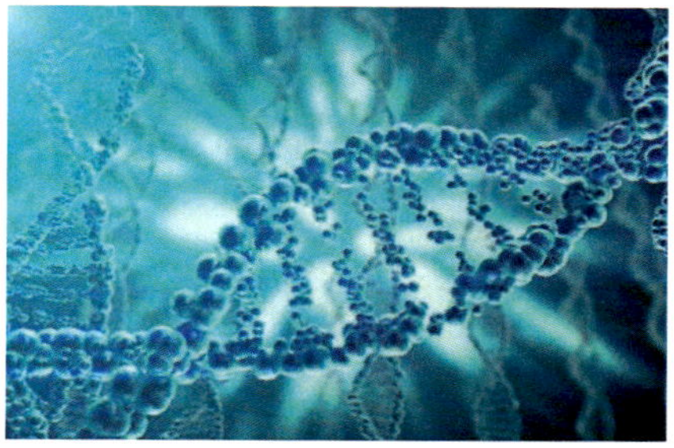
Adenosine deaminase (ADA)	An enzyme of the purine metabolism that catalyzes the irreversible deamination of adenosine and deoxyadenosine to inosine and deoxyinosine, respectively.	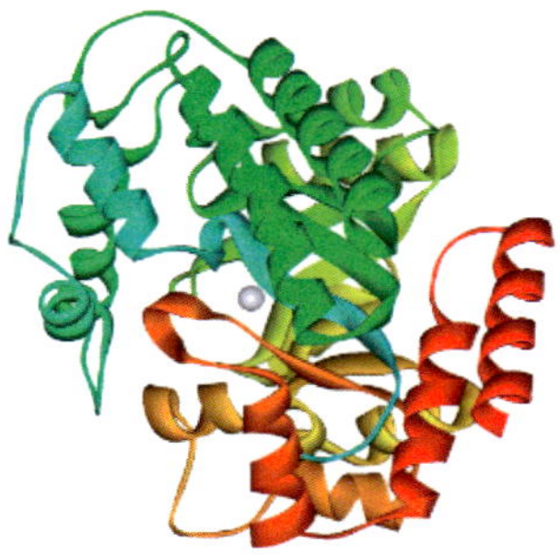
Computed Tomography (CT) scans	Computed tomography scan is a medical imaging technique used to obtain detailed internal images of the body.	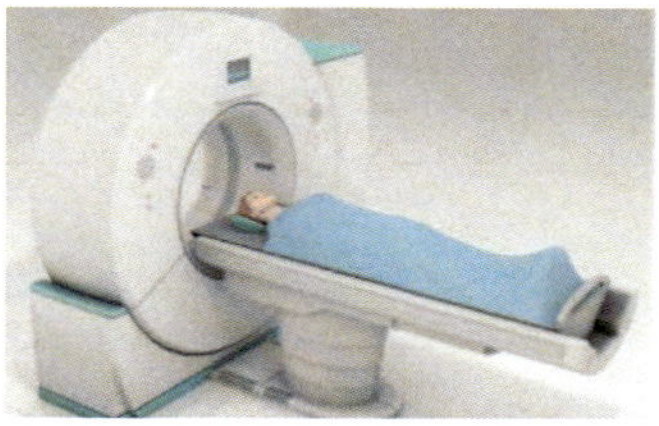
Vascular endothelial growth factor (VEGF)	A potent angiogenic factor and was first described as an essential growth factor for vascular endothelial cells.	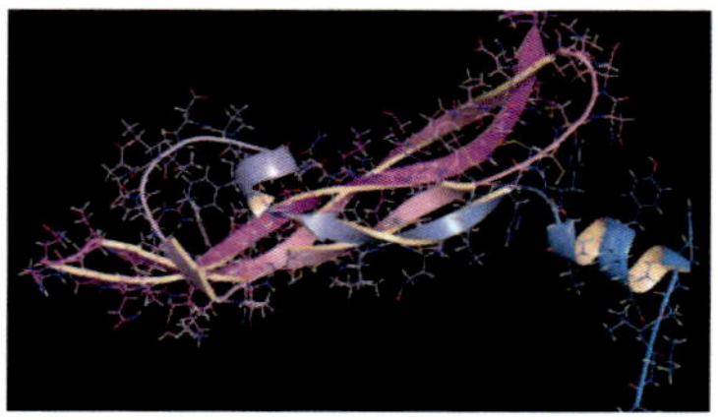

7.1. Pleural Fluid Analysis

The examination of pleural fluid in a laboratory following a thoracentesis, also known as a pleural tap, is called pleural fluid analysis. To remove extra fluid from the area inside the chest cavity but outside the lungs, a thoracentesis is performed. This region typically holds 20 milliliters of transparent or yellow liquid. Coughing and dyspnea are two symptoms that may indicate an overabundance of fluid in this area. A chest X-ray, CT scan, or ultrasound will reveal a pleural effusion, which is an excess of pleural fluid. During a thoracentesis, your doctor will place a hollow needle or catheter between your back's two ribs. The term "intercostal space" refers to this area between two ribs. Usually, local anesthesia is used during the procedure. Your doctor will drain the extra fluid and send it to a lab to ascertain its contents and the most likely reason for the fluid buildup. An examination of a fluid sample that has gathered in the pleural space is known as pleural fluid analysis. The pleura, or lining that covers the outside of the lungs, and the chest wall are separated by this space. Pleural effusion is the term used to describe a condition where fluid accumulates in the pleural space.

In addition to having a physiological role in respiration, pleural fluid is a valuable tool for evaluating and diagnosing illnesses, injuries, and other anomalies. To determine the causes of abnormal pleural fluid collections and pleural effusions, it is helpful to briefly review the anatomy and physiology of normal pleural fluid. The Light criteria is a helpful tool for distinguishing between transudate and exudate, which can subsequently be further assessed using laboratory testing and in relation to the patient's clinical presentation. Assessing the pleural fluid can help identify the underlying cause of the pleural effusion and direct treatment.

Many conditions can cause problems within the pleural cavity and in the pleural fluid. The following are some of the most common:

- **Pleurisy**: pleura inflammation, causing sharp pain with breathing; most commonly caused by a viral infection
- **Pleural Effusion**: excess fluid in the pleural space; commonly from congestive heart failure or malignancy.
- **Pneumothorax**: a buildup of air or gas in the pleural space; commonly from acute lung injury, trauma, or chronic diseases such as chronic obstructive pulmonary disease or tuberculosis
- **Hemothorax**: a buildup of blood in the pleural space; commonly from injury or trauma to the chest

The most frequent causes of transudative pleural effusions in adults are liver cirrhosis and congestive heart failure. The most common causes of exudative pleural effusions are gastrointestinal disorders, lung diseases, and malignant pleural disease. The most frequent causes of pleural effusions in children are pneumonia, cancer, and congenital heart disease. A total white blood cell count of 1.716 x 10(3) cells mL(-1) is the composition of normal pleural fluid. Differential cell counts: 75% macrophages, 23% lymphocytes, and sporadically occurring mesothelial cells (1%–2%), neutrophils (1%–2%), and eosinophils (0%). Interestingly, the percentage of neutrophils in smokers is slightly higher than in nonsmokers (Burgess, 2004; Chernecky and Berger, 2013; Blok, 2019; Broaddus, 2022).

7.1.1. Development

The parietal circulation continuously produces pleural fluid through bulk flow, and the lymphatic system continuously reabsorbs it through the stomata in the parietal pleura. In a healthy individual, the pleural space has a low protein concentration (less than 1.5 g/dL) and only holds 10 to 20 mL of fluid. A pressure gradient causes pleural fluid to be filtered at the parietal pleural level from systemic microvessels to the extrapleural interstitium and then into the pleural space. The lymphatics contribute approximately 75% of the pleural cavity's drainage by opening as stomata directly onto the parietal pleura, with very little absorption occurring through the visceral pleura. Under typical circumstances, the visceral pleura is not responsible for any appreciable pleural fluid drainage. When pleural fluid or another fluid builds up in the pleural space, the body may react by increasing the rate of reabsorption. It takes an increase in absorption rate of about 40 times the reference rate for excess fluid to start building up in the pleural space. Considerable fluid buildup in the pleural cavity typically denotes either excessive pleural fluid production, lymphatic obstruction, or another fluid source, like hemorrhage.

7.1.2. Light's Criteria

Finding the right diagnosis with the least amount of research is the main goal when looking into a pleural effusion. The majority of doctors initially classified an effusion as transudative or exudative based on the pleural protein level before the development of Light's criteria. Gradients of more than 12 g/L in serum and fluid albumin also suggested exudates; however, these criteria are not very sensitive when applied alone. Use of Light's criteria is advised when pleural protein levels are between 25 and 35 g/L. Exudative pleural effusions are defined as follows: (1) total pleural and plasma protein ratios greater than 0.5; (2) pleural and plasma lactate dehydrogenase (LDH) ratios greater than 0.6; and (3) pleural LDH levels greater than two thirds of the normal serum level. Light's criteria have a high sensitivity of 98% in identifying exudative pleural effusions; however, their ability to exclude transudates is still low. As an example, research by Porcel et al. revealed a sensitivity of nearly 100% for exudates, but discovered that roughly one-fifth of diuretic-treated patients with congestive heart failure also fulfilled Light's exudate criteria. Notwithstanding this shortcoming, Light's criteria continue to be more effective than clinical judgment in differentiating between transudates and exudates. A prospective study with n=249 patients that directly compared Light's criteria to clinical suspicion found that the latter was significantly more accurate than the former (84% versus 93%, n<0.01), highlighting the significance of the criteria in everyday clinical practice.

The majority of research to date has concentrated on improving the applicability of Light's criteria's without compromising its ability to discriminate. It has been proposed, for instance, that serum LDH alone does not raise the values of the other two criteria components. A Brazilian study that suggests new criteria to distinguish between the two types of effusions supports this. This study demonstrated a diagnostic yield similar to Light's criteria by measuring only total pleural protein and LDH without the need for serum samples. Numerous non-routine biochemical measurements on pleural fluid have also been produced by other studies, which may help distinguish between transudates and exudates. For example, a pleural fluid bilirubin with a pleural: serum ratio of >0.6 is suggestive of an exudate with a sensitivity and specificity of 90.6% and 96.2%, respectively. A previous study that used both LDH and pleural cholesterol measurements showed comparable sensitivity to differentiate between the two types of effusion, while an early case series showed that pleural fluid cholesterol >60 mg/dL is indicative of an exudative effusion with high sensitivity. Because it increases pleural endothelial permeability, vascular endothelial growth factor (VEGF), a crucial mediator of angiogenesis and vascular permeability, may also be a significant mediator and marker in the identification of exudates. The median VEGF levels in exudates were roughly twice that of transudates in a study involving 79 patients. Furthermore, increased levels of tumor necrosis factor-alpha (TNF-α) are observed in malignant and infectious pleural effusions, but not in transudates. Alkaline phosphatase, creatine kinase, and uric acid are other biochemical parameters that have been studied to help distinguish between transudate and exudate; these parameters had diagnostic accuracies that were lower than the conventional Light's criteria.

A number of these studies have suggested new and different standards that do not require venepuncture, which will save money on tests and diagnostic procedures. To distinguish between the two types of effusion, these criteria's cut-off points differ. With a 96% diagnostic accuracy to date, Light's criteria continue to be reliable and the best way to distinguish pleural transudates from exudates for the time being (Burgess, 2004; Chernecky and Berger, 2013; Blok, 2019; Broaddus, 2022).

7.1.3. Pleural Effusion (Fluid in the Chest)

Fluid accumulation in the area between your lungs and chest cavity is known as pleural effusion, or "water on the lung." Symptoms such as chest pain may manifest, contingent on the underlying cause. The interior of the chest cavity and the exterior of the lungs are covered in thin membranes known as pleura. This lining always contains a tiny amount of liquid to aid in lubricating the lungs as they expand inside the chest during breathing. However, issues may occur if an excessive amount of fluid accumulates, for instance as a result of a medical condition. This is known by doctors as a pleural effusion. Pleural effusion can result from some conditions, but congestive heart failure is the most frequent cause.

- **Symptoms:** Some pleural effusion sufferers experience no symptoms at all. They might be exhibiting signs of a fever or cough that indicate an underlying illness. An X-ray of the chest or a physical examination performed for another reason may reveal that you have pleural effusion. A physician examining you may find that one side of your chest is enlarged and produces a dull tapping sound.

Depending on the cause, a person with pleural effusion may also have:

- chest pain
- cough
- fever
- shortness of breath

See your doctor immediately if you have symptoms of pleural effusion.

7.1.4. Causes

Fluid buildup outside of the lung in the chest cavity results in pleural effusion. It may be exudative or transudative. Increased pressure on the small and large vessels of different organs can lead to leakage, which results in fluid collections filled with protein, a condition known as transudative pleural effusion. It happens in people with cirrhosis or coronary heart disease. Irritation, inflammation, or infection can result in exudative pleural effusion. These may lead to decreased drainage, increased fluid production, or both.

Causes of pleural effusion include:

- congestive heart failure
- cirrhosis or poor liver function
- pulmonary embolism, which is caused by a blood clot and is a blockage in the lung arteries
- complications from open-heart surgery
- pneumonia
- severe kidney disease
- autoimmune diseases, such as lupus and rheumatoid arthritis
- the use of some medications, such as methotrexate, phenytoin, or amiodarone
- radiation therapy
- rupture of the esophagus
- ovarian hyperstimulation syndrome
- certain types of cancer, for instance, lung cancer and breast cancer
- COVID-19

7.1.5. Types

Pleural effusion can be classified as transudative or exudative.

- **Transudative Pleural Effusions:** This type is caused by fluid leaking into the pleural space due to increased pressure in the blood vessels.

It can happen if you:

- o have congestive heart failure
- o have cirrhosis
- o have kidney disease
- o have just started peritoneal dialysis
- o have malnutrition due to low albumin levels in the blood

- **Exudative Effusions:** This happens when a buildup of fluid occurs as the result of:
  - o inflammation
  - o infection
  - o tumors
  - o a lung injury

Conditions that could result in this type of pleural infusion include:

- o tuberculosis
- o cancer
- o inflammatory conditions, such as pancreatitis, lupus, or rheumatoid arthritis
- o complications from heart surgery
- o chylothorax, which results from an obstruction in the lymph vessels
- o pneumonia
- o hemothorax, when blood collects in the pleural cavity

Some conditions, such as pulmonary embolism, can lead to either transudate or exudate pleural effusion.

- **Pleural Effusions and Cancer:** Cancer cells may spread to the pleura or obstruct the normal fluid flow within the pleura to cause pleural effusions. Certain cancer treatments, like radiation therapy or chemotherapy, can also cause fluid accumulation. Pleural effusions are more common in some cancers than in others, such as:
  - o lung cancer
  - o breast cancer
  - o ovarian cancer
  - o leukemia

- o melanoma
- o cervical cancer
- o uterine cancer
- o mesothelioma, which results from exposure to asbestos

Signs and symptoms often include:

- o shortness of breath
- o cough
- o chest pain
- o weight loss

If the doctor determines that repeated drainage is necessary, they may drain the fluid or perform pleurodesis. To do this, a shunt that diverts the fluid from the chest must be inserted. In the event that you are infected or at risk of infection, they might recommend antibiotics. Pain and inflammation may be lessened by steroids or other anti-inflammatory drugs. They will also talk about alternative cancer treatment plans. Individuals receiving cancer treatment may also have weakened immune systems, which increases their vulnerability to infections or other side effects.

7.1.6. Treatment

The treatment and outcome will depend on the cause of the pleural effusion.

- **Draining Fluid:** A small tube inserted into the chest or a needle used to remove fluid from the chest cavity are two methods used to treat pleural effusion.
- **Antibiotics:** If the pleural effusion is due to infectious causes, antibiotics are essential.
- **Pleurodesis:** is the permanent apposition between the parietal pleura and the visceral pleura induced by: 1) "natural" stimuli of an infectious, inflammatory or traumatic type, 2) Deliberate introduction of substances into the pleural cavity, chemical pleurodesis (CP) and 3) Surgical procedures performed on the pleural sheets, surgical pleurodesis (SP). The simplest form of deliberate pleurodesis would be CP, removal of the fluid and introduction of the sclerosing substance; the most complex, SP, would be the parietal pleurectomy
- **Surgery:** If the problem is not resolved with conservative management (drainage, chemical pleurodesis, antibiotics, etc.), surgical debridement or thoracoscopic decortication is the alternative.

7.1.7. Diagnosis

Some possible tests include:

- Chest ultrasound
- CT scan
- Thoracentesis, where the doctor removes some pleural fluid for analysis
- Bronchoscopy
- Pleural biopsy

7.1.8. Risks and Complications

Pleural effusions may present as simple or complex. Simple pleural effusions are fluid-filled and show no symptoms of inflammation or infection. They are less likely to result in long-term lung issues. On the other hand, fluid in complicated pleural effusions has a high level of inflammation or infection. They need to be treated right away, and chest drainage is often necessary. Pleural effusion may indicate more serious symptoms in certain conditions.

Researchers discovered in 2021 that patients with COVID-19 who experienced pleural effusion had a higher risk of serious inflammation and complications, which may have an impact on their prognosis.

- **Treatment Can Also Lead to Complications:** Pain and discomfort are common minor side effects of more invasive treatments, and they usually go away over time. The severity of the ailment, the cause, and the chosen course of treatment will all affect more severe consequences.

Serious complications can include:

- o pulmonary edema or fluid in the lungs, which can result from draining fluid too quickly during thoracentesis
- o partial collapsed lung
- o infection or bleeding
- o empyema, when there is pus in the pleural space
- o trapped lung, when a layer forms around the lung that prevents it from expanding

These complications, while serious, are rare. Your doctor will help determine the most effective treatment option and discuss the benefits and risks of each procedure (Burgess, 2004; Chernecky and Berger, 2013; Blok, 2019; Broaddus, 2022).

7.1.9. Organ Systems Involved

The area that lies between the lungs and the internal thoracic wall is known as the pleural cavity, and it contains the pleural fluid. An intricate network of parietal and visceral layers makes up the fibrous mesothelial membrane lining the pleural cavity. Inside the thoracic cavity is the parietal layer, while the outside of the lungs is covered by the visceral layer. These continuous layers have no communication between the left and right pleural cavities, meeting to form a double layer at the hilum of each lung. It is possible to distinguish between the two pleural layers in terms of the pleural cavity innervation. Whereas the parietal layer is innervated by somatic fibers and is extremely sensitive, the visceral pleura, which is autonomic fiber innervated, is typically insensitive to irritation and inflammation. The four sections of the parietal innervation—the cervical, costal, mediastinal, and peripheral pleural zones—have different and clinically relevant presentations in the context of physiologic insult. Innervated by the first thoracic spinal nerve, the cervical pleura can refer pain to the inner aspect of the upper limb when it becomes inflamed. The thoracic nerves covering the area innervate the costal pleura, which can refer pain to the thorax above. As the C4 dermatome distributes down the fibrous pericardium, the phrenic nerve innervates the mediastinal pleura and may refer pain to the ipsilateral shoulder. The anterior abdominal wall may experience pain referred by the lower six thoracic nerves to the peripheral diagrammatic pleura.

The blood supply to the parietal pleura is supplied by the musculophrenic, internal thoracic, and intercostal arteries. The venous drainage of the parietal pleura is supplied by the intercostal veins. The parietal pleura's lymphatics empty into the diaphragmatic, posterior mediastinal, parasternal, and intercostal nodes. The lymphatic drainage of the visceral pleura passes through the hilar lymph nodes, while the venous and blood supply originate from the bronchial vessels. Three areas remain vulnerable that may be clinically relevant in the event of trauma to the lungs and pleura: (1) above the medial end of the first ribs, (2) below the costal-xiphisternal angle on the right side, and (3) below the costovertebral angles. The bony thorax serves as the anatomical protection of the pleural cavities. Via the parietal pleural stomata and lymphatics, pleural fluid leaves the pleural space after entering through the systemic capillaries in the parietal pleurae.

7.1.10. Function

During respiration, the fluid serves as a lubricant to enable the two pleura layers to move easily past one another. The subatmospheric pressure of the pleural fluid keeps the thoracic cavity and lungs at a negative pressure, which is essential for inhalation and keeps the lungs from collapsing. The fluid that lies between the layers of the pleura, the membranes that surround the lungs and line the cavity, is known as pleural fluid. Pleural cavity or pleural space is the term used to describe the area that holds the fluid. A tiny quantity of a thin, serous fluid that serves as a lubricant during breathing makes up normal pleural fluid. Viral infections, traumatic injuries, and other factors can alter the volume of pleural fluid, which can result in respiratory issues and other unfavorable circumstances.

Numerous medical conditions have the potential to impact both the pleural cavity and the pleural fluid. Among them are:

- Pleural effusion is a condition wherein excess fluid accumulates in the pleural space. There are many causes of pleural effusions, including congestive heart failure, pulmonary embolism, kidney conditions, cancer, and autoimmune diseases such as lupus and rheumatoid arthritis. Approximately 1.5 million people in the U.S. are affected by pleural effusion each year.
- When a buildup of fluid contains cancer cells, it is called a malignant pleural effusion. While this most commonly occurs with during stage 4 lung cancer, it can also occur with other cancers that have spread (metastasized) from other parts of the body, including the breast and ovaries.

7.1.11. Pathophysiology

Changes in fluid and solute homeostasis lead to the development of pleural effusions; the mechanism causing these changes determines whether the effusion is transudative (low protein content) or exudative (high protein content). A transudate effusion is brought on by an imbalance between the hydrostatic and oncotic pressures inside the capillaries. An exudative effusion is characterized by a change in the local inflammatory factors that cause a pleural fluid buildup.

When the rate of pleural fluid production outpaces the rate of reabsorption, fluid builds up in the pleural space. When filtration rate surpasses maximum lymph flow, exudative type effusion occurs, resulting in an effusion with a higher-than-normal protein content. Increased pleural liquid protein concentration results in the formation of exudate by increasing the protein permeability of the systemic capillaries. Exudative pleural effusions are typically brought on by malignancy, granulomatous diseases like coccidioidomycosis or tuberculosis, collagen vascular diseases, infections like pneumonia, and other inflammatory conditions. Hypooncotic fluid (lower protein content) is caused by an increase in both capillary and mesothelial water permeability. Transudate forms if filtration surpasses the maximum lymph reabsorption through the parietal stomata. Transudative pleural effusions can arise from cirrhosis, nephrotic syndrome, malnourishment, and congestive heart failure. The final three conditions show a hypoalbuminemia-related drop in colloid oncotic pressure. Increased capillary permeability brought on by the release of inflammatory mediators and cytokines from the platelet-rich thrombi may be the cause of the localized pleural fluid effusion observed following a pulmonary embolism.

7.1.12. Clinical Significance

Since the treatments for exudative and transudative etiologies differ greatly, the diagnosis of the etiology is crucial. A more thorough investigation is nearly always necessary for exudative effusions, and this may involve an emergent thoracotomy, a biopsy, or cytopathology studies. Any patient who has an exudative effusion should have an etiology determined. On the other hand, transudative effusions typically don't need to be treated; instead, the underlying cirrhosis or heart failure should be the focus of therapy. Malignant pleural effusion is a frequent condition that has a dismal prognosis. Malignant pleural effusions usually present as dyspnea and a unilateral, large pleural effusion. Differentiating between benign and malignant pleural effusions can be aided by CT and ultrasound imaging.

Management of pleural effusion should be as follows:

- Diagnostic or therapeutic thoracentesis or chest tube drainage
- Obtain pleural fluid and serum studies of protein and LDH
- If indicated consider additional pleural fluid studies such as cell count, differential, cultures, or triglycerides
- Evaluate fluid using the Light criteria to determine if it is exudative
- Narrow differential diagnosis based on whether transudative or exudative

7.2. Peritoneal Fluid Analysis

A liquid called peritoneal fluid lubricates the abdominal cavity. It is present in the spaces between the peritoneal layers that line the abdominal wall in tiny amounts (usually 5–20 mL). When an organ is being digested or moved, the peritoneal fluid helps to moisten its exterior and lessen friction. Peritoneal inflammation (peritonitis) and/or an excessive build-up of peritoneal fluid (peritoneal effusion or ascites) can be brought on by several illnesses and disorders. A series of examinations known as peritoneal fluid analysis assess this fluid to identify the reason for the elevated fluid.

The two main reasons that fluid may collect in the abdominal cavity are:

- An imbalance between the pressure within blood vessels—which drives fluid out of blood vessels—and the amount of protein in blood—which keeps fluid in blood vessels. The fluid that accumulates in this case is called a transudate. Transudates are most often caused by congestive heart failure, nephrotic syndrome, or hepatic cirrhosis.
- An injury or inflammation of the peritoneum, in which case the fluid is called an exudate. This type of fluid may be the result of conditions such as infection, malignancies (metastatic cancer, lymphoma, mesothelioma), pancreatitis, ruptured gallbladder, or autoimmune disease.

It is crucial to identify the type of fluid (transudate or exudates) present as this helps identify the potential causes of inflammation or fluid accumulation. To differentiate between transudates and exudates, medical professionals and laboratory technicians perform a preliminary battery of tests that includes cell count, serum and fluid albumin levels, and fluid appearance. If the fluid confirms one diagnosis over the other, more testing might be carried out to identify the exact illness or condition causing ascites. While peritoneal fluid analysis is crucial, abdominocentesis is not required if additional clinical findings point to the need for surgery. Enterocentesis rarely causes complications, but after a distended bowel puncture, peritonitis and abdominal wall cellulitis can occur.

7.2.1. How Is It Used?

The diagnosis of ascites, or fluid accumulation in the abdomen, and peritoneal inflammation, or peritonitis, can be aided by peritoneal fluid analysis. An initial battery of tests is used to distinguish between the two types of fluid that may be produced, transudate and exudate, as there are two main causes for fluid accumulation.

These tests typically include:

- Fluid albumin level—the serum-ascites albumin gradient (SAAG) calculation (serum albumin level minus the fluid albumin level) may be used to differentiate between transudates and exudates. A SAAG level of 1.1 g/dL or greater suggests the presence of a transudate and less than 1.1 g/dL, an exudate.
- Cell count and differential
- Appearance

A transudate is an accumulation of fluid that occurs when there is an imbalance between the pressure inside blood vessels, which pushes fluid out of the vessel, and the amount of protein in the blood, which retains fluid in the vessel. The most common causes of transudates are hepatic cirrhosis, nephrotic syndrome, and congestive heart failure. Further testing on the fluid usually isn't required if it turns out to be a transudate. Exudate: An abnormal collection of fluid (referred to as an exudate) may result from peritoneal injuries or inflammation. Exudates can be seen in cases of pancreatitis, infections, cancer, ruptured gallbladders, or autoimmune diseases.

Laboratory tests may be performed to determine one of the following conditions:

- Infectious diseases caused by viruses, bacteria, or fungi.
- Inflammatory conditions – peritonitis due to certain chemicals, irradiation, or rarely an autoimmune disorder
- Malignancies – such as mesothelioma, tumor of the liver (hepatoma), lymphoma, or metastatic cancer
- Pancreatitis – due to certain drugs, infections, blockages, and circulating lipids (fats)

Additional testing on exudate fluid may include:

- Peritoneal fluid glucose, amylase, tumor markers, bilirubin, creatinine, lactate dehydrogenase (LD)
- Microscopic examination – may be performed if infection or cancer is suspected; a laboratory professional may use a special centrifuge (cytocentrifuge) to concentrate the fluid's cells on a slide. The slide is treated with a special stain and evaluated for abnormal cells, such as malignant cells (cancer cells).
- Gram stain – for direct observation of bacteria or fungi under a microscope
- Bacterial culture and susceptibility testing – ordered to detect the presence of any microbes that have grown in the culture and to guide antimicrobial therapy
- Less commonly ordered tests for

infectious diseases, such as tests for viruses, mycobacteria (AFB testing in identifying tuberculosis), and parasites

- Adenosine deaminase - rarely ordered for detecting tuberculosis in peritoneal fluid

7.2.2. Test Result Interpretation

Test results can help distinguish between types of peritoneal fluid and help diagnose the cause of fluid accumulation. The initial set of tests performed on a sample of peritoneal fluid helps determine whether the fluid is a transudate or exudate. Findings may include:

1. **Transudate:** Most ascitic fluids are transudates and are caused by either congestive heart failure or hepatic cirrhosis. Typical fluid analysis results include:
    - Physical characteristics—fluid generally appears clear or straw-colored
    - Protein—less than 3 g/dL
    - Albumin level—low (typically evaluated as the difference between serum albumin and peritoneal fluid albumin, termed serum-ascites albumin gradient, or SAAG; values above 1.1 g/dL are considered evidence of a transudate.)
    - Lactate dehydrogenase (LD) fluid/serum ratio—less than 0.6
    - Glucose—equal to the glucose level in the blood
    - Cell count—few cells are present, usually lymphocytes
    - Specific gravity—less than 1.015
2. Exudate:
    - Physical characteristics—fluid may appear cloudy
    - Protein—greater than 3 g/dL
    - Albumin level—higher than in transudates (typically with a SAAG less than 1.1 g/dL)
    - Lactate dehydrogenase (LD) fluid/serum ratio—greater than 0.6
    - Glucose—less than 60 mg/dL
    - Cell count—increased
    - Specific gravity—greater than 1.015

Exudates can be the result of many different illnesses, and additional testing is typically necessary to make a diagnosis. Exudates can be brought on by pancreatitis, infections, trauma, and different cancers. A medical professional may request any of the following tests based on the suspected cause and expected outcomes.

- **Physical Characteristics:** the normal appearance of a peritoneal fluid sample is usually straw-colored and clear. Abnormal appearances may give clues to conditions or diseases present and may include:
    - o Yellow with liver disease, milky from obstruction of the lymphatic system, and greenish from bile
    - o Reddish peritoneal fluid may indicate the presence of blood, most often due to trauma.
    - o Cloudy peritoneal fluid may indicate the presence of microbes and/or white blood cells (WBCs), pointing to an infection. It may also indicate lymph system blockage or trauma.

- **Chemical Tests**: tests that may be performed in addition to albumin may include:
  - Glucose—typically about the same as blood glucose levels; may be lower with infection
  - Amylase—increased with pancreatitis
  - Tumor markers—to identify the type of malignancy
- **Microscopic Examination**: may be performed if infection or cancer is suspected; normal peritoneal fluid has small numbers of WBCs but no red blood cells (RBCs) or microbes. Results of an evaluation of the different kinds of cells present may include:
  - Total cell counts—WBCs and RBCs in the sample are enumerated. Increased WBCs may be seen with infections and malignant conditions.
  - WBC differential—determination of percentages of different types of WBCs; an increased number of neutrophils may be seen with bacterial infections.
  - Cytology—a special centrifuge (cytocentrifuge) concentrates a small sample of cells that is then treated with a special stain to be examined under a microscope for abnormal cells and for white blood cell differentiation. The differential can help determine whether the cells are the result of an infection or the presence of a tumor.
- **Infectious Disease Tests**: tests may be performed to look for microbes if an infection is suspected.
  - Gram stain—for direct observation of bacteria or fungi under a microscope; there should be no microbes present in peritoneal fluid.
  - Bacterial culture and susceptibility testing—if bacteria are present, susceptibility testing can be performed to guide antimicrobial therapy. If there are no microbes present, it does not rule out an infection; they may be present in small numbers or their growth may be inhibited because of prior antibiotic therapy.
  - Fungal tests—if a culture is positive, the fungus or fungi causing the infection will be identified in the report and susceptibility testing may be done to guide therapy.
  - Adenosine deaminase—a markedly elevated level in peritoneal fluid in a person with symptoms that suggest tuberculosis means it is likely that person has a *Mycobacterium tuberculosis* infection in that region of the body. This is especially true when there is a high prevalence of tuberculosis in the geographic region where a person lives.

Other less common tests for infectious diseases may be performed to identify a virus, mycobacteria (such as the mycobacterium that causes tuberculosis), or a parasite as the cause of an infection and fluid accumulation.

7.3. Approaches of Pericardial Fluid Testing

The serous fluid that the pericardium's serous layer secretes into the pericardial cavity is known as pericardial fluid. There are two layers in the pericardium: an inner serous layer and an outer fibrous layer. The pericardial cavity, into which the pericardial fluid is secreted, is enclosed by two membranes on this serous layer. The fluid is comparable to the brain's cerebrospinal fluid, which also acts as a cushion and permits some movement in the organ. The membrane that surrounds the heart is called the pericardium, and it has two layers. A fluid that lies in between the pericardium's membranes is called pericardial fluid, which is produced by pericardial membranes. The fluid lubricates the heart's motion and lowers friction while the organ pumps blood. Pericardial effusion, or excessive accumulation of pericardial fluid, and/or pericarditis, an inflammation of the pericardium, are caused by a variety of conditions and diseases. A series of examinations known as pericardial fluid analysis assess this fluid in an effort to identify the reason for the elevated fluid.

The two main reasons for fluid accumulation in the pericardial space are:

- An imbalance between the pressure within blood vessels—which drives fluid out of blood vessels—and the amount of protein in blood—which keeps fluid in blood vessels. The fluid that accumulates in this case is called a transudate. Transudates are most often caused by congestive heart failure or cirrhosis.
- An injury or inflammation of the pericardium, in which case the fluid that accumulates is called an exudate. Conditions such as infections, malignancies (metastatic cancer, lymphoma, mesothelioma), or autoimmune disease may cause the accumulation of exudate.

It is crucial to distinguish between transudate and exudate to limit the range of potential causes of pericardial fluid accumulation. To differentiate between transudates and exudates, medical professionals and laboratory technicians perform a preliminary battery of tests that includes measurements of cells, albumin or protein levels, and fluid appearance. Further testing may be carried out to identify the exact ailment causing pericarditis and/or pericardial effusion if the fluid is found to be one or the other.

7.3.1. Testing Details

The diagnosis of pericarditis, an inflammation of the pericardium, and pericardial effusion, a build-up of fluid surrounding the heart, can be aided by pericardial fluid analysis. Fluid accumulation can be caused by either pericardial inflammation or an imbalance in blood vessel pressure. To distinguish between the two types of resultant fluids, known as transudate and exudate, an initial set of tests is performed. These tests include fluid protein or albumin level, cell count, and appearance.

- **Transudate:** Fluid buildup can occur from an imbalance between the blood's protein content, which keeps fluid in the blood vessel, and the blood vessel's internal pressure, which forces fluid out of the vessel. Transudates are typically brought on by cirrhosis or congestive heart failure. Further testing on the fluid usually isn't required if it turns out to be a transudate.
- **Exudate:** injury or inflammation of the pericardium may cause abnormal collection of fluid (called

an exudate). Exudates are associated with a variety of conditions and diseases. If the fluid is an exudate, then several additional tests may be ordered to help diagnose the specific condition, which may include:

- o Infectious diseases – caused by viruses, bacteria, or fungi. Infections may originate in the pericardium or spread there from other places in the body. For example, pericarditis may follow a respiratory infection or a chest cold.
- o Bleeding – bleeding disorders and/or trauma can lead to blood in the pericardial fluid.
- o Inflammatory conditions – pericarditis may follow a heart attack, radiation treatment, or be part of autoimmune disorders such as rheumatoid arthritis and lupus.
- o Cancer – such as mesothelioma that has arisen in the pericardium or metastatic cancer that has spread to it.

Additional testing on exudate fluid may include:

- Pericardial fluid glucose
- Microscopic examination
- Cytology
- Gram stain
- Bacterial culture and susceptibility testing
- Adenosine deaminase—rarely, this test may be used to help detect tuberculosis (TB).
- Less commonly ordered tests for infectious diseases, such as tests for viruses, mycobacteria (AFB smear and culture), and parasites.

7.3.2. Test Result Interpretation

The results of tests can be used to diagnose the cause of fluid accumulation and to differentiate between different types of pericardial fluid. Whether pericardial fluid is an exudate or a transudate is ascertained by the first series of tests conducted on the sample.

- **Transudate:**
  - o Physical characteristics—fluid appears clear
  - o Protein or albumin level—low
  - o Cell count—few cells are present
- **Exudate:** Exudates can be caused by a variety of conditions and diseases. Initial test results may show:
  - o Physical characteristics—fluid may appear cloudy
  - o Protein or albumin level—high
  - o Cell count—increased

Additional test results and their associated causes may include:

- **Physical Characteristics:** the normal appearance of a sample of pericardial fluid is straw-colored and clear. Abnormal results may give clues to the conditions or diseases present and may include:
  - o Milky appearance—may point to lymphatic system involvement.
  - o Reddish pericardial fluid may indicate the presence of blood.
  - o Cloudy, thick pericardial fluid may indicate the presence of microorganisms and/or white blood cells.

- **Chemical tests** – in addition to protein or albumin, a glucose test may be performed. Glucose in pericardial fluid samples is typically about the same as blood glucose levels. It may be lower with infection.
- **Microscopic Examination** – normal pericardial fluid has small numbers of white blood cells (WBCs) but no red blood cells (RBCs) or microorganisms. Results of an evaluation of the different kinds of cells present may include:
    - o Total cell counts—quantity of WBCs and RBCs in the sample. Increased WBCs may be seen with infections and other causes of pericarditis.
    - o WBC differential—determination of percentages of different types of WBCs. An increased number of neutrophils may be seen with bacterial infections.
    - o Cytology—after being centrifuged, a sample is stained with a particular dye and checked under a microscope to look for any abnormal cells. When metastatic cancer or mesothelioma is suspected, this may be carried out. The presence of specific aberrant cells, such as immature blood cells or tumor cells, can reveal the type of cancer that is present.
- **Infectious Disease Tests** – routine tests may be performed to look for microorganisms if infection is suspected:
    - o Gram stain—for direct observation of bacteria or fungi under a microscope. There should be no organisms present in pericardial fluid.
    - o Bacterial culture and susceptibility testing—if bacteria are present, susceptibility testing can be performed to guide antimicrobial therapy. If there are no microorganisms present, it does not rule out an infection. Bacteria may be present in small numbers or their growth may be inhibited because of prior antibiotic therapy.
    - o Adenosine deaminase—it is probable that a person with symptoms suggestive of tuberculosis has a Mycobacterium tuberculosis infection in the pericardium if there is a noticeably elevated level in the percardial fluid. This is particularly true if the person lives in an area where tuberculosis is highly prevalent.

Other less common tests for infectious diseases may be performed. Those tests may identify pericardial fluid accumulation due to a viral infection, mycobacteria (such as the mycobacterium that causes tuberculosis), or a parasite (Burgess, 2004; Chernecky and Berger, 2013; Blok, 2019; Broaddus, 2022).

7.3.3. Composition of Pericardial Fluid

The pericardial fluid, like the pleura fluid, is a plasma ultrafiltrate with particular properties. According to volumetric research, the pericardial fluid volume is approximately 20–60 mL (average 15–35 mL). The fluid distribution inside the cavity is heterogeneous, according to pericardial fluid coloring studies. In particular when supine, the greatest quantity is found inside the superior and transversal sinuses, the atrioventricular and intraventricular sulcus, and the superior ventricle. The pericardial fluid is continuously stirring up, according to certain pharmacokinetic studies, so the supplement's composition remains constant regardless of position.

A heterogeneous cell population has been observed in studies conducted on human normal pericardial fluid in relation to the cell population. The cells that make up the tissue include mesothelial cells, basophils (1%), eosinophils (1.7%), lymphocytes (53%) and glanulocytes (31%). Therefore, "lymphocytosis" in pericardial fluid should always be taken seriously and should only be classified as pathological when it accounts for more than 60% of the total cell population.

Like other serosal cavity fluids, the pericardial fluid is regarded as a plasma ultrafiltration product.

7.3.4. Physiology

The pericardium contributes in important functions. In is necessary for: (1) lubricating the moving surfaces of the heart, (2) stabilizing the heart anatomic position, (3) isolating the heart from the adjacent anatomical structures, prohibiting the adhesion formation, the inflammatory or neoplastic extention, (4) limiting heart dilatation during diastole, reducing the endomyocardial tension, (5) preventing cardiac hypertrophy in pressure overload conditions, (6) reducing the right ventricular impulse work in left ventricular overload conditions, (7) the ventriculoatrial blood retrogression prevention during high end-diastolic ventricular pressures, (8) the preservation of the negative endothoracic pressure, which is crucial for the atria blood filling, (9) the nervous stimulation response and regulation of the cardiac frequency and arterial blood pressure, (10) the formation of a hydrostatic compensation system ensuring that end-diastolic pressure remains the same at all hydrostatic levels and the Frank–Starling mechanism is functional.

7.4. Pleural, Peritoneal and Pericardial Effusions: A Biochemical Approach

Numerous circumstances can lead to the pathological buildup of serous fluids in the peritoneal, pericardial, and pleural spaces. The accurate and timely diagnosis is crucial for patient management, which is why biochemical analysis of extravascular bodily fluids is regarded as an important tool in the process. Determining the gross appearance of serous fluids, distinguishing between transudative and exudative effusions, and performing additional specialized biochemical testing to determine the effusion etiology are all part of the biochemical evaluation process. In a clinical laboratory, standard samples for analysis include blood, urine, and cerebrospinal fluid. On the other hand, sometimes the assessment of serous extravascular fluids (i.e., peritoneal, pericardial, and pleural) is required. Biochemical analysis of these samples can direct the clinician to the definitive diagnosis and treatment options while also giving him useful information about the fluid's etiology (Tarn and Lipworth, 2001).

7.4.1. Pleural Effusions

Excessive fluid formation and its accumulation in the pleural space lead to pleural effusions. Pleural effusions are most frequently caused by heart failure, cancer, pneumonia, tuberculosis, and pulmonary embolism. It is important to identify the cause of pleural effusions in patients so that the right course of treatment can be started. The clinical assessment of pleural effusions heavily relies on the patient's medical history and physical examination. The presence of a pleural effusion is then confirmed by radiological, ultrasound, or computed tomography (CT) chest scans. Thoracentesis is the extraction of pleural fluid with a syringe or needle, used for therapeutic or diagnostic purposes. To obtain the blood sample required for additional effusion evaluation, it should be combined with pleural fluid sampling (within 30 minutes of obtaining the sample), i.e., the distinction between exudative and transudative effusions. Biochemical analyses offer crucial diagnostic information in the majority of pleural effusion cases, particularly when no underlying diagnosis is evident. Pleural fluid (PF) analysis can be done using a variety of tests, either as the only diagnostic procedure or in conjunction with other procedures to help identify the etiology of the effusion (Romero et al., 1993)

7.4.1.1. Appearance of Pleural Fluid

The etiology of pleural effusion can be inferred from fluid appearance, despite the fact that it is a nonspecific tool for PF evaluation. The vast majority of transudates and exudates are straw-colored, clear, odorless, and viscous fluids. A uniformly red appearance combined with a peripheral PF hematocrit of 1-20% reduces the range of possible diagnoses to trauma, embolism, and malignancy. Hemothorax is indicated by a PF hematocrit that is greater than half of the peripheral hematocrit. Both the presence of cells and debris and a high lipid concentration in PF can contribute to its turbidity. After centrifuging turbid PFs, a clear supernatant shows that turbidity is caused by cells and debris, which may point to the existence of empyema. Otherwise, a high lipid concentration following centrifugation is likely the cause of any turbidity that remains, indicating the presence of either pseudochylothorax or chylothorax. However, PF triglyceride analysis is a more conclusive test, and PF is chyle if concentrations > 1–2 mmol/L. A black fluid indicates an Aspergillus infection, while anchovy-brown fluid may indicate an amebic liver abscess.

7.4.1.2. Differentiation of Exudates from Transudates

Determining whether pleural effusions are transudative or exudative is the first step in the biochemical evaluation process (Figure 7.1). Cirrhosis and heart failure are two examples of systemic non-inflammatory diseases that can result in transudative pleural effusions. They react to underlying disease treatment. Increased capillary permeability and fluid accumulation are the results of an inflammatory or malignant process that affects the pleura, leading to exudative effusions. Exudates are frequently caused by pulmonary emboli, cancer, pneumonia, and tuberculosis. A definitive diagnosis can only be made after a thorough diagnostic examination.

For the past 40 years, Light's criteria have been widely used in clinical practice to distinguish between transudates and exudates (Table 7.1). In the initial research, Light et al. demonstrated a 99% sensitivity and 98% specificity in detecting exudates. Subsequent research replicated the original sensitivity of Light's criteria, but with lower specificities (65–86%), leading to higher rates of transudate misclassification into exudates. Despite this drawback, it was reported that Light's criteria were more effective at differentiating between transudates and exudates than clinical judgment alone.

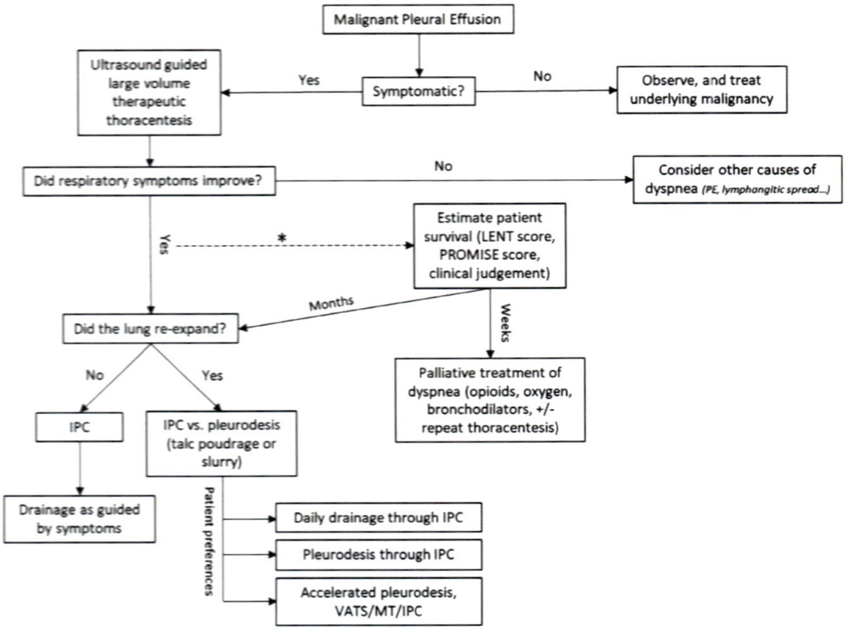

Figure 7.1. *Biochemical analysis of pleural effusions: IPC (indwelling pleural catheter), VATS (video assisted thoracoscopic surgery), MT (medical thoracoscopy). * The role of prognostication scores in clinical practice is still unclear, and physicians' prediction of survival is not very accurate; therefore, a "predicted" short survival should be interpreted with caution.*

Source: Jacobs B, Sheikh G, Youness HA, Keddissi JI, Abdo T. Diagnosis and Management of Malignant Pleural Effusion: A Decade in Review. Diagnostics. 2022; 12(4):1016. https://doi.org/10.3390/diagnostics12041016.

Table 7.1. Light's Criteria for the Differentiation of Pleural Effusions

Light's Criteria	Pleural Fluid Only Three Test Combination
Pleural fluid to serum total protein > 0.5	Total protein > 3g/dL
Pleural fluid to serum lactate dehydrogenase (LDH) ratio > 0.6	Cholesterol > 55mg/dL
Pleural fluid LDH > two-thirds upper limit of normal	LDH > two-thirds the upper limit of normal

Source: Nicholson MJ, Manley C, Ahmad D. Thoracentesis for the Diagnosis and Management of Pleural Effusions: The Current State of a Centuries-Old Procedure. Journal of Respiration. 2023; 3(4):208-222. https://doi.org/10.3390/jor3040020.

The goal of several studies has been to increase Light's criteria's cost-effectiveness without sacrificing its diagnostic precision. Measuring only PF protein and PF lactate dehydrogenase (LD) produced better diagnostic results when compared to Light's requirements. An early study on PF cholesterol revealed that concentrations greater than 1 point 6 mmol/L could be used as a single, affordable test to replace Light's criteria for distinguishing between exudative and transudative effusions. Subsequent research, however, did not support these findings. To distinguish the two types of effusion, more biochemical parameters—and their combinations—have been studied. While the PF cholesterol > 1.2 mmol/L and/or PF LD > 200 U/L showed similar diagnostic accuracy to Light's criteria for the differentiation of PFs, the measurement of cholesterol and LD in PF as an alternative to Light's criteria for the identification of exudates without requiring blood sampling. It has been observed recently that transudative pleural effusions have higher concentrations of ischemia-modified albumin (IMA) than tuberculous effusions. Measurements of pleural IMA demonstrated good diagnostic performances in transudate/exudate differentiation, though they did not outperform Light's criteria. For this reason, other biochemical markers like uric acid, creatine kinase, and alkaline phosphatase (ALP) have also been studied. When measured against Light's criteria, their diagnostic performances were lower.

According to estimates, the use of diuretics in patients with congestive heart failure (CHF) may lead to the incorrect classification of up to 25% of cardiac-related pleural effusions as exudatives. According to reports, diuretic therapy in CHF patients causes fluid to shift out of the pleural space, which raises the concentrations of different PF components, such as PF protein and PF LD. As a result, exudative diagnostic criteria may be met by transudative pleural effusions linked to CHF. Patients receiving diuretic treatment had a marked decrease in the misclassification of transudative effusions following the introduction of the serum effusion albumin gradient (SEAG), which is computed as the difference between serum and PF albumin concentration. A transudate-class effusion is identified if the SEAG is greater than 12 g/L. It is not recommended to use the albumin gradient alone to differentiate between transudates and exudates due to its low sensitivity. Therefore, SEAG computation is advised if the clinical appearance points to a transudative effusion, especially in cases of CHF or cirrhosis, but the PF meets Light's criteria for exudative effusion. Recent research has demonstrated elevated concentrations of N-terminal brain natriuretic peptide precursor (NT-proBNP) in PF and serum of patients suffering from pleural effusion and CHF. NT-proBNP values ≥ 1500 ng/L in pleural fluid have a sensitivity and specificity of 91% and 93%, respectively, in distinguishing pleural effusions due to heart failure from those caused by other etiologies. Further research proved that for the identification of cardiac-related pleural effusions, pleural NT-proBNP determination was superior to Light's criteria. It is important to exercise caution when interpreting NT-proBNP results, as patients with renal failure and the elderly have physiologically elevated NT-proBNP concentrations.

The meta-analysis was conducted to compare the discriminative properties of various biochemical markers used in the identification of exudative effusions. Only in PF specimens were the combinations of two or three tests conducted (i.e., In addition to saving diagnostic costs and avoiding the need for blood sampling, the combined use of PF LD and PF cholesterol or PF LD, PF cholesterol, and PF protein) demonstrated diagnostic performances comparable to modified Light's criteria. By comparing the results to a cut-off point, all of the aforementioned tests divide effusions into transudative and exudative categories. Sensitivity and specificity are used to characterize each test's diagnostic performance. Because sensitivity and specificity values do not indicate the likelihood of disease in the event of a positive test result, their application to specific patients in clinical practice is limited. Furthermore, combining several tests with a single cut-off point for each test raises sensitivity but lowers specificity, suggesting the need for more (and frequently superfluous) testing to confirm the diagnosis. A Bayesian method that measures diagnostic confidence overcomes the drawbacks of binary testing. According to this theory, a test can only affect a subject's pre-test probability of being an exudate or transudate, not distinguish between the two. To estimate the post-test probability of exudative effusions, multilevel likelihood ratios for tests commonly used to distinguish between transudates and exudates were reported. But the ease of use and familiarity of Light's criteria ought to be weighed against the addition of new and laborious techniques for separating exudates from transudates (Ebnezer, 2003; Pisetsky, 2020).

7.4.2. Evaluation of Exudative Effusions

Finding the cause of a pleural effusion is the next difficult task after it has been classified as an exudate. Exudative effusions may require further testing based on their clinical presentation (Figure 7.1). This includes testing for indicators of tuberculous pleuritis, additional biochemical testing, cytological analysis, smears and cultures to identify infection, and total and differential cell counts. For the most part, exudates contain more leukocytes than 500 × 106 / L. Differential leukocyte count in post-fibrosis (PF) indicates the stage of the inflammatory response and reduces the range of possible diagnoses, despite its limited diagnostic utility. Acute inflammatory processes affecting the pleura, such as those caused by parapneumonia, pulmonary embolism, viral infections, gastrointestinal disorders, and tuberculous pleuritis, are indicated by neutrophil predominance. A subacute or chronic process is indicated by the predominance of mononuclear cells. A pleural eosinophilia (at least 10% of eosinophils) is primarily caused by blood or air in the pleural space, while pleural lymphocytosis is suggestive of malignant or tuberculous pleuritis (i.e., cancer or a pneumothorax). The pH range of exudative matter is 7.440–7.300. Many factors can induce local alkalosis and alter the pH levels of the PF, including systemic acidosis, infections with Proteus, and local anesthetics injected into the pleural space. Consequently, the clinical context should always be taken into consideration when interpreting PF pH results. In patients with parapneumonic effusion, a pH value below 7.200 (and/or PF LD greater than three times the upper serum reference limit) suggests the necessity of fluid drainage. In patients with malignant effusions, a pH level below 7.300 indicates a lower prognosis and a less favorable reaction to chemical pleurodesis. Low PF glucose concentration (< 3.4 mmol/L) suggests the presence of malignant disease, tuberculosis, or complicated parapneumonic effusion when PF pH is unavailable.

Triglyceride and cholesterol levels can be measured to aid in the diagnosis of pseudochylothorax and chylothorax. The accumulation of lymph or chyle in the pleural space following a thoracic duct leak—most commonly as a result of trauma, surgery, or cancer—is known as a chylothorax. The buildup of cholesterol, lecithin, and/or globulin-rich fluid in long-term PFs causes a pseudochylothorax. Concentrations of PF triglycerides greater than 1.2 mmol/L are indicative of chylothorax. PF cholesterol levels are typically measured concurrently to rule out the presence of pseudochylothorax. < 5.2 mmol/L are associated with chylothorax. PF triglycerides < 0.6 mmol/L and PF cholesterol >There are 5:1 mmol/L in pseudochylothorax. However, the use of lipoprotein analysis to detect chylomicrons in PF is the gold standard for diagnosing chylothorax.

In clinical practice, PF microscopic examination and PF cultures are typically used in combination to establish the diagnosis of tuberculous pleurisy. It has been reported that the sensitivity of these traditional techniques to diagnose tuberculous pleural effusions is less than 50%. Consequently, a number of biochemical indicators have been suggested to aid in the diagnosis of tuberculous pleurisy. Both adenosine deaminase (ADA) and interferon-γ (IFN-γ) are released during the immune response to mycobacterial antigens in the pleura and have been thoroughly investigated. It has been demonstrated that IFN-γ is a sensitive and specific marker for tuberculous pleural effusion diagnosis. Researchers found that the results showed 89% sensitivity and 97% specificity, respectively. An enzyme called ADA is thought to reflect the activity of immune cells and is involved in the catabolism of purines. It is regarded as a nonspecific indicator of inflammation and is released by activated neutrophils, macrophages, and lymphocytes. With a reported sensitivity of 92% and specificity of 90% at a commonly used cutoff point of 40 U/L, elevated ADA activity in PF is a sensitive and specific marker for the diagnosis of tuberculous pleuritis, especially in high-prevalence areas. Even though both biomarkers have excellent diagnostic performance, ADA is more frequently utilized in clinical practice because it is less expensive and IFN-γ does not have a clear cutoff point. However, results should be interpreted in light of clinical and microbiologic findings, as none of these PF biomarkers is specific for tuberculous pleuritis.

In the context of tuberculous pleural effusions, other biomarkers such as PF neopterin, leptin, lysozyme, interleukine (IL)-6, IL-1β, IL-8, and others have been investigated. Their implementation into standard clinical practice is hindered by their expensive nature and inconsistent diagnostic results. Many scoring systems that use clinical and laboratory data have been proposed to overcome the limitations of individual tests in the differentiation of malignant and tuberculous pleural effusions. They don't seem to do poorly on any one test. Even though cytological examination of suspected malignant PFs is quick and effective in diagnosing cancer, up to 40% of patients may receive falsely negative results. The cytology diagnostic performances are associated with the type of tumor, the tumor burden in the pleural space, and the competency of the cytologist (1). While single PF tumor markers like CYFRA 21-1, CA 125, CA 15-3, and carcinoembryonic antigen (CEA) have been studied as noninvasive methods for pleural malignancy diagnosis, the results obtained are inconsistent, and the low sensitivity limits the utility. Combinations of tumor markers, such as CEA, CA 125, and CYFRA 21-1 or CEA, CA 15-3, CYFRA 21-1, and CA 125, have been investigated in an attempt to increase sensitivity. It was shown that these combinations might be useful adjunctive instruments in the detection of malignant PF, enhancing the diagnostic utility of PF cytology. However, because it is not cost-effective, routinely determining tumor markers in the diagnosis of malignant pleural effusions is not advised. As an alternative diagnostic tool that signals the need for a pleural biopsy, the determination of tumor markers may be useful in cases of suspicious malignant pleural effusion and negative cytological findings, or in the absence of an obvious primary source (Porcel and Light, 2006).

A serum reference range exceeding values or a ratio of PF to serum AMY > 1 indicates high activity of amylase (AMY) in PF. Patients with esophageal rupture, malignant disease, liver cirrhosis, and pancreatic pseudocysts all have elevated PF AMY. If these indicators are absent, the standard measurement of AMY in PFs is useless. A urinothorax can be diagnosed with increased PF creatinine concentrations (PF/serum creatinine ratio > 1). With pronounced urine odor, low glucose concentrations, and low pH, the PF typically exhibits transudative symptoms. Rarely, an effusion can develop from cerebrospinal fluid (CSF) accumulation in the pleural space. Determining the presence of β2-transferrin, which is typically exclusively found in CSF, and the extremely low protein concentration in the PF both point to the presence of CSF. Serum immunological analyses lack additional diagnostic information when performed with PF immunological tests, such as measuring rheumatoid factor (RF) levels or the antinuclear antibody (ANA) titer. TNF-α, procalcitonin, IL-8, IL-6, pleural C-reactive protein, and TNF-α are among the characteristics of PF analysis that distinguish infection from inflammation in the complicated versus non-complicated context. With high sensitivity and specificity for parapneumonic effusion, pleural CRP is elevated in non-malignant exudates relative to malignant ones. Additional research revealed that parapneumonic versus tuberculous or malignant effusions can be distinguished with 100% accuracy using a PF CRP cut-off value of 53 mg/L. Combining IL-8 and CRP measurement can accurately and specifically distinguish between complex and simple parapneumonic effusions (El-Gabalawy and Tanner, 2021).

7.4.3. Peritoneal Effusions

The pathological accumulation of fluid in the peritoneal cavity is called a peritoneal effusion, also known as ascites. Liver cirrhosis, cancer, congestive heart failure, tuberculosis, nephrotic syndrome, pancreatic illness, and dialysis are among the common causes. The possible etiology of ascites formation can be inferred from the history and physical examination. Studies using abdominal radiography, ultrasound, and CT can be used to identify tiny amounts of peritoneal fluid and determine the potential cause of ascites. On the other hand, diagnostic paracentesis, when a patient presents with new-onset ascites, needs to be hospitalized because of ascites, or when there is an unexplained decline in clinical findings, the removal of peritoneal fluid is advised. The quickest and least expensive way to diagnose ascites is through abdominal paracentesis combined with the proper ascitic fluid biochemical analysis.

7.4.3.1. Appearance of Peritoneal Fluid

Ascites is a transparent, straw-colored fluid that typically indicates cirrhosis. If a traumatic tap is not the cause, bloody ascitic fluid may indicate pancreatitis, malignancy, or abdominal trauma. When traumatic taps cause ascitic fluid to appear bloody, the fluid usually clears up and/or clots when left to stand following paracentesis. Abdominal infections are the usual cause of purulent ascites, which is characterized by a rise in polymorphonuclear (PMN) leukocytes. The color of ascitic fluid in cases of complicated hemorrhagic pancreatitis can vary from tea-colored to black. Acute pancreatitis, cholecystitis, and intestinal or gallbladder perforations are the usual causes of bile stained ascites. Because of their high triglyceride content, lymph effusions often present as turbid or milky ascites. A few drops of ether added to chylous ascites can help clear its turbidity. Even though pseudochylous ascites doesn't clear up with ether, it still looks turbid. A black ascites is a characteristic of malignant melanoma.

7.4.3.2. Differentiation of Exudates from Transudates

The first step in the biochemical assessment of ascites, similar to pleural effusion analysis, is to distinguish between transudative and exudative effusions (Figure 7.2). This idea is predicated on the idea that ascites, which are produced when exudate from peritoneal surfaces affected by tumors or inflammatory processes, have elevated protein concentrations. On the other hand, the fluid that results from transudation in systemic conditions like nephrotic syndrome, heart failure, or cirrhosis has low protein concentrations. The ascites protein cut-off, which falls between 25 and 30 g/L, has historically been used to classify ascites as transudative or exudative. Nevertheless, this method produced low sensitivity and a high rate of misclassifications. Moreover, ascites of mixed origin are not addressed. e. caused by something other than portal hypertension, an underlying illness. Furthermore, it was noted that peritoneal fluid protein concentrations in healthy women often exceed 40 g/L, well into the exudative range. Research suggests a modification of the original Light's criteria for the diagnosis of exudative ascites. A lack of reproducibility between studies has prevented the routine application of other biochemical parameters, such as ascitic/serum bilirubin ratio, ascitic cholesterol, and ascitic/serum cholesterol ratio, which have been studied for the purpose of distinguishing between transudative and exudative ascites. Furthermore, a useful model that accurately classified 70% of unknown cases of malignant ascites was studied. This model included measurements of total protein, LD, TNF-α, complement C4, and haptoglobin in ascitic fluid. Though encouraging, these findings require more development in the clinical context prior to being incorporated into standard clinical practice. The classic division of ascites into transudates and exudates has been replaced with the physiologically grounded serum ascites albumin gradient (SAAG) system.

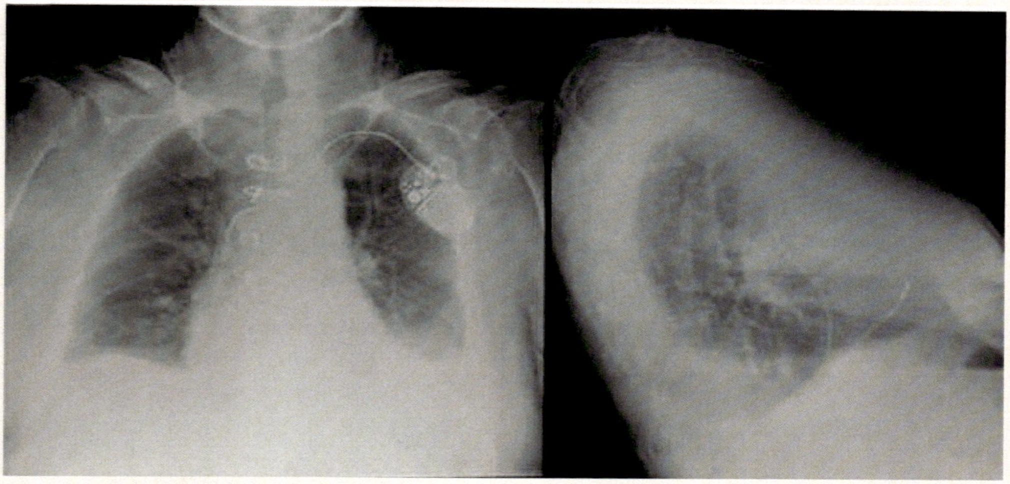

Figure 7.2. *Posteroanterior (PA) and lateral chest radiography demonstrating a left sided pleural effusion.*

Source: Nicholson MJ, Manley C, Ahmad D. Thoracentesis for the Diagnosis and Management of Pleural Effusions: The Current State of a Centuries-Old Procedure. Journal of Respiration. 2023; 3(4):208-222. https://doi.org/10.3390/jor3040020.

It has been shown that the difference in albumin concentration between the serum and ascites is known as SAAG, and it is directly correlated with portal pressure measurements. Accordingly, patients with normal portal pressure are found to have SAAG values < 11 g/L, whereas those with ≥ 11 g/L suggest the presence of portal hypertension. In a sizable prospective investigation, the diagnostic accuracy of ascitic total protein concentration and SAAG in differentiating ascites from portal hypertension was 56% and 97%, respectively. The reasons for this notable discrepancy in accuracy were as follows: ascitic total protein concentrations are directly correlated with serum protein concentrations but indirectly correlated with portal pressure, whereas SAAG directly correlates only with portal pressure. These influencing factors vary in their contribution to the highly variable ascitic total protein concentration in cirrhosis patients. The conventional transudate/exudate concept was replaced with the SAAG concept due to its superiority (McGrath and Anderson, 2001).

It's crucial to be aware of a few methodological problems with albumin measurement. Serum albumin levels of less than 11 g/L should be anticipated in cirrhosis patients. In this instance, method assay range may result in inaccurate SAAG calculation results owing to assay inaccuracy in the low range, or SAAG calculation may not be possible at all. Because of lipid fraction interference, albumin concentrations in cases of chylous ascites may be artificially elevated. Additionally, because globulins influence colloid osmotic pressure and have an inverse relationship with SAAG, hyperglobulinemia (> 50 g/L) can produce a false negative correlation with SAAG values. It's still unknown if the amount of time that passes between ascites and serum samples matters when calculating SAAG.

7.4.3.3. Specific Analyses for Ascites Evaluation

For a more thorough assessment of the etiology of ascites, particular biochemical analyses may prove beneficial following the division of the condition into two main categories (Figure 7.2). The development of spontaneous bacterial peritonitis (SBP) should be monitored in all ascitic fluid samples. The optimal threshold for diagnosing SBP is a PMN leukocyte count in ascitic fluid of at least 250 × 106 / L. Despite not being specific, it is a very sensitive SBP indicator. For the purpose of diagnosing SBP, an ascitic PMN count of ≥ 500 × 106 / L is deemed specific. Without waiting for the results of microbiology tests, all patients with suspected SBP must start antibiotic treatment right away due to the poor prognosis. Leukocyte esterase strip testing was looked into as a potential diagnostic tool for cirrhotic patients with ascites to help shorten the time it takes to diagnose SBP. Comparing urine strip tests to the gold standard, very high sensitivity and specificity were observed.

Furthermore, it has been proposed that the quickness, affordability, and accessibility of urine test strips may help treat SBP patients more effectively, particularly when inflammatory cell clumping occurs in ascitic fluid specimens. The ascites etiology cannot be fully understood by analyzing the amount of glucose present in ascitic fluid. Serum and ascitic fluid glucose concentrations are similar. However, due to leukocyte or bacterial consumption, low glucose has been linked to SBP, carcinomatosis, and tuberculous peritonitis. There is a strong correlation between a decreased ascites protein concentration and a higher risk of SBP development. To diagnose pancreatic ascites, ascitic fluid with AMY activity ≥ 2000 U/L is helpful. Together with leakage into the peritoneum, ruptured pseudocysts, and mesenteric thrombosis, elevated ascitic AMY activity is also observed in these settings. In cases where cytological results are unclear, the diagnostic value of various tumor markers has been assessed for the diagnosis of malignant ascites. Comparing them to comparable analyses in serum, they are typically thought to have minimal clinical significance. When distinguishing ascites from urine, measurements of the concentrations of urea and creatinine in ascitic fluid can be helpful. Urine is present when there is a difference in the concentrations of ascitic fluid urea and creatinine and serum urea and creatinine that are higher than when serum is drawn simultaneously. Rare but dangerous, chylous ascites can result from abdominal surgery, abdominal cancers, inflammatory illnesses, abdominal infections, or trauma. High triglyceride concentration (greater than 2.25

mmol/L or higher than in corresponding serum) is a distinguishing factor between pseudochylous effusions and chylous ascites.

However, the measurement of triglyceride levels in serum and ascites at the same time is required, since the triglyceride concentration in lymphatic fluid is linked to the patient's nutritional status. On the other hand, triglyceride concentrations in ascites greater than 1.2 mmol/L are thought to be indicative of chylous ascites.

An optimal ADA cut off point of ≥ 39 U/L was found in a systematic review that examined the utility of ADA in ascitic fluid as a diagnostic tool in peritoneal tuberculosis, involving 254 patients. With a sensitivity of 100% and specificity of 97%, peritoneal tuberculosis was found to have an exceptional diagnostic efficiency. Other parameters found in ascitic fluid, such as total bilirubin in biliary leak cases, ALP in intestinal obstruction or perforation cases, ammonia in appendix rupture cases, lactic acid in bacterial peritonitis cases, and GGT in patients with alcoholic cirrhosis, may be clinically relevant in certain circumstances.

7.4.4. Pericardial Effusions

The buildup of fluid in the pericardial space as a result of pericarditis or pericardium injury is known as pericardial effusions. Exudative pericardial effusions are caused by pericardial inflammatory, infectious, malignant, or autoimmune processes, whereas transudative effusions are typically linked to heart failure, hypoalbuminemia, post-radiation therapy, and renal insufficiency.

While pericardial effusions can be diagnosed with echocardiography, their etiology cannot be conclusively ascertained with this test. The removal of pericardial fluid, or pericardiocentesis, serves both therapeutic and diagnostic functions.

7.4.4.1. Appearance of Pericardial Fluid

Pale yellow, transparent pericardial fluid is present. An infection or cancer is indicated by turbid fluid. Mucus with blood in it may have a hematologic or malignant cause. Because of chylopericardium, the appearance is milky.

7.4.4.2. Differentiation of Exudative from Transudative Pericardial Effusions

In contrast to the widely accepted biochemical assessment of pleural effusions, there is a dearth of information regarding the diagnostic utility of biochemical tests for the assessment of pericardial fluid. Meyers et al., examined in a retrospective study the accuracy with which different biochemical tests could categorize effusions as transudates or exudates. Fluid LD > 300 U/L, fluid/serum total protein ratio > 0.5, and fluid total protein concentrations > 30 g/L can be used to distinguish between exudative and transudative pericardial effusions. Fluid/serum LD ratio > 0.6 (87%) yielded the best diagnostic accuracy in terms of identifying exudates. It is important to note that retrospective research may produce skewed findings and conclusions, so it is important to interpret these results cautiously. When Light's criteria were used to differentiate between pericardial effusions in a prospective study, the diagnostic efficiency was 94%, and the sensitivity and specificity of the method for identifying exudates were 98% and 72%, respectively. Similar to the differentiation of pleural effusions, it has been reported that patients on diuretic therapy were misclassified from transudative to exudative pericardial fluid when using Light's criteria. When applied to the assessment of pleural effusions, the SEAG concept outperformed Light's criteria in patients taking diuretics, yielding a sensitivity of 90% and specificity of 89% for the identification of pericardial exudates. With a sensitivity of 88% and specificity of 56%, pericardial effusion cholesterol concentrations ≥ 1.2 mmol/L produced an 83% diagnostic efficiency in identifying pericardial exudates. Improved diagnostic results were obtained when the fluid/serum cholesterol ratio was calculated. A cut-off set at 0.3 produced a diagnostic efficiency of 88%, sensitivity of 91%, and specificity of 83%. Still, Ben-Horin et al. examined the physiological pericardial fluid composition in a small group of patients chosen for elective open heart surgery. It was discovered that the concentrations of small molecules i.e., creatinine, urea, uric acid, and glucose) matched those in serum. On the other hand, total protein concentrations were 0.6 of their serum levels, and the pericardial fluid's LD concentration was 2.5 times higher than serum's. It was discovered that the pericardial fluid/serum LD ratio, pericardial fluid LD, and the pericardial fluid/serum total protein ratio did not meet satisfactory standards for discriminatory accuracy. Given these results, care must be taken when applying Light's criteria to the interpretation of pericardial fluid LD and total protein, as pericardial transudates may contain levels of these parameters in the exudative range.

7.4.4.3. Evaluation of Exudative Pericardial Effusions

Particularly in regions with high prevalence, measuring ADA in pericardial effusions has shown to be a quick and reliable method of diagnosing tuberculous pericarditis. The diagnostic utility of ADA measurement in tuberculous pericarditis diagnosis yields 88% sensitivity and 83% specificity at a cut-off value set at 40 U/L. Researchers have looked into using neuron specific enolase and CEA to detect malignant pericardial effusions. The limited number of patients studied limits the diagnostic utility of tumor markers, despite their promising nature.

7.4.5. Preanalytical and Analytical Considerations

The preanalytical phase of recommendations for serous fluid testing is not available, so serous fluid collection, handling, and processing should be done in accordance with the protocols for serum or plasma specimens.

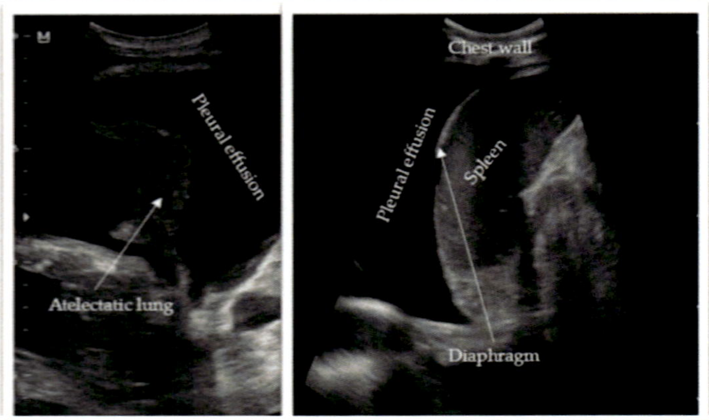

Figure 7.3. *Thoracic ultrasonography demonstrating an anechoic pleural effusion with surrounding structures.*

Source: Nicholson MJ, Manley C, Ahmad D. Thoracentesis for the Diagnosis and Management of Pleural Effusions: The Current State of a Centuries-Old Procedure. Journal of Respiration. 2023; 3(4):208-222. https://doi.org/10.3390/jor3040020.

Samples of serous fluid should be collected, then promptly transported to the laboratory by placing them in the proper containers. Within 30 minutes of serous fluid sampling, serum samples should be obtained for the computation of ratios and gradients (Figure 7.3).

To address the challenges clinical laboratories encounter when analyzing serous fluid, the Clinical and Laboratory Standards Institute (CLSI) created C49-A(Burgess, 2004; Chernecky and Berger, 2013; Blok, 2019; Broaddus, 2022) (Table 7.2)

Table 7.2. Demonstrating the Most Likely Etiologies of Pleural Effusions Based on their Ultrasonographic Appearance

Effusion Type	Anechoic	Complex Non-septated	Complex Septated	Echogenic
Transudative	X	X		
Exudative	X	X	X	X
Hemorrhagic				X

Source: Nicholson MJ, Manley C, Ahmad D. Thoracentesis for the Diagnosis and Management of Pleural Effusions: The Current State of a Centuries-Old Procedure. Journal of Respiration. 2023; 3(4):208-222. https://doi.org/10.3390/jor3040020.

A Closer Look

Functions of the Pericardium

The pericardium is a double-layered sac that encloses the heart and the roots of the great vessels, serving several crucial functions in protecting and supporting the cardiovascular system. Structurally, the pericardium consists of two layers: the fibrous pericardium, which is the outer layer composed of tough, fibrous tissue, and the serous pericardium, which is the inner layer consisting of two sublayers, the parietal and visceral layers. The parietal layer lines the inner surface of the fibrous pericardium, while the visceral layer, also known as the epicardium, covers the surface of the heart.

One of the primary functions of the pericardium is to provide physical protection to the heart. The fibrous pericardium, with its dense and resilient connective tissue, acts as a tough protective barrier that protects the heart from external mechanical forces and trauma. It helps maintain the heart's position within the thoracic cavity, preventing excessive movements that could potentially damage the delicate structures of the heart or its associated blood vessels. Additionally, the pericardium's protective role extends to minimizing friction between the heart and surrounding structures during cardiac contractions, facilitating smooth and efficient cardiac function.

Moreover, the pericardium plays a vital role in maintaining the structural integrity and shape of the heart. By enclosing the heart within a confined space, the pericardium prevents overdistension of the heart chambers, ensuring optimal cardiac function and preventing excessive stretching of the myocardium, which could compromise cardiac performance. Furthermore, the pericardium helps distribute the forces generated during cardiac contractions evenly across the heart's surface, promoting uniform myocardial contraction and relaxation throughout the cardiac cycle.

The pericardium also serves as a lubricated surface that facilitates the heart's movements within the thoracic cavity. The serous pericardium secretes a small amount of serous fluid into the pericardial cavity, forming a thin film that reduces friction between the heart and the surrounding structures, such as the mediastinum and the lungs, during cardiac contractions and movements. This lubricating effect allows the heart to move smoothly within the pericardial sac, minimizing energy expenditure and preventing wear and tear on the heart's surface.

Additionally, the pericardium plays a role in regulating cardiac function by providing a barrier against infections, inflammation, and pathological processes. While the fibrous pericardium offers mechanical protection, the serous pericardium acts as a barrier that limits the spread of infectious agents, inflammatory mediators, or malignant cells to the heart and surrounding structures. It helps maintain the sterile environment of the pericardial cavity, preventing infections such as pericarditis, which can impair cardiac function and lead to serious complications if left untreated.

Summary

- Pleural fluid analysis is the analysis of pleural fluid in the laboratory that occurs after a pleural tap, or thoracentesis. A thoracentesis is a procedure used to drain excess fluid from the space outside of the lungs but inside the chest cavity. Normally, this area contains about 20 milliliters of clear or yellow fluid.
- Pleural fluid is continuously produced by the parietal circulation in the way of bulk flow, while it is also continuously reabsorbed by the lymphatic system via the stomata in the parietal pleura.
- Pleural effusion, also called water on the lung, happens when fluid builds up in the space between your lungs and chest cavity. You may have symptoms, such as chest pain, depending on the cause. Thin membranes, called pleura, cover the outside of the lungs and the inside of the chest cavity.
- Pleural effusions can occur when cancer cells spread to the pleura or block the flow of normal fluid within the pleura. Fluid may also build up due to certain cancer treatments, such as radiation therapy or chemotherapy.
- The pleural fluid is contained in the pleural cavity, which is the space between the internal thoracic wall and the lungs. The pleural cavity is lined by a fibrous mesothelial membrane that is made up of a parietal and visceral layer.
- The fluid functions as a lubricant to allow the two layers of the pleura to glide smoothly past each other during respiration. The pressure of the pleural fluid is subatmospheric and maintains the negative pressure between the lungs and thoracic cavity, which is necessary for inhalation while also preventing the lungs from collapsing.
- Pleural effusions develop when changes in fluid and solute homeostasis occur, and the mechanism causing these changes determines whether it will be an exudative (high protein content) or transudative (low protein content) effusion.
- Diagnosis of the etiology is essential, as the treatments for exudative and transudative etiologies differ significantly. Exudative effusions almost always require a further investigative workup, which may include cytopathology studies, biopsy, or even an emergent thoracotomy
- Peritoneal fluid is a liquid that acts as a lubricant in the abdominal cavity. It is found in small quantities (generally 5-20 mL) between the layers of the peritoneum that line the abdominal wall. Peritoneal fluid acts to moisten the outside of the organs and to reduce the friction of organ movement during digestion and movement.

References

1. Blok, B. K. (2019). Thoracentesis. In J. R. Roberts, C. B. Custalow, & T. W. Thomsen (Eds.), Roberts & Hedges' *Clinical Procedures in Emergency Medicine and Acute Care* (7th ed., chap. 9). Philadelphia, PA: Elsevier.

2. Broaddus, V. C., & Light, R. W. (2022). Pleural effusion. In V. C. Broaddus, J. D. Ernst, T. E. King, et al. (Eds.), *Murray and Nadel's Textbook of Respiratory Medicine* (7th ed., chap. 108). Philadelphia, PA: Elsevier.
3. Burgess, L. J. (2004). Biochemical analysis of pleural, peritoneal and pericardial effusions. *Clinical Chimica. Acta., 343*, 61–84. http://dx.doi.org/10.1016/j.cccn.2004.02.002 (accessed on 21 May 2024).
4. Chernecky, C. C., & Berger, B. J. (2013). Paracentesis (peritoneal fluid analysis) - diagnostic. In C. C. Chernecky & B. J. Berger (Eds.), *Laboratory Tests and Diagnostic Procedures* (6th ed., pp. 849–851). St. Louis, MO: Elsevier Saunders.
5. Ferraz Maranhao, B. H., da Silva Junior, C. T., da Silva Chibante, A. M., & Perez Cardoso, G. (2010). Determination of total proteins and lactate dehydrogenase for the diagnosis of pleural transudates and exudates: redefining the classical criterion with a new statistical approach. *Jornal. Brasileiro. de Pneumologia., 36*, 468–474.
6. Hamm, H., Brohan, U., Bohmer, R., & Missmahl, H. P. (1987). Cholesterol in pleural effusions. *Chest, 92*, 296–302. http://dx.doi.org/10.1378/chest.92.2.296 (accessed on 21 May 2024).
7. Hassan, T., Al-Alawi, M., Chotirmall, S. H., & McElvaney, N. G. (2012). Pleural fluid analysis: standstill or a work in progress? *Pulmonary Medicine, 2012*, Article ID 716235.
8. Kwo, P. Y. (2018). Clinical features of liver disease. In R. Saxena (Ed.), *Practical Hepatic Pathology: A Diagnostic Approach* (2nd ed., chap. 2). Philadelphia, PA: Elsevier.
9. Light, R. W. (2002). Pleural effusion. *New England Journal of Medicine, 346*, 1971–1977. http://dx.doi.org/10.1056/NEJMcp010731 (accessed on 21 May 2024).
10. Light, R. W. (2011). Pleural effusions. *Medical Clinics of North America, 95*, 1055–1070. http://dx.doi.org/10.1016/j.mcna.2011.08.005 (accessed on 21 May 2024).
11. McGrath, E. E., & Anderson, P. B. (2011). Diagnosis of pleural effusion: a systematic approach. *American Journal of Critical Care, 20*, 119–128. http://dx.doi.org/10.4037/ajcc2011685 (accessed on 21 May 2024).
12. Mehta, S., & Fallon, M. B. (2022). Cirrhosis of the liver and its complications. In E. J. Wing & F. J. Schiffman (Eds.), *Cecil Essentials of Medicine* (10th ed., chap. 44). Philadelphia, PA: Elsevier.
13. Percy, A. (2021). Procedures. In K. Kleinman, L. Mcdaniel, & M. Molloy (Eds.), *The Harriet Lane Handbook* (22nd ed., chap. 4). Philadelphia, PA: Elsevier.
14. Porcel, J. M., & Light, R. W. (2006). Diagnostic approach to pleural effusion in adults. *American Family Physicians, 73*, 1211–1220.
15. Romero-Candeira, S., Hernandez, L., Romero-Brufao, S., Orts, D., Fernandez, C., & Martin, C. (2002). Is it meaningful to use biochemical parameters to discriminate between transudative and exudative pleural effusions? *Chest, 122*, 1524–1529. http://dx.doi.org/10.1378/chest.122.5.1524 (accessed on 21 May 2024).
16. Romero, S., Candela, A., Martin, C., Hernandez, L., Trigo, C., & Gil, J. (1993). Evaluation of different criteria for the separation of pleural transudates from exudates. *Chest, 104*, 399–404. http://dx.doi.org/10.1378/chest.104.2.399 (accessed on 21 May 2024).
17. Roth, B. J., O'Meara, T. F., & Hal Cragun, W. (1990). The serum-effusion albumin gradient in the evaluation of pleural effusions. *Chest, 98*, 546–549. http://dx.doi.org/10.1378/chest.98.3.546 (accessed on 21 May 2024).

18. Segura, R. M. (2004). Useful clinical biological markers in diagnosis of pleural effusions in children. *Paediatric Respiratory Reviews, 5*(Suppl A), S205–S212. http://dx.doi.org/10.1016/S1526-0542(04)90039-5 (accessed on 21 May 2024).

19. Tarn, A. C., & Lapworth, R. (2001). Biochemical analysis of pleural fluid: what should we measure? *Annals of Clinical Biochemistry, 38*, 311–322. http://dx.doi.org/10.1258/0004563011900812 (accessed on 21 May 2024).

Chapter 8

SYNOVIAL FLUID ANALYSIS

Contents

Introduction

A diagnostic technique called synovial fluid analysis is used to evaluate the condition of the joints, mainly in cases of joint-related illnesses like gout, infection, and arthritis. This fluid, which is present in the cavities of synovial joints, is essential for providing the cartilage with nutrition, shock absorption, and lubrication. Its composition analysis helps formulate a suitable treatment plan and offers important insights into the underlying pathology. Assessing the presence of inflammation in the joint is one of the main goals of synovial fluid analysis. Increases in the quantity of leukocytes, or white blood cells, in the synovial fluid are frequently the outcome of inflammatory diseases such as rheumatoid arthritis. White blood cells called neutrophils are especially suggestive of acute inflammation, whereas lymphocytes might point to a chronic inflammatory process. The presence of these cells aids in the diagnosis of the particular form of arthritis and aids in the tracking of disease activity over time, as does the evaluation of their quantity and morphology. Evaluating the viscosity and clarity of the synovial fluid is another important part of the analysis process. Similar to egg whites, healthy synovial fluid is clear and viscous. A hazy appearance could be a sign of an infectious or inflammatory process if it contains bacteria, cells, or other debris. Microscopic examination may confirm the diagnosis of crystal-induced arthritis, including pseudogout and gout, by revealing the presence of distinctive crystals in the synovial fluid.

Additional diagnostic information is provided by synovial fluid biochemical analysis. Moreover, synovial fluid analysis helps rule out other possible causes of joint pain, like joint trauma or bleeding. Visually or through laboratory testing, the presence of blood in the synovial fluid may indicate hemorrhagic conditions such as hemarthrosis or traumatic injury.

Orientation and Directional Terms

Term	Definition	Illustration
Morphology	Morphology is the study of words, including the principles by which they are formed, and how they relate to one another within a language.	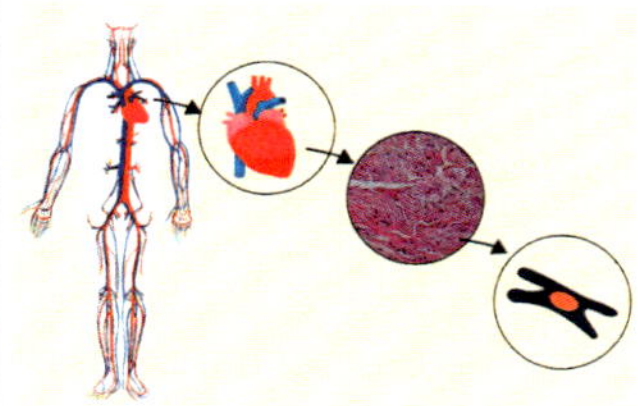
Hemarthrosis	Hemarthrosis is a condition of articular bleeding, that is into the joint cavity.	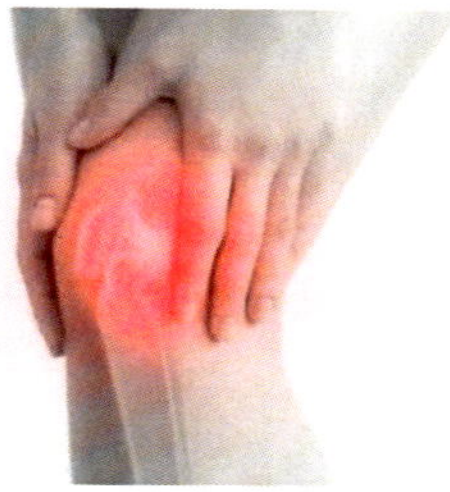
Arthrocentesis	Arthrocentesis, is the clinical procedure performed to diagnose and, in some cases, treat musculoskeletal conditions.	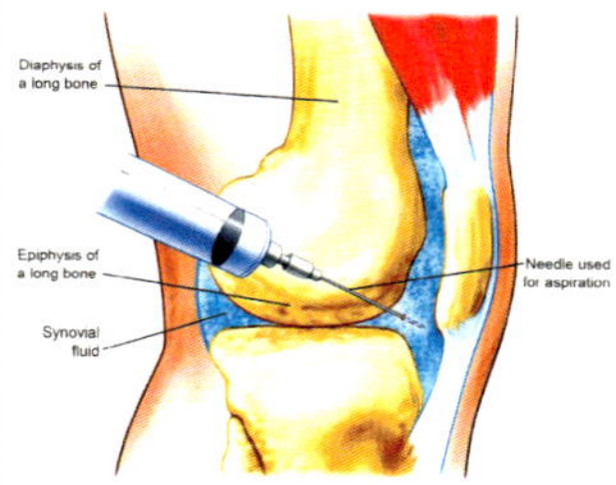
Clopidogrel	Clopidogrel is an antiplatelet medicine. It prevents platelets (a type of blood cell) from sticking together and forming a dangerous blood clot.	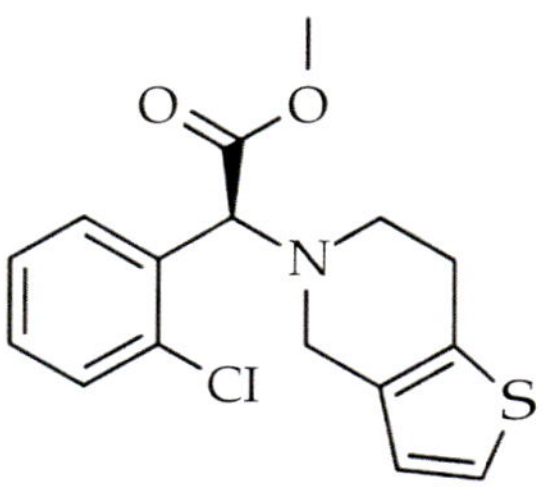
Rheopectic	Rheopecty is the rare property of some non-Newtonian fluids to show a time-dependent change in viscosity; the longer the fluid undergoes shear, the higher its viscosity.	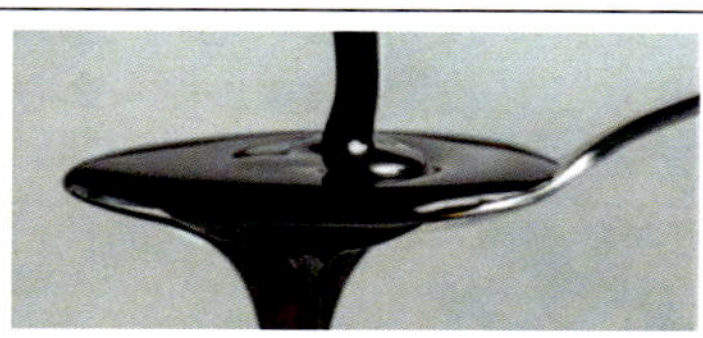

8.1. Overview of Synovial Fluid Analysis

In the cavities of synovial joints, there is a viscous, non-Newtonian fluid known as synovial fluid, or synovia. The main function of synovial fluid, which has a consistency similar to egg white, is to lessen friction that develops between the articular cartilage of synovial joints when an object moves. A tiny portion of the transcellular fluid, which makes up extracellular fluid, is synovial fluid.

Synovial fluid analysis typically involves the following components:

1. **Clinical Evaluation:** Analysis of synovial fluid is frequently carried out in tandem with a comprehensive clinical evaluation that includes a physical examination and a medical history. Interpreting synovial fluid analysis results and directing additional diagnostic and therapeutic interventions depend on clinical findings such as range of motion, stiffness, swelling, and joint pain.
2. **Arthrocentesis:** The initial stage of synovial fluid analysis is aspirating synovial fluid using arthrocentesis, a minimally invasive technique that involves inserting a needle into the joint cavity. Arthrocentesis is usually guided by imaging methods like fluoroscopy or ultrasound and can be carried out in a sterile environment under local anesthesia.
3. **Synovial Fluid Appearance:** The appearance of synovial fluid is examined visually after arthrocentesis. Normal synovial fluid has an egg white-like viscosity and is clear and colorless. Modifications in the appearance of synovial fluid, such as turbidity, cloudiness, or blood presence, may point to an infection or underlying joint pathology.
4. **Synovial Fluid Analysis:** The collected synovial fluid is then sent to the laboratory for analysis. Synovial fluid analysis includes several components:
   - i. **Cell Count and Differential:** The total white blood cell (WBC) count and differential count (percentage of different types of white blood cells) are performed to assess the degree of inflammation within the joint. An elevated WBC count, particularly neutrophils, suggests active inflammation or infection.
   - ii. **Microscopic Examination:** Synovial fluid is examined under a microscope to detect the presence of crystals (e.g., urate crystals in gout, calcium pyrophosphate crystals in pseudogout), which may indicate crystal-induced arthritis.
   - iii. **Biochemical Analysis:** Biochemical tests measure various components of synovial fluid, including protein, glucose, lactate, and uric acid levels. Abnormalities in these parameters can provide additional diagnostic information and aid in distinguishing between different types of joint disorders.
   - iv. **Microbiological Culture:** Synovial fluid is cultured

to identify the causative organism in cases of suspected infectious arthritis. Bacterial, fungal, and viral cultures are performed to isolate and identify pathogens, guiding antimicrobial therapy.

5. **Interpretation and Diagnosis:** The patient's clinical presentation and additional diagnostic findings are taken into consideration when interpreting the synovial fluid analysis results. Analysis of synovial fluid aids in diagnosis, distinguishes between different joint disorders (e.g., infectious arthritis, crystal-induced arthritis), determine the degree of the illness, and direct the course of treatment.

8.1.1. Purpose of Synovial Fluid Analysis

A synovial fluid analysis may be ordered to diagnose or rule out the following conditions:

- **Autoimmune Disorders:** In some autoimmune disorders, including rheumatoid arthritis, lupus, and psoriatic arthritis, the immune system damages healthy tissues of the joints.
- **Septic Arthritis:** Septic arthritis is an infection caused by microbes such as bacteria or fungi that lead to acute inflammation in one or more joints.
- **Goutor Pseudogout:** Gout and pseudogout are painful forms of arthritis, caused by the accumulation of uric acid or calcium crystals in the joint.
- **Bleeding in the Joint:** Also called hemarthrosis, an accumulation of blood in the joint can be caused by an injury to the joint, cancer, hemophilia, and other health conditions.

Changes in the volume and composition of synovial fluid can be attributed to bacterial, fungal, or viral penetration, inflammation, or trauma. It is essential to aspirate and analyze synovial fluid when patients present with acutely painful joints and have suspicions of infection, inflammation, or non-inflammatory causes of effusion. This will help with diagnosis and direct the course of treatment.

8.1.1.1. What Does the Test Measure?

A synovial fluid analysis may involve a number of tests conducted on the fluid that has been removed from the joint. Three general categories can be used to group the tests performed as part of the synovial fluid analysis: microscopic assessment, chemical analysis, and gross assessment.

A physician's examination of synovial fluid for qualities like volume, clarity, color, and viscosity is referred to as a gross assessment of synovial fluid.

Chemical assessment of synovial fluid often includes the following tests:

Chemical Analysis of Synovial Fluid		
Test Name	**What It Measures**	**Why**
Glucose Testing	The amount of glucose	Glucose levels are lower in certain conditions, including autoimmune disorders or septic arthritis.

Lactate	The amount of lactate	High levels of lactate are associated with infection.
Total Protein	The amount of protein	Elevated protein concentration can indicate an inflammatory or bleeding disorder.
Uric Acid Testing	The amount of uric acid	The presence of uric acid indicates gout.

Several tests are performed as part of a microscopic assessment of synovial fluid to further assess a patient's symptoms. A crystal analysis, which is a microscopic evaluation, looks for crystals in the synovial fluid under a microscope equipped with a particular filter. If crystals are found in the synovial fluid, the makeup and structure of the crystals can support specific diagnoses further. The additional tests carried out as part of a microscopic evaluation differ based on the suspected reason behind a patient's symptoms.

The microscopic assessment of synovial fluid routinely includes the following tests:

Microscopic Assessment of Synovial Fluid		
Test Name	**What It Measures**	**Why**
White Blood Cell (WBC) Count and Differential	Presence and type of WBCs	WBC levels become elevated in response to infections, septic arthritis, gout, and pseudogout.
Gram Stain	Presence and type of microbes	Positive Gram stains can help diagnose septic arthritis and infection.
Bacterial Culture	Presence and type of microbes	The presence of certain microbes may indicate infection.

8.2. Features of Synovial Fluid

The synovial membrane, which lines the inside of synovial joints, secretes synovial fluid into the joint cavity. Synovial fluid is an ultrafiltrate of plasma that is composed of both blood plasma-derived proteins and proteins produced by joint tissue cells. The fluid includes lubricin (proteoglycan 4; PRG4) secreted by the surface chondrocytes of the articular cartilage, hyaluronan secreted by fibroblast-like cells in the synovial membrane, and interstitial fluid filtered from blood plasma. This fluid fills all empty spaces in the articular cartilage surface by seeping into microcavities and irregularities and forming a thin layer (approximately 50μm) at the surface. Articular cartilage fluid functions as a synovial fluid reserve in an efficient manner. To keep a layer of fluid on the cartilage surface during movement, the synovial fluid inside the cartilage is mechanically squeezed out (also known as "weeping lubrication").

The functions of the synovial fluid include:

- reduction of friction — synovial fluid lubricates the articulating joints
- shock absorption — as a dilatant fluid, that possesses rheopectic properties, becoming more viscous under applied pressure; the synovial fluid in diarthrotic joints becomes thick the moment shear is applied to protect the joint and subsequently, thins to

normal viscosity instantaneously to resume its lubricating function between shocks.

- nutrient and waste transportation — the fluid supplies oxygen and nutrients and removes carbon dioxide and metabolic wastes from the chondrocytes in the surrounding cartilage
- molecular sieving - pressure within the joint forces hyaluronan in the fluid against the synovial membrane forming a barrier against cells migrating into, or fluid migrating out of, the joint space. This function is dependent on the molecular weight of the hyaluronan.

A viscous, transparent, colorless fluid called synovial fluid fills the joint cavity, nourishing and lubricating the articular cartilage and enabling easy joint movement. Water, electrolytes, proteins, and other molecules make up its complex composition, which helps it to have lubricating and shock-absorbing qualities.

The structure of synovial fluid is characterized by its components and their functions:

1. **Water:** The primary component of synovial fluid is water, which accounts for approximately 80-90% of its volume. Water provides lubrication and hydration to the articular surfaces, reducing friction and allowing for smooth movement within the joint.
2. **Hyaluronic Acid (HA):** Hyaluronic acid is a high molecular weight glycosaminoglycan that gives synovial fluid its viscous and elastic properties. It forms a gel-like matrix within the synovial fluid, providing lubrication and shock absorption, as well as contributing to the viscoelasticity of the joint.
3. **Proteoglycans:** Proteoglycans are large protein molecules bound to glycosaminoglycan chains, including hyaluronic acid. They help maintain the structural integrity of the synovial fluid and contribute to its lubricating properties by attracting and retaining water molecules within the joint cavity.
4. **Albumin and Globulins:** Synovial fluid contains various proteins, including albumin and globulins, which play roles in maintaining osmotic balance, transporting nutrients, and modulating immune responses within the joint. These proteins also contribute to the viscosity and lubricating properties of synovial fluid.
5. **Cytokines and Growth Factors:** Synovial fluid contains a variety of cytokines, growth factors, and other signaling molecules that regulate inflammation, tissue repair, and homeostasis within the joint. These molecules help coordinate the immune response to injury or infection and modulate the activity of cells involved in joint maintenance and repair.
6. **Lipids:** Synovial fluid contains small amounts of lipids, including phospholipids and fatty acids, which contribute to the lubrication of articular surfaces and help maintain the integrity of the synovial membrane.
7. **Electrolytes:** Synovial fluid contains electrolytes such as sodium, potassium, chloride, and calcium,

which help maintain osmotic balance, pH, and fluid composition within the joint cavity.

The dynamic structure of synovial fluid is impacted by a number of variables, such as age, joint health, and the presence of disease. The lubricating and shock-absorbing qualities of synovial fluid can change as a result of modifications in its composition and structure brought on by injury, inflammation, or disease processes. Comprehending the composition and structure of synovial fluid is crucial in clarifying its function in joint pathology and health, as well as in creating interventions to cure disorders related to joints.

8.2.1. Composition

The vascularized connective tissue that makes up synovial tissue is sterile and does not have a basement membrane. There are two different cell types: type A and type B. Type A is derived from blood monocytes and its function is to clear the synovial fluid of wear-and-tear debris. Hyaluronan is produced by type B. Hyaluronic acid, lubricin, collagenases, and proteinases make up synovial fluid. The viscosity coefficient is not a constant and the fluid is not linearly viscous, indicating non-Newtonian flow characteristics in synovial fluid. Due to its anti-thixotropic properties, synovial fluid becomes more viscous quickly in response to sudden pressure increases, such as those caused by mechanical shocks. Hyaluronic acid, or hyaluronan, is a polymer of disaccharides consisting of D-glucuronic acid and D-N-acetylglucosamine connected by alternating beta-1,4 and beta-1,3 glycosidic bonds that is found in normal synovial fluid at a concentration of 3-5 mg/ml. The synovial membrane produces hyaluronan, which is then secreted into the joint cavity to lubricate the surfaces between the synovium and cartilage and to increase the viscosity and elasticity of articular cartilages.

Lubricin, also called PRG4, is a second lubricating substance secreted by synovial fibroblasts and found in synovial fluid. It is primarily in charge of the so-called boundary-layer lubrication, which lessens friction between the opposing cartilage surfaces. Additionally, there is some evidence that it controls the growth of synovial cells. Phagocytic cells are also present, which eliminate bacteria and debris resulting from typical joint wear and tear.

8.2.2. Clinical Significance

- **Collection:** Synovial fluid may be collected by syringe in a procedure termed arthrocentesis, also known as joint aspiration.
- **Classification:** Synovial fluid may be classified into normal, noninflammatory, inflammatory, septic, and hemorrhagic:

Classification of Synovial Fluid in an Adult Knee Joint					
	Normal	**Non-inflammatory**	**Inflammatory**	**Septic**	**Bleeding**
Volume (ml)	<3.5	>3.5	>3.5	>3.5	>3.5
Viscosity	High	High	Low	Mixed	Low
Clarity	Clear	Clear	Cloudy	Opaque	Mixed
Color	Colorless/straw	Straw/yellow	Yellow	Mixed	Red

WBC/mm^3	<200	<2,000	5,000-75,000	>50,000	Similar to blood level
Polys (%)	<25	<25	50-70	>70	Similar to blood level
Gram stain	None	None	None	+ (S aureus & Streptococcus) - (Neisseria gonorrhoeae)	None

Glucose (mg/dl) concentration in synovial fluid is nearly equal to serum.

Source: https://en.wikipedia.org/wiki/Synovial_fluid.

- **Synovial Fluid Viscosity**
  - o Normal
    - § Traumatic arthritis
    - § Degenerative (Osteo) arthritis
    - § Pigmented villonodular synovitis
  - o Normal or Decreased:
    - § Systemic lupus erythematosus
  - o Decreased:
    - § Rheumatic fever
    - § Rheumatoid arthritis
    - § Gout
    - § Pyogenic (Septic) arthritis
    - § Tubercular arthritis
    - § Less of lubrication in joints
- **Pathology**

  Many synovial fluid types are associated with specific diagnoses:
  - o Noninflammatory (Group I)
    - § Osteoarthritis, degenerative joint disease
    - § Trauma
    - § Rheumatic fever
    - § Chronic gout or pseudogout
    - § Scleroderma
    - § Polymyositis
- Systemic lupus erythematosus
    - § Erythema nodosum
    - § Neuropathic arthropathy (with possible hemorrhage)
    - § Sickle-cell disease
    - § Hemochromatosis
    - § Acromegaly
    - § Amyloidosis
  - o Inflammatory (Group II)
    - § Rheumatoid arthritis
    - § Reactive arthritis
    - § Psoriatic arthritis
    - § Acute rheumatic fever
    - § Acute gout or pseudogout
    - § Scleroderma
    - § Polymyositis
    - § Systemic lupus erythematosus
    - § Ankylosing spondylitis
    - § Inflammatory bowel disease arthritis
    - § Infection (viral, fungal, bacterial) including Lyme disease
    - § Acute crystal synovitis (gout)
  - o Septic (Group III)
    - § Pyogenic bacterial infection
    - § Septic arthritis

- o Hemorrhagic
  - § Trauma
  - § Tumors
  - § Hemophilia/coagulopathy
  - § Scurvy
  - § Ehlers-Danlos syndrome
  - § Neuropathic arthropathy

8.2.3. Analysis

The concentration of glucose (mg/dl) in synovial fluid is almost the same as that of serum. Around 1940, cadaver-derived fluid was used to analyze the cytology and biochemistry of human synovial fluid by comparing its properties to those of other synovial fluids, such as that of cows.

- **Chemistry:** An antiquated method for figuring out whether there is an inflammatory infiltrate is the mucin clot test. Acetic acid is added to the synovial fluid specimen for this test. This should cause the hyaluronic acid to congeal and form a "mucin clot" in a healthy specimen. A mucin clot does not form when inflammation is present because the hyaluronic acid is broken down. In septic arthritis, lactate levels are elevated and typically exceed 250 mg/dL. In lupus and rheumatoid arthritis, complement factors are reduced.
- **Microscopy:** The synovial fluid is examined under a microscope to check for crystals and cell count. Crystals include calcium pyrophosphate, hydroxyapatite, corticosteroid, and monosodium urate crystals. When gout or gouty arthritis occurs, monosodium urate crystals can be seen. They are needle-shaped, negatively birefringent crystals that range in length from 2 to 20μm. The crystals exhibit negative birefringence, making them appear blue in perpendicular light and yellow in parallel light.

  Pseudogout, also called calcium pyrophosphate deposition disease, or CPPD, is characterized by the presence of calcium pyrophosphate crystals. These crystals are rhomboids or rod-shaped, with lengths ranging from 2 to 20μm and positive birefringence (yellow under perpendicular light, blue under parallel light). Crystals of hydroxyapatite are tiny and negatively birefringent. They are typically only visible when stained with Alizarin Red S. After a therapeutic corticosteroid injection into the joint space, corticosteroid crystals may be observed. They have a jagged, blunt appearance with varying birefringence.
- **Cracking Joints:** A synovial joint experiences a negative pressure and an increase in joint capsule volume when its two articulating surfaces separate from one another. Because there is not enough synovial fluid in the joint to completely fill its expanding volume, gases that are dissolved in it—mostly carbon dioxide—are released and swiftly fill the empty space, causing a bubble to form very quickly. We call this process cavitation. Synovial joint cavitation produces a high-frequency "cracking" sound.

8.2.4. Etymology and Pronunciation

The term *synovia* came to English around 1640 (the anglicized form *synovial* is first recorded in the mid 18th century) from Neo-Latin, where it was coined perhaps by Paracelsus from Greek *συν-* "with" and Latin *ovum* "egg" and *-ia* because it resembles egg white in consistency and external appearance.

The synovial membrane is more accurately referred to as the less confusing term synovium, which is a much more recent pseudo-Latin coinage. Its etymology is not explained by medical dictionaries, and neither do general dictionaries record it. However, it appears to be derived from the term synovia, i.e., The term synovia was mistakenly reinterpreted as the plural of the previously nonexistent term synovium due to its obfuscated etymology, which included mixed Greek and Latin elements. This may have been done in analogy with other plural terms for liquids, such as waters for amniotic fluid. The non-Latinate plural synoviums is preferable to the pseudo-Latin term synovia if one is determined to use it for the synovial membrane.

8.3. Infectious (Septic) Arthritis

Septic arthritis, another name for infectious arthritis, is a serious joint infection that is caused by pathogens invading the synovial space. This invasion can result in swelling, pain, inflammation, and possibly irreversible joint damage. All ages can be affected by septic arthritis, although immunocompromised patients, the elderly, and newborns are more likely to experience it. Early diagnosis and treatment are crucial to avoiding systemic infection and long-term joint problems.

Septic arthritis is most frequently caused by bacterial pathogens, with adult Streptococcus species and Gram-negative bacteria trailing behind Staphylococcus aureus as the most common organism. Gram-negative bacteria like *Escherichia coli* and Group B *Streptococcus* are commonly linked to infections in children, particularly in newborns. The bacteria can enter the joint by contiguous spread from nearby tissues, hematogenous spread from far-off infection sites, or direct inoculation after trauma or surgery.

Acute joint pain, swelling, erythema, and restricted range of motion are the hallmarks of septic arthritis's clinical presentation. These symptoms are frequently accompanied by systemic infection symptoms like fever, chills, and malaise. Usually, when the affected joint is palpated, it feels tender and warm to the touch. Septic arthritis in babies can manifest as vague symptoms like irritability, inability to bear weight, or fever without apparent cause.

Imaging studies, laboratory testing, and clinical evaluations are all used in the diagnosis of septic arthritis. An essential diagnostic procedure is synovial fluid analysis, which is done via arthrocentesis to collect synovial fluid for analysis. To determine the pathogen causing the inflammation, the synovial fluid is analyzed using cell count, differential, Gram stain, and culture. Analysis of synovial fluid from septic arthritis usually shows positive cultures for the pathogen and increased white blood cell counts, mostly neutrophils. To evaluate for joint effusion, soft tissue swelling, and evidence of bony erosions or joint space narrowing, imaging studies such as plain radiographs, ultrasounds, or magnetic resonance imaging (MRI) may be used. These findings may suggest underlying joint damage and help with treatment planning.

Empirical antibiotic therapy against suspected pathogens must be started as soon as possible to treat septic arthritis. Then, based on culture and sensitivity results, the therapy must be customized. Depending on the results of culture, empirical therapy frequently consists of broad-spectrum antibiotics that are effective against Streptococcus species and Staphylococcus aureus. Antifungal or antimycobacterial medications may be recommended in cases of suspected fungal or mycobacterial arthritis. To remove purulent material and lessen the bacterial burden within the joint, joint drainage techniques like arthrocentesis or surgical irrigation and debridement may be required in addition to antibiotics. If left untreated, septic arthritis can cause severe joint damage, systemic consequences like sepsis or bacteremia, and permanent functional impairment. Therefore, to maximize results and avoid irreversible joint damage in patients with septic arthritis, early recognition, prompt diagnosis, and aggressive management are crucial. Rehab and physical therapy are essential in restoring joint function and mobility, and long-term follow-up is frequently required to monitor for recurrent infections, joint instability, and functional limitations.

An infection in a joint results in infectious arthritis. Another name for it is septic arthritis. It happens when a joint or the fluid around a joint becomes infected due to a bacterial or viral infection. We refer to this fluid as synovial fluid. Usually, this infection starts in another part of the body and travels to the joint tissue through the bloodstream. Injections, open wounds, and surgery are other possible entry points for the infection into the body. Usually, infectious arthritis affects just one joint. The disease usually affects a large joint, like the shoulder, hip, or knee. It happens more frequently in young people, the elderly, and drug addicts.

8.3.1. Symptoms of Infectious Arthritis

The symptoms of infectious arthritis can vary depending on your age and the medications you're taking. The symptoms may include:

- severe pain that worsens with movement
- swelling of the joint
- warmth and redness around the joint
- a fever
- chills
- fatigue
- weakness
- decreased appetite
- a rapid heart rate
- irritability

Septic arthritis, another name for infectious arthritis, manifests as a variety of symptoms that indicate joint infection and inflammation. Depending on the causative pathogen, age of the patient, and underlying medical conditions, the clinical presentation may differ.

However, common symptoms of infectious arthritis include:

1. **Joint Pain:** The hallmark symptom of infectious arthritis is severe joint pain, which is often sudden in onset and may worsen with movement or weight-bearing. The pain is typically localized to the affected joint and may be accompanied by tenderness to touch.
2. **Joint Swelling:** Inflammation of the synovial membrane leads to joint swelling, causing the affected joint to appear enlarged, red, and warm to the touch. The swelling is often accompanied by a feeling of fullness or tightness in the joint.
3. **Limited Range of Motion:** Joint inflammation and swelling can

restrict the normal range of motion, leading to stiffness and difficulty moving the affected joint. Patients may experience decreased flexibility and find it challenging to perform activities of daily living.

4. **Fever:** Systemic symptoms such as fever, chills, and malaise are common in infectious arthritis and may indicate systemic spread of infection. Fever is often present in cases of bacterial arthritis and may be accompanied by other signs of systemic inflammation.
5. **Localized Symptoms:** In addition to joint-related symptoms, patients with infectious arthritis may experience localized symptoms such as warmth, redness, and tenderness over the affected joint. These symptoms are indicative of inflammation and may be more pronounced in acute cases.
6. **Systemic Symptoms:** In severe cases or when the infection spreads beyond the joint, patients may experience systemic symptoms such as fatigue, weakness, and loss of appetite. These symptoms suggest a more widespread infection and may require urgent medical attention.
7. **Joint Dysfunction:** If left untreated, infectious arthritis can lead to joint dysfunction and permanent damage, resulting in chronic pain, deformity, and functional impairment. Timely diagnosis and management are essential to prevent long-term complications and preserve joint function.

It's crucial to remember that diagnosing infectious arthritis can be difficult because its symptoms can mimic those of other joint conditions. To confirm the diagnosis and direct the proper course of treatment, a comprehensive clinical evaluation that includes a history, physical examination, and diagnostic tests like synovial fluid analysis, imaging studies, and blood tests is required. Early diagnosis and treatment of infectious arthritis are essential to avoid long-term disability, systemic complications, and joint damage.

8.3.2. Risk Factors for Infectious Arthritis

Certain people are more likely to get infectious arthritis than others. The risk factors include:

- having joint problems such as arthritis, gout, or lupus
- having a history of joint surgery
- having certain skin conditions
- having open wounds
- abusing illegal drugs or alcohol
- taking drugs that suppress the immune system
- having a weakened immune system
- having cancer
- smoking
- having diabetes

Although infectious arthritis, also referred to as septic arthritis, can affect people of any age, it is more frequently seen in particular groups of people and in particular situations.

Several risk factors increase the likelihood of developing infectious arthritis:

1. **Immunocompromised Conditions:** Individuals with weakened immune systems due to conditions such as HIV/AIDS, cancer undergoing chemotherapy, diabetes mellitus, chronic kidney disease, or

autoimmune disorders are at increased risk of developing infectious arthritis. Impaired immune function reduces the body's ability to fight off infections, making it more susceptible to joint infections.

2. **Joint Trauma or Surgery:** Trauma to a joint, such as a fracture, dislocation, or penetrating injury, increases the risk of bacterial entry into the joint space, leading to infectious arthritis. Similarly, invasive joint procedures or surgeries, including arthroscopy, joint replacement surgery, or intra-articular injections, can introduce pathogens into the joint and predispose to infection.
3. **Age:** Infectious arthritis can affect individuals of all ages, but certain age groups are at higher risk. In infants and young children, particularly those under one year of age, the risk of septic arthritis is increased due to the immaturity of their immune systems and higher susceptibility to infections. In older adults, age-related changes in joint structure and function, along with comorbidities such as diabetes and immunosenescence, can predispose to joint infections.
4. **Preexisting Joint Conditions:** Chronic joint diseases such as rheumatoid arthritis, osteoarthritis, gout, or previous joint trauma increase the risk of developing infectious arthritis. Inflammation, joint damage, and alterations in the synovial membrane associated with these conditions provide a favorable environment for bacterial colonization and invasion.
5. **Intravenous Drug Use:** Individuals who inject drugs intravenously are at increased risk of developing infectious arthritis, particularly from bacteria such as Staphylococcus aureus or Streptococcus species. Contaminated needles and skin flora can introduce pathogens into the bloodstream, leading to hematogenous spread and joint infection.
6. **Skin Infections or Wounds:** Skin infections such as cellulitis, abscesses, or open wounds increase the risk of bacterial dissemination into the bloodstream and subsequent joint infection. Bacteria can enter the joint through breaks in the skin, resulting in localized joint inflammation and septic arthritis.
7. **Prosthetic Joints:** Individuals with prosthetic joints, such as total hip or knee replacements, are at increased risk of developing prosthetic joint infections (PJI) leading to septic arthritis. Bacteria can adhere to the prosthetic surface and form biofilms, making them resistant to host defenses and antimicrobial therapy.
8. **Underlying Medical Conditions:** Certain medical conditions such as obesity, peripheral vascular disease, chronic kidney disease, and cirrhosis are associated with impaired wound healing, vascular insufficiency, and increased susceptibility to infections, predisposing to infectious arthritis.
9. **Hematologic Disorders:** Conditions that affect the blood, such as sickle

cell disease or hemophilia, can increase the risk of septic arthritis due to impaired circulation, tissue oxygenation, and immune function.

10. **Inflammatory Bowel Disease:** Individuals with inflammatory bowel disease, including Crohn's disease and ulcerative colitis, are at increased risk of developing septic arthritis due to chronic inflammation, immunosuppressive therapy, and gastrointestinal infections.

It is crucial to comprehend these risk factors to identify those who are more likely to develop infectious arthritis and to put preventive measures, early detection, and effective management strategies into place to lessen the morbidity and mortality linked to this potentially fatal condition.

8.3.3. Diagnostic Value of Synovial Fluid Analysis in Differentiating Infectious vs. Non-infectious Joint Diseases

To distinguish between infectious and non-infectious joint diseases, synovial fluid analysis is an essential diagnostic tool. It offers important information that helps with treatment choices and enhances patient outcomes.

Synovial fluid analysis is crucial for determining the pathogen responsible for infectious joint diseases. Analysis of synovial fluid may also show elevated levels of inflammatory markers, suggestive of an ongoing infection, such as erythrocyte sedimentation rate (ESR) and C-reactive protein (CRP). Furthermore, synovial fluid stained with Gram staining may offer quick preliminary identification of bacterial pathogens, facilitating the early start of focused antibiotic therapy.

On the other hand, synovial fluid analysis usually shows a sterile inflammatory response without evidence of microbial invasion in non-infectious inflammatory arthritis, such as psoriatic arthritis (PsA) or rheumatoid arthritis (RA). There may be elevated white blood cell counts, primarily lymphocytes, which are indicative of the autoimmune arthritis's chronic inflammatory process. Furthermore, the diagnosis of non-infectious inflammatory arthritis is further supported by the presence of autoantibodies in synovial fluid, such as rheumatoid factor (RF) and anti-cyclic citrullinated peptide (anti-CCP) antibodies.

Another useful tool for distinguishing infectious from non-infectious joint diseases is synovial fluid biochemical analysis. Due to bacterial metabolic activity, synovial fluid glucose levels are frequently reduced in septic arthritis; in non-infectious inflammatory arthritis, however, glucose levels are usually within normal range. Evaluation of synovial fluid lactate levels may also be useful in differentiating between infectious and non-infectious etiologies; elevated lactate levels are indicative of bacterial infection. Moreover, the presence of synovial fluid can offer important hints for diagnosis. Synovial fluid in cases of infectious arthritis may seem turbid or purulent, which is indicative of the presence of cellular debris and pus. On the other hand, synovial fluid from non-infectious inflammatory arthritis frequently appears clear to somewhat hazy and lacks purulence.

Overall, by evaluating cellular, biochemical, and microbiological parameters, synovial fluid analysis is essential in distinguishing between infectious and non-infectious joint diseases.

8.3.3.1. Non-infectious Joint Diseases

The term "non-infectious joint diseases" refers to a broad category of illnesses that cause pain, stiffness, and functional impairment in the joints due to inflammation, degeneration, or structural abnormalities. All ages are susceptible to these conditions, which are frequently chronic in nature and necessitate long-term management techniques to reduce symptoms and maintain joint function. Osteoarthritis (OA), rheumatoid arthritis (RA), gout, and juvenile idiopathic arthritis (JIA) are among the most prevalent non-infectious joint diseases. Each of these conditions has a distinct pathophysiology and clinical presentation.

The most common type of arthritis, osteoarthritis (OA), also called degenerative joint disease, mostly affects older adults. It is characterized by osteophyte formation, joint inflammation, and progressive articular cartilage degradation, which results in joint stiffness, pain, and decreased range of motion. Age, obesity, joint injury, and genetic predisposition are risk factors for osteoarthritis (OA). Joint degeneration and cartilage breakdown are caused by many factors, including mechanical stress, abnormal joint loading, and biochemical changes within the joint microenvironment, though the precise cause of osteoarthritis (OA) is still unknown. The goals of OA management strategies are to reduce pain, enhance joint function, and impede the advancement of the disease by combining non-pharmacological interventions (e.g., physical activity, and weight control) and pharmaceutical treatments (e.g., intra-articular injections, and analgesics).

The inflammatory synovium that characterizes rheumatoid arthritis (RA), a chronic autoimmune disease, causes joint pain, swelling, and progressive joint damage. Although it can affect many joints throughout the body, RA mainly affects the tiny joints in the hands and feet. Dysregulated immune responses play a role in the pathophysiology of RA, as immune cells attack and target the bone, cartilage, and synovium in afflicted joints. The development of RA is influenced by genetic, environmental, and hormonal factors, which result in erosive joint changes, synovial hyperplasia, and chronic inflammation. Disease-modifying antirheumatic medications (DMARDs), biologic therapies, and targeted immunomodulatory agents are used in combination to treat RA with the goals of reducing inflammation, symptomatic relief, and preventing joint damage.

A metabolic disorder called gout is typified by the accumulation of crystals called monosodium urate in the joints, which causes recurrent bouts of acute inflammatory arthritis. Although it usually affects the big toe, gout can also affect the ankles, knees, and wrists. Gout risk factors include food-related issues (e.g., foods high in purines, alcohol), metabolic syndrome, obesity, and genetic predisposition. Because of poor uric acid metabolism or excretion, elevated serum uric acid levels cause urate crystals to form in the joints, which in turn cause inflammation. Acute flare-ups of gout are typified by an abrupt onset of intense joint pain, swelling, and redness; anti-inflammatory drugs are frequently needed to alleviate symptoms. Gout treatment for the long term focuses on lowering serum uric acid levels through lifestyle changes (e.g., exercise, and weight reduction) and medication treatments (e.g., urate-lowering substances). A collection of chronic inflammatory joint diseases that affect children under 16 and last longer than six weeks is known as juvenile idiopathic arthritis (JIA). JIA includes several subtypes, each with unique clinical characteristics and disease trajectories, such as oligoarticular, polyarticular, systemic, enthesitis-related, and psoriatic arthritis. Although the precise cause of JIA is still unknown, a combination of immunological, environmental, and genetic factors are thought to be involved. Joint pain, edema, stiffness, and decreased physical function are common symptoms in children with JIA, and these symptoms can have a serious negative influence on their long-term results and quality of life. Through a multidisciplinary approach involving medication, physical therapy, and routine monitoring by pediatric rheumatologists, treatment for juvenile idiopathic arthritis (JIA) aims to control inflammation, preserve joint function, and prevent disease complications.

Non-infectious joint diseases are a broad category of illnesses that cause pain, stiffness, and functional impairment in the joints due to joint inflammation, degeneration, or structural abnormalities. These conditions, which include juvenile idiopathic arthritis, gout, osteoarthritis, and rheumatoid arthritis, present serious obstacles for both patients and medical professionals and call for all-encompassing management plans that are customized to meet the needs of each patient. Prolonged investigation into the fundamental mechanisms of non-infectious joint diseases and the creation of targeted treatments have the potential to enhance prognoses and quality of life for those afflicted with these crippling ailments. (El-Gabalawy and Tanner, 2021)

8.4. Role of Synovial Fluid Analysis in Early Diagnosis of Rheumatic Diseases

The early detection of rheumatic diseases, a collection of illnesses marked by inflammation and damage to the joints, muscles, ligaments, and tendons, is greatly aided by the analysis of synovial fluid. Timely intervention can greatly enhance patient outcomes and quality of life, which is why early detection of these diseases is so important. Because synovial fluid, the lubricating fluid found in joint cavities, comes into direct contact with the affected tissues and is sensitive to changes in the joint microenvironment, it acts as a repository for diagnostic data. The ability of synovial fluid analysis to identify inflammatory markers in the joint space is one of the main advantages in the early diagnosis of rheumatic diseases. An analysis of synovial fluid in diseases like rheumatoid arthritis (RA), an autoimmune disease marked by persistent inflammation of the synovium, can show increased levels of inflammatory cells, especially neutrophils and lymphocytes. The existence of these cells and the evaluation of their number and shape offer important hints for differentiating RA from other types of arthritis and help start the right treatment plans early in the course of the illness.

Additionally, synovial fluid analysis improves diagnostic accuracy by enabling the identification of particular biomarkers linked to rheumatic diseases. For example, even in the early stages of RA, the presence of antibodies against the cyclic citrullinated peptide (anti-CCP) and rheumatoid factor (RF) in synovial fluid is highly suggestive of the disease. Similarly, the diagnosis of gout—a type of arthritis brought on by the deposition of monosodium urate crystals in the joints—is confirmed by the presence of uric acid crystals in synovial fluid. Clinicians can minimize joint damage and initiate disease-modifying therapies promptly by using these biomarkers to make timely and accurate diagnoses.

The ability of synovial fluid analysis to distinguish between infectious and non-infectious causes of joint inflammation is another important feature in the early diagnosis of rheumatic diseases. Analysis of synovial fluid in conditions like septic arthritis, a bacterial infection of the joint, can show the presence of bacteria on microbiological culture and elevated white blood cell counts with a neutrophil predominance. On the other hand, analysis of synovial fluid in non-infectious inflammatory arthritis (RA, psoriatic arthritis) usually reveals a sterile inflammatory response without microbiological invasion. This distinction is important because it helps determine the best course of treatment. For example, infectious arthritis requires immediate antibiotic therapy to prevent joint destruction and systemic complications.

Moreover, synovial fluid analysis makes it easier to track a patient's response to treatment and the state of their rheumatic diseases. Through the serial evaluation of synovial fluid parameters, including cell counts, inflammatory markers, and biomarker levels.

8.4.1. Synovial Fluid Biomarkers for Disease Diagnosis and Prognosis

Synovial fluid biomarkers have become important diagnostic and surveillance instruments for a range of joint-related conditions, providing information about the underlying pathophysiology and supporting individualized therapeutic strategies. The synovial fluid of afflicted joints contains a variety of molecules, including proteins, nucleic acids, and metabolites, which are biomarkers. The patterns of expression of these molecules are indicative of distinct disease processes that take place within the joint microenvironment.

Rheumatoid factor (RF) is a synovial fluid biomarker that has been extensively researched. It is an autoantibody that targets the Fc portion of immunoglobulin G). Increased levels of radiofrequency (RF) in synovial fluid have a strong correlation with rheumatoid arthritis (RA), an autoimmune disease marked by progressive joint destruction and persistent synovial inflammation. RF indicates the prognosis and severity of the disease and is used as a diagnostic marker for RA. Similarly, antibodies against the cystic citrullinated peptide (anti-CCP) have been found in synovial fluid; these antibodies are highly specific for RA and help in the early diagnosis and prognosis of the disease.

Apart from autoantibodies, synovial fluid contains cytokines and chemokines that are important mediators of inflammation and tissue damage in a variety of joint diseases. The pathophysiology of RA and other inflammatory arthropathies is linked to several pro-inflammatory cytokines, including interleukin-1 (IL-1), interleukin-6 (IL-6), and tumor necrosis factor-alpha (TNF-α). Specific measurements of these cytokines in synovial fluid inform and direct treatment choices, especially when it comes to biologic therapies that target cytokine signaling pathways. Furthermore, new synovial fluid biomarkers linked to particular disease processes have been identified thanks to recent developments in molecular biology techniques. For example, it has been discovered that the synovial fluid of patients suffering from osteoarthritis (OA) and rheumatoid arthritis (RA) displays dysregulated expression patterns of microRNA (miRNA) molecules, which are small non-coding RNAs involved in post-transcriptional gene regulation. These miRNAs are promising candidates for disease diagnosis and therapeutic targeting because they regulate important pathways that underlie joint inflammation, cartilage degradation, and synovial hyperplasia.

Another new field of study that aims to find biomarkers indicative of metabolic alterations taking place in diseased joints is metabolomic profiling of synovial fluid. Researchers can uncover metabolic signatures linked to various joint diseases and acquire insights into disease-specific metabolic pathways by examining the makeup of metabolites in synovial fluid. Metabolomic biomarkers may be used to identify new therapeutic targets for intervention, track the effectiveness of treatments, and diagnose diseases.

Synovial fluid biomarkers provide useful information for prognostication and diagnosis of a variety of joint-related conditions, such as inflammatory arthropathies, OA, and RA. Through the identification of molecular signatures of disease within the joint microenvironment, these biomarkers aid in the early detection of disease, direct therapeutic choices, and open the door to patient-specific personalized medicine approaches. Prolonged investigations into the discovery and validation of new synovial fluid biomarkers have the potential to enhance rheumatology patients' prognosis, diagnosis, and treatment.

8.4.1.1. Prognosis

When it comes to the course and result of joint-related conditions, the prognosis in synovial fluid analysis refers to the predictive value of biomarkers and other factors found in the synovial fluid of affected joints. In addition to lubricating and nourishing the joints, synovial fluid also acts as a storehouse of diagnostic data indicative of the underlying pathophysiology taking place in the joint microenvironment.

Angiogenic factors found in synovial fluid, in addition to biomarkers for inflammation and tissue remodeling, are involved in prognosticating disease. Patients with inflammatory arthropathies have higher levels of vascular endothelial growth factor (VEGF) and angiopoietin-1 (Ang-1), two substances involved in angiogenesis and neovascularization within the synovium. A worse prognosis is indicated by increased angiogenic activity, which is linked to worsening joint inflammation, synovial hyperplasia, and progressive joint damage (Ebnezer, 2003; Pisetsky, 2020; El-Gabalawy and Tanner, 2021).

Moreover, prognostic evaluations and treatment choices can be influenced by synovial fluid biomarkers linked to treatment response. For instance, cytokine levels after treatment with biologic agents or disease-modifying anti-rheumatic medications (DMARDs) can be used as surrogate markers of treatment efficacy and to forecast long-term results. In a similar vein, tracking the expression of microRNAs (miRNAs) in synovial fluid may be useful in identifying patients who will benefit from particular therapies and have improved prognoses.

For joint-related conditions, the prognosis in synovial fluid analysis includes a thorough evaluation of biomarkers and other variables indicative of disease severity, progression, and response to treatment. Through the utilization of synovial fluid analysis, physicians can obtain valuable insights for prognostic assessments, customize treatment plans to meet the unique requirements of each patient, and enhance the prognosis of patients suffering from joint diseases. In the field of rheumatology, ongoing research efforts to validate and improve synovial fluid biomarkers have the potential to improve prognostic accuracy and improve patient care.

8.4.2. Synovial Fluid Analysis in Pediatric Rheumatology

In pediatric rheumatology, synovial fluid analysis is a useful diagnostic tool that helps with the assessment and treatment of a range of joint-related conditions in kids and teenagers. Juvenile idiopathic arthritis (JIA), systemic lupus erythematosus (SLE), juvenile dermatomyositis (JDM), and systemic vasculitides are among the many conditions that fall under the umbrella of pediatric rheumatic diseases. These conditions can have a wide range of clinical manifestations and can be difficult to diagnose. Critical information obtained from synovial fluid analysis aids clinicians in determining the specific causes of joint inflammation, evaluating the state of the disease, and formulating personalized treatment plans for pediatric patients.

Among the main uses of synovial fluid analysis in pediatric rheumatology is the assessment of suspected inflammatory arthritis, especially juvenile idiopathic arthritis (JIA), which is the most prevalent chronic rheumatic disease in children. Analyzing synovial fluid helps define its cellular and biochemical makeup and confirm the existence of synovial inflammation. When joint inflammation (JIA) occurs, synovial fluid usually has an inflammatory profile, with higher levels of pro-inflammatory cytokines like TNF-α and interleukin-6 (IL-6) and higher counts of white blood cells. Furthermore, autoantibodies like rheumatoid factor (RF) and antinuclear antibodies (ANA) in synovial fluid may offer additional diagnostic hints that help with JIA subtype subclassification and prognostication.

Moreover, the analysis of synovial fluid helps differentiate between infectious and non-infectious causes of inflammation in the joints of pediatric patients, which is crucial for directing the right course of treatment.

Synovial fluid analysis is helpful not only in diagnosis but also in evaluating disease activity and therapy response in pediatric rheumatic diseases.

Because it offers diagnostic, prognostic, and therapeutic insights into joint-related disorders in children and adolescents, synovial fluid analysis is essential to pediatric rheumatology. Clinicians can diagnose pediatric patients with rheumatic diseases accurately, evaluate disease activity, track treatment response, and enhance patient outcomes by utilizing the data gathered from synovial fluid analysis. Prolonged investigation and clinical application of synovial fluid analysis have the potential to enhance our comprehension of pediatric rheumatology and improve patient treatment in this specialized domain.

8.4.3. The Role of Synovial Fluid Analysis in Sports Medicine

In sports medicine, synovial fluid analysis has a variety of applications that help with joint-related injuries and ailments that athletes frequently face. These include assessment, diagnosis, and treatment. Because athletes are more likely to sustain a variety of joint injuries, synovial fluid analysis offers important diagnostic data that helps with treatment choices and speeds up a player's return to the field. The assessment of acute joint injuries, such as traumatic joint effusions and ligamentous injuries, is one of the main uses of synovial fluid analysis in sports medicine. Synovial fluid analysis can assist clinicians in distinguishing between inflammatory effusions, which may indicate underlying joint pathology such as osteoarthritis or synovitis, and traumatic effusions, which are the result of acute joint trauma or hemorrhage, following a sports-related injury. The evaluation of blood, protein levels, and synovial fluid cell counts can help determine the extent of the injury and direct the right course of treatment, which may include surgery, rest, or rehabilitation.

Furthermore, synovial fluid analysis plays a critical role in the diagnosis and follow-up of overuse injuries as well as chronic joint diseases that are common in athletes, including inflammatory arthritis and osteoarthritis. Analysis of synovial fluid in athletes with osteoarthritis may show increased levels of inflammatory cytokines and products of cartilage degradation, revealing information about the severity and course of the disease. Similarly, synovial fluid analysis can help athletes with inflammatory arthritis optimize their therapy and minimize the negative effects on their athletic performance by verifying the diagnosis, evaluating the disease's activity, and tracking their response to treatment.

Moreover, synovial fluid analysis helps with the diagnosis and treatment of crystal-induced arthritis, which includes pseudogout and gout, which can affect athletes as a result of joint trauma or metabolic imbalances. Synovial fluid can be examined under a microscope to identify distinctive crystals, such as calcium pyrophosphate crystals in pseudogout or monosodium urate crystals in gout. This identification helps to confirm the diagnosis and guide treatment decisions, which may include dietary adjustments, medication therapy, and lifestyle changes.

Synovial fluid analysis is useful not only for diagnosis but also for therapeutic interventions and rehabilitation plans for athletes recovering from joint injuries. Through evaluation of the biochemical and inflammatory characteristics of synovial fluid, we can customize treatment plans to target distinct pathophysiological processes that underlie joint damage and inflammation. For example, synovial fluid findings may guide the administration of intra-articular injections of hyaluronic acid or corticosteroids to reduce joint pain and inflammation and promote healing. In a similar vein, athletes can have customized return-to-sport protocols and rehabilitation plans depending on the degree of inflammation in their joints as well as the existence of underlying joint pathology identified by synovial fluid analysis. In general, synovial fluid analysis contributes significantly to sports medicine by offering prognostic, therapeutic, and diagnostic information about joint-related ailments and injuries that athletes may experience.

Through the incorporation of synovial fluid analysis into the clinical assessment of athletes, medical professionals can maximize therapeutic approaches, reduce time spent away from sports, and foster both long-term joint health and athletic effectiveness. Prolonged investigation and clinical application of synovial fluid analysis have the potential to progress sports medicine procedures and improve player outcomes at all competitive levels.

8.4.5. Synovial Fluid Analysis in the Era of Precision Medicine

In the age of precision medicine, synovial fluid analysis is a game-changer for joint-related disease diagnosis and treatment, utilizing cutting-edge molecular and genomic technologies to customize patient-specific regimens. Precision medicine seeks to maximize therapeutic outcomes and minimize side effects by providing individualized care based on the distinct genetic, molecular, and environmental factors influencing disease pathogenesis and treatment response.

Finding disease-specific biomarkers and molecular signatures that guide diagnosis, prognosis, and treatment choices is one of the main uses of synovial fluid analysis in precision medicine. Clinicians can diagnose patients more quickly and accurately by identifying biomarkers indicative of particular joint diseases, such as gout, osteoarthritis, or rheumatoid arthritis, by molecularly analyzing the composition of synovial fluid. Moreover, based on the molecular profiles and underlying disease mechanisms of each patient, molecular profiling of synovial fluid allows for patient stratification into discrete subgroups, which in turn makes it easier to select customized targeted therapies.

Additionally, for patients undergoing precision medicine interventions, synovial fluid analysis is essential for tracking disease activity and treatment response. Clinicians can monitor changes in disease activity, forecast treatment response, and modify treatment regimens by serially evaluating synovial fluid biomarkers. For instance, tracking the expression levels of pro-inflammatory cytokines in synovial fluid, such as interleukin-6 (IL-6) or tumor necrosis factor-alpha (TNF-α), may help determine the degree of disease activity and direct the choice of biologic therapies that target particular cytokine pathways. Furthermore, the analysis of synovial fluid aids in the identification of new therapeutic targets and the advancement of precision medicine techniques for conditions pertaining to the joints. Through the clarification of the molecular mechanisms that underlie joint inflammation, cartilage degradation, and synovial hyperplasia, scientists can ascertain targets that are amenable to medication and create tailored treatments that target particular pathways implicated in the etiology of disease. Examples of potential precision medicine interventions for rheumatic diseases include inhibitors of pro-inflammatory cytokines, matrix metalloproteinases (MMPs), or microRNAs (miRNAs) found through synovial fluid analysis.

Moreover, synovial fluid analysis facilitates the integration of multi-omics data, such as transcriptomics, proteomics, metabolomics, and genomics, to offer a thorough grasp of the pathophysiology of disease and the effectiveness of treatment. Researchers can find novel biomarkers for disease diagnosis and prognosis, predict treatment outcomes, and identify molecular signatures associated with disease subtypes by examining the intricate interactions between genes, proteins, and metabolites in the synovial fluid.

In the age of precision medicine, synovial fluid analysis is a potent diagnostic and therapeutic tool for conditions relating to the joints. It provides information on the etiology of the disease, the efficacy of treatment, and the need for individualized care. (Ebnezer, 2003; Pisetsky, 2020).

A Closer Look

Synovial Fluid

Synovial fluid is a crucial component of the musculoskeletal system, playing a pivotal role in joint function and health. It is a viscous, transparent fluid found in the cavities of synovial joints, such as the knees, elbows, and shoulders. Composed mainly of water (around 80%), synovial fluid also contains electrolytes, proteins (like albumin and globulin), hyaluronic acid, and lubricin.

The primary function of synovial fluid is to reduce friction between the articular cartilage surfaces of bones during movement. This lubrication allows for smooth and pain-free joint motion, essential for everyday activities and physical performance. Furthermore, synovial fluid nourishes the cartilage, providing it with oxygen and nutrients while removing metabolic waste products.

Synovial fluid composition can vary depending on factors such as age, joint health, and certain medical conditions. For example, in osteoarthritis, the composition may change, leading to a decrease in viscosity and lubricating properties, resulting in joint pain and stiffness.

Analysis of synovial fluid is valuable in diagnosing joint-related diseases and conditions. Techniques such as arthrocentesis (joint aspiration) can provide samples for evaluation, including tests for cell count, glucose levels, and the presence of crystals or microorganisms, aiding in the identification and treatment of joint disorders. In essence, synovial fluid is not merely a lubricant but a complex biological fluid crucial for joint function, maintenance, and health, highlighting its significance in orthopedic medicine and rheumatology.

Summary

- Synovial fluid analysis is a diagnostic procedure used to assess the health of the joints, primarily in cases of joint-related disorders such as arthritis, gout, and infection.
- Synovial fluid analysis is a diagnostic procedure used to evaluate the composition of synovial fluid, the lubricating fluid found within joint cavities, for diagnostic and therapeutic purposes.
- A synovial fluid analysis is performed when pain, inflammation, or swelling occurs in a joint, or when there's an accumulation of fluid with an unknown cause.
- During arthrocentesis, you will be lying down or sitting in a position that makes it easy for the health care provider to access your joint. A needle attached to a sterile syringe is then carefully inserted into the joint space.
- The inner membrane of synovial joints is called the synovial membrane and secretes synovial fluid into the joint cavity. Synovial fluid is an ultrafiltrate from plasma, and contains proteins derived from the blood plasma and proteins that are produced by cells within the joint tissues.
- Microscopic analysis of synovial fluid is performed to evaluate for cell count and crystals. Crystals include monosodium urate crystals, calcium pyrophosphate, hydroxyapatite and corticosteroid crystals.
- Infectious arthritis, also known as septic arthritis, is a serious joint infection characterized by the invasion of pathogens, such as bacteria, viruses, or fungi, into the synovial space, leading to inflammation, pain, swelling, and potentially irreversible joint damage.
- Synovial fluid analysis plays a pivotal role in the early diagnosis of rheumatic diseases, a group of conditions characterized by inflammation and damage to the joints, muscles, ligaments, and tendons.
- Synovial fluid biomarkers have emerged as valuable tools for diagnosing and monitoring various joint-related diseases, offering insights into the underlying pathophysiology and aiding in personalized treatment approaches.
- Synovial fluid analysis in the era of precision medicine represents a paradigm shift in the diagnosis and management of joint-related disorders, leveraging advanced molecular and genomic technologies to tailor treatment strategies to the individual characteristics of patients.

References

1. Blewis, M. E., Nugent-Derfus, G. E., Schmidt, T. A., Schumacher, B. L., & Sah, R. L. (2007). A model of synovial fluid lubricant composition in normal and injured joints. *European Cell Materials, 13*(1), 26–39.
2. Courtney, P., & Doherty, M. (2009). Joint aspiration and injection and synovial fluid analysis. *Best Practice & Research Clinical Rheumatology, 23*(2), 161–192.
3. Ebnezer, J. (2003). *Essentials of Orthopedics for Physiotherapists.* Delhi: Jaypee Brothers Medical Publishers (P) Ltd, Edition 1/e, DOI. 10.5005/jp/books/10292.

4. El-Gabalawy, H. S., & Tanner, S. (2021). Synovial fluid analyses, synovial biopsy, and synovial pathology. In G. S. Firestein, R. C. Budd, S. E. Gabriel, I. B. McInnes, & J. R. O'Dell (Eds.), *Firestein & Kelley's Textbook of Rheumatology* (11th ed., Chap. 56). Philadelphia, PA: Elsevier.

5. Miyaguchi, M., Kobayashi, A., Kadoya, Y., Ohashi, H., Yamano, Y., & Takaoka, K. (2003). Biochemical change in joint fluid after isometric quadriceps exercise for patients with osteoarthritis of the knee. *Osteoarthritis and Cartilage, 11*(4), 252–259.

6. Pisetsky, D. S. (2020). Laboratory testing in the rheumatic diseases. In L. Goldman & A. I. Schafer (Eds.), *Goldman-Cecil Medicine* (26th ed., Chap. 242). Philadelphia, PA: Elsevier.

Chapter

9

ANALYSIS OF VAGINAL SECRETIONS

Contents

Introduction

Understanding vaginal secretions is crucial for assessing reproductive health and diagnosing potential issues. Vaginal discharge, a natural phenomenon, serves various physiological functions, including maintaining vaginal pH, preventing infections, and supporting fertility. Its characteristics, such as consistency, color, odor, volume, and pH level, can fluctuate throughout the menstrual cycle due to hormonal changes. Typically, it ranges from clear to milky white, with a mild musky odor. However, deviations from the norm may indicate underlying concerns.

Analyzing vaginal secretions involves a comprehensive assessment of these characteristics. Consistency provides insights into hormonal status, with thinner, clearer discharge often indicating ovulation. Changes in color, such as pinkish or brownish tinges, may signal the presence of blood, possibly related to menstruation or abnormalities. Odor, typically mild, can become stronger with infections like bacterial vaginosis or sexually transmitted infections. Volume variations, influenced by factors like sexual arousal or pregnancy, can be indicative of hormonal fluctuations or infections.

The pH level of vaginal secretions, usually acidic, plays a critical role in maintaining a healthy vaginal environment by inhibiting harmful bacterial growth. Disruptions in pH balance may lead to infections or discomfort. Microscopic examination of vaginal secretions can reveal the presence of abnormal cells, pathogens, or clues to hormonal imbalances. Specific tests, such as wet mounts or cultures, aid in identifying infections and guiding appropriate treatment.

Monitoring changes in vaginal secretions empowers individuals to detect abnormalities early and seek timely medical intervention. While some variations are normal, persistent alterations in color, consistency, odor, or volume warrant professional evaluation. By understanding and analyzing vaginal secretions, individuals can proactively manage their reproductive health and well-being.

Orientation and Directional Terms

Term	Definition	Illustration
Vaginal fornix	Vaginal fornix is the widest part at the end of the vaginal canal and is composed of anterior, posterior and lateral parts.	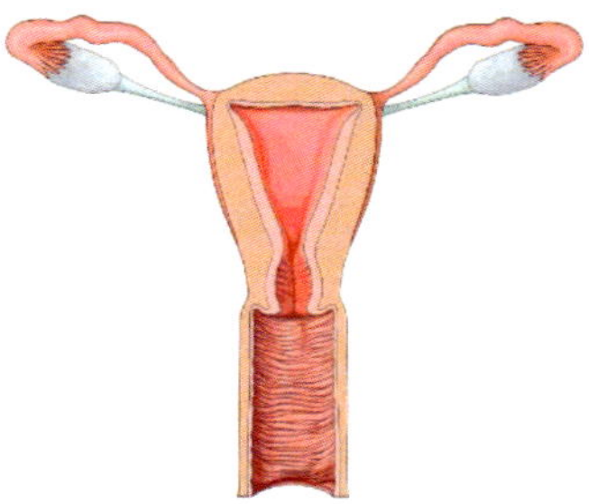
Vulvovaginitis	Vulvovaginitis or vaginitis is swelling or infection of the vulva and vagina. Vaginitis is a common problem that can affect women and girls of all ages.	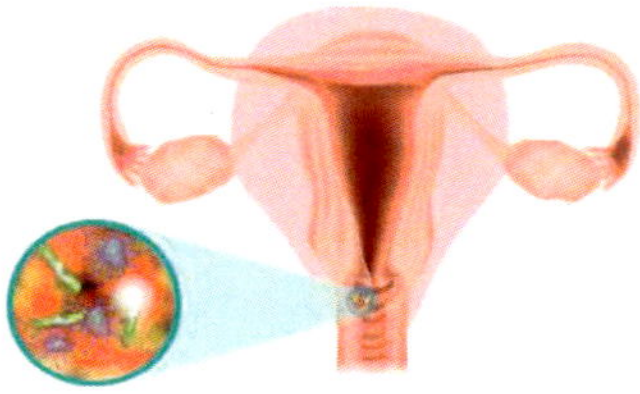
Abnormal Cells	Abnormal cells are caused by the human papillomavirus (HPV). An abnormal cervical screening test result means that you have changes in the cells covering the neck of your womb (cervix). These changes are not cancer. The cells often go back to normal by themselves.	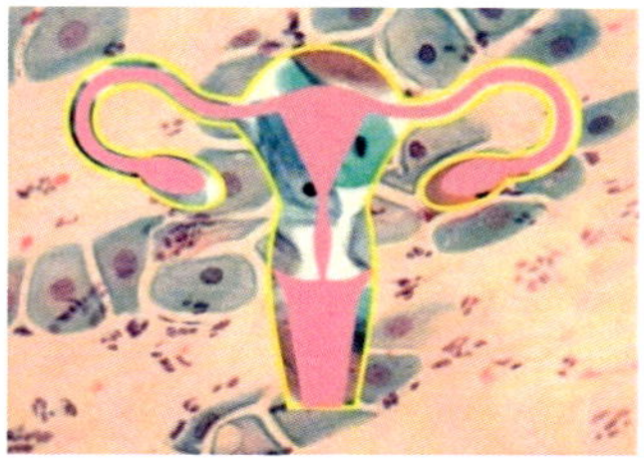
Dyspareunia	Dyspareunia is genital pain during or after sexual intercourse. Painful sexual intercourse can be felt externally on the vulva or internally in the vagina, uterus or pelvis.	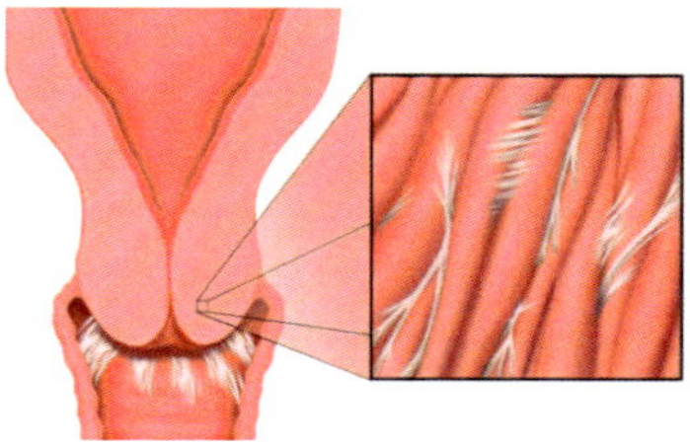
Trichomoniasis	Trichomoniasis is a common sexually transmitted infection caused by a parasite. In women, trichomoniasis can cause a foul-smelling vaginal discharge, genital itching and painful urination. Men who have trichomoniasis typically have no symptoms.	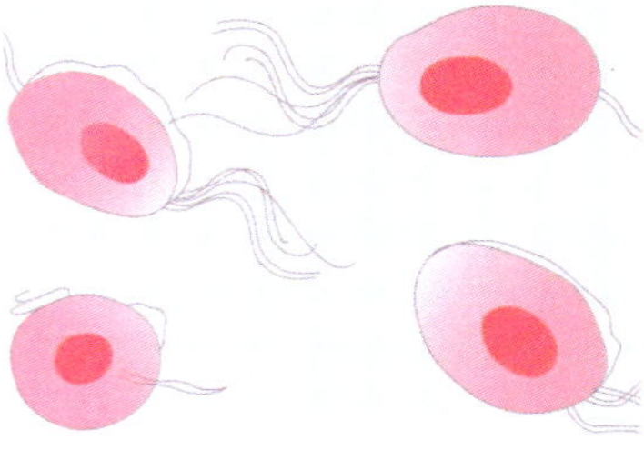

9.1. Specimen Collection and Handling

The recovery and detection of microorganisms and other cellular components are maximized by the proper collection and handling of vaginal secretion specimens. The cause of vaginitis or vulvovaginitis can be identified based on the presence, absence, or combination of elements seen under a microscope.

Vaginal secretions are collected by a medical professional during a pelvic exam. The vaginal fornices are accessed using a nonlubricated speculum that has only been moistened with warm water. Because they frequently contain antimicrobial agents, speculum lubricants should be avoided. The tool used to collect specimens is typically a sterile, polyester-tipped (e.g., Dacron) swab on a plastic shaft or a sterile wire loop as an alternative. While wooden shafts have been toxic to Chlamydia trachomatis, cotton has been toxic to Neisseria gonorrhoeae, making the choice of sampling device crucial. To collect vaginal secretions from the posterior vaginal fornix and the vaginal pool, the medical professional uses one or more swabs or a collection loop.

Following collection, the labeled specimen needs to be brought as soon as possible to the laboratory in a biohazard bag with a requisition slip attached. Apart from the customary patient identification details on the request sheet, a suitable medical history encompassing the patient's menstrual cycle, exposure to sexually transmitted infections, and utilization of vaginal lubricants, creams, and douches must be furnished.

Tests on vaginal secretion specimens should be performed as soon as possible. If a delay in transport or analysis is unavoidable, these specimens should be kept at room temperature. Refrigeration adversely affects the recovery of *N. gonorrheae* and the detection of the trophozoite *Trichomonas vaginalis*, whose identification depends on observing its characteristic "flitting" or jerky motility. However, for detection of *C. trachomatis* or viruses (e.g., herpes simplex virus), refrigeration is preferred to prevent overgrowth of the normal bacterial flora.

When a medical professional looks at the vaginal secretions right away after collection (i.e., provider-performed microscopy testing), the microscopic examinations are carried out by immersing the swab directly into 0.5 mL to 1.0 mL of sterile physiologic saline (0.9% NaCl). An alternative method involves rolling a swab of vaginal secretions directly onto a microscope slide with a tiny drop of sterile physiological saline on it for microscopic observation.

9.1.1. pH

To absorb the secretions, one can place commercial pH paper directly on the vagina's lateral wall and leave it there for approximately one minute. The pH value is then ascertained by comparing the pH paper's color change with a color chart. As an alternative, vaginal secretions can be collected with a swab, and the liquid sample is then quickly expressed onto pH paper. Because of its high alkaline pH, it is crucial to avoid contact with any cervical discharge, regardless of the technique employed. It should be noted that a sampling swab's pH value cannot be determined using that swab after it has been immersed in saline (pH ~7) because the saline has changed it.

The pH range for vaginal secretions should be between 3 and 4 points. Lactobacilli are the main bacteria in a healthy vagina, and the main metabolic byproduct of these bacteria is lactic acid, which keeps the pH of the vagina normally acidic. Research has shown that some lactobacilli also generate hydrogen peroxide, which improves the vagina's naturally acidic environment even more. Part of the reason hydrogen peroxide has bactericidal properties is that it inhibits the growth of certain natural bacteria, like Gardnerella vaginalis. In actuality, bacterial vaginosis is linked to a decrease in or complete absence of lactobacilli that produce hydrogen peroxide.

Table 9.1. Overview of Studies Performed on Human CVF

Study	Samples	Part of Sample Analyzed	Separation Method	MS Method
Venkataraman et al., 2005	Undiluted CVF collected in cup from healthy women (postmenarcheal, pre-menopausal)	Cationic fraction	2D-PAGE (1D: AU-PAGE; 2D: Tricine- SDS-PAGE)	MALDI-TOF-TOF
Di Quinzio et al., 2007	Swabs from pregnant women (37 weeks gestation)	Only protein spots identified common to five gels	2D-PAGE (1stD: IEF; 2ndD SDS-PAGE) followed by RP-LC	MALDI-TOF or ESI-linear IT
Dasari et al., 2007	Swabs from pregnant women (18,5 weeks gestation as mean)	Whole CVF	1D-SDS-PAGE followed by offline 2D(SCX/RP)-LC	ESI-Q-TOF
Tang et al., 2007	Washings from clinically normal women; 7 washings from women infected with *Candida* spp.	Whole CVF	2D-PAGE (1stD: IEF; 2ndD SDS-PAGE)	MALDI-TOF-TOF
Shaw et al., 2007	Gauze from healthy women	Whole CVF	1D-SDS-PAGE or SCX-LC both followed by RP-LC	ESI-linear IT
Pereira et al., 2007	Swabs from pregnant women (15.8–35.9 weeks gestation)	Whole CVF	2D-DIGE or MudPIT(SCX/RP)-LC	ESI-Q-TOF
Klein et al., 2008	Swabs from pregnant women (30.5 weeks gestation as mean)	Whole CVF	RP-LC	ESI-IT
This study: From: Comprehensive proteomic analysis of human cervical-vaginal fluid using colposcopy samples	Washings from HPV-infected women	Whole CVF	Ultrafiltration or C_4-LC protein fractionation/ C_{18}-LC peptide separation	MALDI-TOF-TOF

Source: Zegels, G., Van Raemdonck, G.A., Coen, E.P. et al. Comprehensive proteomic analysis of human cervical-vaginal fluid using colposcopy samples. Proteome Sci 7, 17 (2009). https://doi.org/10.1186/1477-5956-7-17.

As it helps with the differential diagnosis of vaginitis, the measurement of the vaginal pH is a valuable diagnostic tool (Table 9.1). A pH of more than 4.5 is linked to trichomoniasis, atrophic varicella, and bacterial vaginosis. A pH of less than 4.5 is considered normal, though candidiasis can also cause it.

9.2. Microscopic Examinations

Microscopic examinations should be performed as soon as possible on vaginal secretion specimens, particularly for detection of *T. vaginalis*, for which identification depends solely on observing actively motile organisms. The vaginal swab is placed into a tube containing approximately 1.0 mL of sterile physiologic saline (0.9% NaCl) and is agitated or twirled for a few seconds to release the secretions from the swab.

Using a vaginal swab, two microscope slides are usually prepared. A direct wet mount examination is conducted on one slide, while the amine or "whiff" test and a 10% KOH preparation are conducted on the second slide. The preparation of a third slide for Gram stain may also be necessary, depending on the laboratory protocol. The saline suspension created with the vaginal swab is used to prepare each slide. Using a disposable transfer pipette or, alternatively, pressing and rolling the moistened swab on the microscope slide to express liquid onto the slide, a drop of this suspension is placed onto a clean, labeled microscope slide. Usually, the KOH and wet mount slides are prepared simultaneously with the slide for Gram stain, if desired.

9.2.1. Wet Mount Examinations

A coverslip is placed on the drop of saline-suspended specimen to prepare the direct wet mount slide, being careful not to trap air bubbles. Bright field or phase-contrast microscopy is used to examine this slide at low power (×100) and high power (×400) magnifications. Low-power magnification is used to examine the specimen's overall distribution as well as the type, quantity, and presence of clumping in the epithelial cells. The elements are then quantified using high-power magnification and criteria akin to those mentioned in Table 9.2. When found in wet mount preparations of vaginal secretions, the following components are usually recognized and reported: yeast, hyphae/pseudohyphae, trichomonads, red blood cells, white blood cells, clue cells, and squamous epithelial cells. Prevalent bacterial morphotypes may also be reported in certain institutions where wet preps are carried out in the microbiology department.

Table 9.2. Quantification Criteria for Microscopic Examinations

Results	Number of Cells or Organisms	Viewing Area
Rare	<10	Per slide
Occasional	<1	Per 10 hpf
1+ (Few)	<1	Per hpf
2+ (Few)	1–5	Per hpf
3+ (Mod)	6–30	Per hpf
4+ (Many)	>30	Per hpf

Source: https://basicmedicalkey.com/analysis-of-vaginal-secretions/#s0060.

- **Blood Cells:** White blood cells can be seen in vaginal secretions in healthy individuals in quantities ranging from a few per preparation to multiple cells per high-power field of view. This variation is frequently linked to a woman's menstrual cycle because ovulation and menses are times when more white blood cells are produced. Red blood cells, on the other hand, are typically absent unless the specimen was taken close to or during menstruation. This emphasizes how every vaginal fluid specimen result needs to be accompanied by the patient's current medical history.

- **Bacterial Flora:** The vagina has a complex bacterial flora with the characteristically large rods of lactobacilli accounting for 50% to 90% of the microbes in a healthy vagina. These morphologically distinct, large, nonmotile, Gram-positive rods produce lactic acid as their major metabolic waste product, which is principally responsible for the acidic (pH 3.8–4.5) environment of a healthy vagina (Figure 9.1). In addition, a subset of these lactobacilli produce hydrogen peroxide, which helps maintain balance in the vaginal flora by preventing the proliferation of other bacteria, in particular, *G. vaginalis* and *Prevotella bivia*. Any decrease in the number of lactobacilli relative to the number of squamous epithelial cells present in the preparation is an indication of an imbalance in the microbial flora. Whereas small numbers of other bacterial morphotypes may be observed in normal vaginal secretions, the presence of increased numbers or a preponderance of them is considered abnormal. These morphotypes include small, nonmotile, Gram-variable coccobacilli (e.g., *G. vaginalis*); thin, curved, Gram-variable, motile rods (e.g., *Mobiluncus* spp.); Gram-positive cocci (e.g., *Peptostreptococcus* spp., staphylococci, and streptococci); Gram-negative cocci (e.g., *Enterococcus* spp.); and Gram-negative rods (e.g., *Prevotella* spp., *Porphyromonas* spp., *Bacteroides* spp., coliforms).

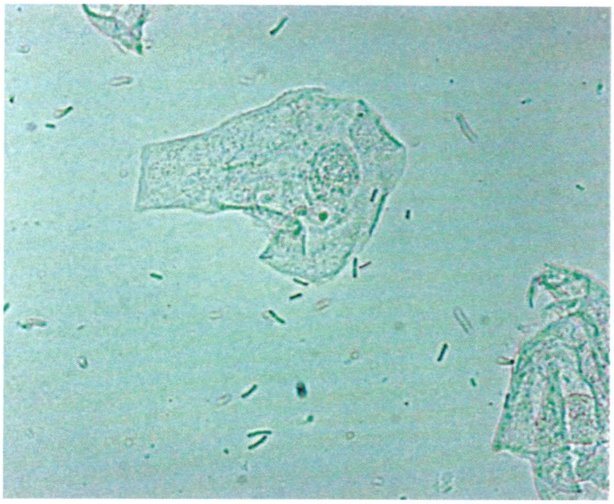

Figure 9.1. *Large rods characteristic of Lactobacillus spp. surrounding a typical squamous epithelial cell from a healthy vagina.*

Source: *https://basicmedicalkey.com/analysis-of-vaginal-secretions/#s0060.*

- **Yeast:** An occasional yeast or blastoconidium can be present in normal vaginal secretions. Because of the visual similarity of yeast and red blood cells, the KOH preparation, which lyses red blood cells, is useful in distinguishing these two entities. Yeast cells are typically 10 μm to 12 μm in diameter and are Gram positive. Increased numbers (1 + or greater) of yeast or the presence of hyphae or pseudohyphae is considered abnormal and indicates candidiasis (i.e., a fungal or yeast infection) (Figure 9.2).

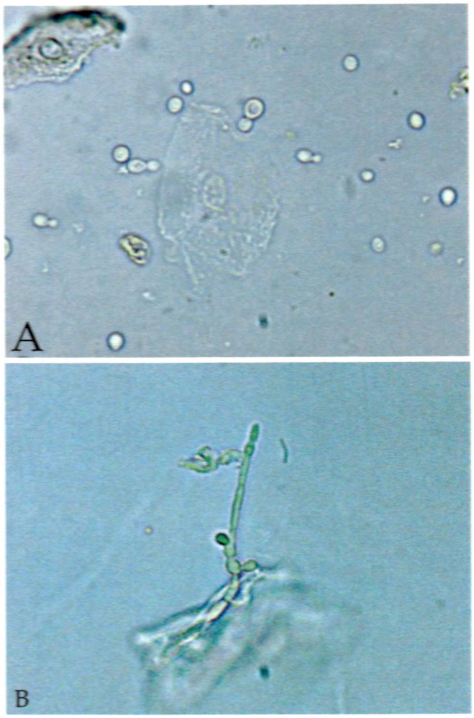

Figure 9.2. *Yeast and pseudohyphae in the wet mount of a vaginal secretion specimen. A, Budding yeast (blastoconidia) and two squamous epithelial cells. B, Pseudohyphae.*

Source: https://basicmedicalkey.com/analysis-of-vaginal-secretions/#s0060.

- **Epithelial Cells:** The vagina is a fibromuscular tube with thick walls that is lined with stratified squamous epithelium. Therefore, a sizable number of squamous epithelial cells are recovered when the vaginal mucosa is swabbed during the collection of vaginal secretions. These cells are easily recognized by their large (30–60 mm), thin, flat, flagstone-shaped appearance. They are predominant in wet mounts from a healthy vagina. They have a large amount of cytoplasm, which becomes finely granulated as the cell ages, and a small, centrally located nucleus (Figure 9.3). The shaggy appearance of clove cells, which are created when many tiny bacteria stick to the membranes of epithelial cells, is not the same as the intracellular keratohyalin granulation brought on by cell degeneration (Figure 9.4). Because so many bacteria are attached to them, clue cells—a diagnostic marker of bacterial vaginosis—appear soft and finely stippled with hazy cellular borders. The nuclei may be hidden within these bacterially-filled, unkempt-looking cells. Although the bacteria do not have to fill the entire cell to qualify as a clue cell, they must cover at least 75% of the cell surface and penetrate the cytoplasmic boundaries of the cell. These cells are sometimes referred to as "bearded." The intracellular keratohyalin granulation of normal degenerating squamous cells is not mistaken for adherent bacteria of clue cells due to the skill and expertise of the microscopist. This distinction is made easier by two microscopic traits: (1) keratohyalin granules vary in size, and (2) they are typically bigger and more flexible than bacteria. Keep in mind that epithelial cells with a lot of big lactobacilli rods covering them are not clue cells.

The vaginal mucosa's luminal squamous epithelium and its surface are home to parabasal cells. Thus, normal vaginal secretions contain either none or very few parabasal cells. On the other hand, specimens from postmenopausal women or during menstruation may contain higher numbers. These cells are round to oval in shape, with clear cytoplasmic borders, and range in diameter from 15 to 40 μm (Figure 9.5).

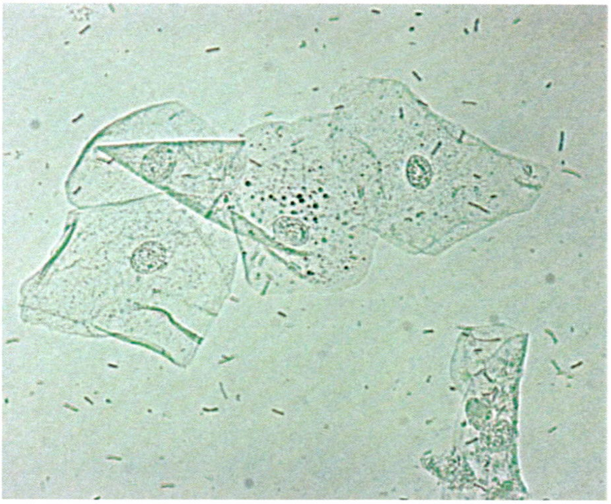

Figure 9.3. *Several squamous epithelial cells from a healthy vagina. Keratohyalin granulation is most pronounced in the centrally located cell. Numerous large rods characteristic of Lactobacillus spp. are also present.*

Source: https://basicmedicalkey.com/analysis-of-vaginal-secretions/#s0060.

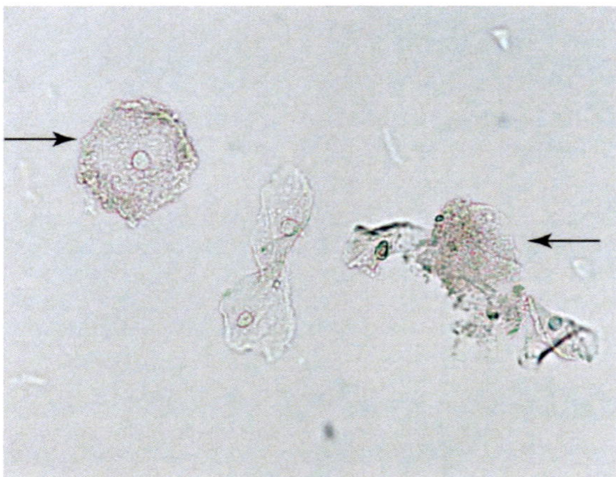

Figure 9.4. *Two clue cells (arrows) and several normal squamous epithelial cells in the wet mount of a vaginal secretion specimen.*

Source: https://basicmedicalkey.com/analysis-of-vaginal-secretions/#s0060.

These cells are similar in size and shape to the transitional epithelial cells of the urinary system, but they have a smaller nucleus-to-cytoplasm ratio (1:1 to 1:2). Women with atrophic vaginitis and desquamative inflammatory vaginitis typically have higher numbers of parabasal cells in their vaginal secretions.

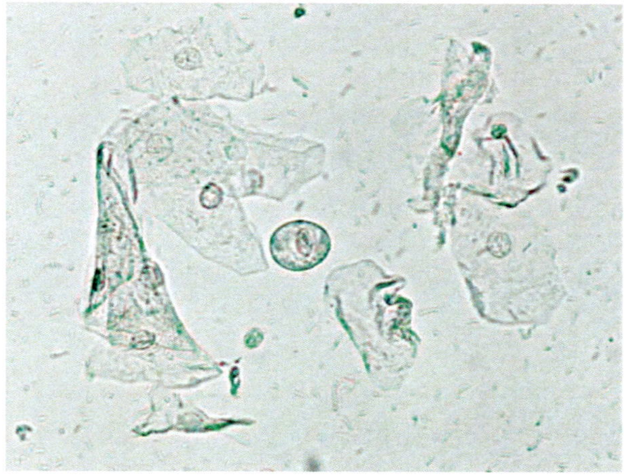

Figure 9.5. *A single parabasal cell surrounded by numerous squamous epithelial cells.*

Source: https://basicmedicalkey.com/analysis-of-vaginal-secretions/#s0060 (Paavonen, 1983).

9.2.2. KOH Preparation and Examination

A straightforward and efficient laboratory technique for diagnosing a variety of vaginal infections, including fungal infections (like Candida) and bacterial vaginosis (BV), is the preparation of potassium hydroxide (KOH) and examination for vaginal secretions. This procedure is also referred to as the KOH test or KOH mount. Using a sample of vaginal discharge combined with a potassium hydroxide solution, a wet mount slide is prepared in this procedure. Below is a detailed guide that will walk you through the KOH preparation and examination process:

1. Collection of Vaginal Discharge Sample:
   - Begin by obtaining a vaginal discharge sample using a sterile cotton swab or a vaginal speculum during a pelvic examination.
   - Gently insert the swab or speculum into the vaginal canal and collect a sample of discharge from the cervix or vaginal walls.
   - Ensure that the sample is representative of the vaginal discharge, including any abnormal texture, color, or odor.
2. **Preparation of KOH Solution:**
   - Prepare a 10% potassium hydroxide (KOH) solution by diluting commercial KOH solution with distilled water. This can be achieved by mixing one part of 10% KOH solution with nine parts of distilled water.
   - Ensure proper labeling of the container containing the KOH solution to prevent misidentification.
3. Mixing the Sample with KOH Solution:
   - Transfer a small amount of the collected vaginal discharge sample onto a clean glass slide using a sterile applicator stick or loop.
   - Add one or two drops of the prepared 10% KOH solution to the vaginal discharge sample on the slide.
   - Gently mix the vaginal discharge and KOH solution using the applicator stick or loop to ensure thorough mixing.
4. Covering the Sample:
   - Place a coverslip over the mixture of vaginal discharge and KOH solution to create a wet mount slide.
   - Apply gentle pressure to the coverslip to spread the mixture evenly and minimize air bubbles.
5. Examination Under Microscope:
   - Place the prepared wet mount slide on the stage of a light microscope.
   - Begin examination using low magnification (e.g., 10x or 20x objective lens) to locate areas of interest and obtain an overall view of the sample.
   - Gradually increase the magnification (e.g., 40x or 100x objective lens) to observe finer details and identify microorganisms or cellular structures.
6. Interpretation of Findings:
   - **Candida Species (Yeast):** In cases of vaginal candidiasis (yeast infection), the KOH preparation may reveal the presence of budding yeast cells, hyphae, or pseudohyphae. These structures are often visible as elongated or branching filaments on the slide.
   - **Bacterial Vaginosis (BV):** The KOH preparation may also aid in the diagnosis of bacterial vaginosis by detecting clue cells, which are epithelial cells

covered with bacteria. Clue cells are indicative of BV and appear as cells with blurred borders and adherent bacteria on microscopic examination.

- **Other Microorganisms:** The KOH mount may also reveal the presence of other microorganisms, such as Trichomonas vaginalis (protozoan parasite) or clue cells coated with bacterial biofilms, which are associated with various vaginal infections.

7. Documentation and Reporting:
   - Record any relevant findings observed during microscopic examination, including the presence of microorganisms, cellular abnormalities, or other diagnostic features.
   - Prepare a concise report summarizing the results of the KOH preparation and examination, along with any additional diagnostic tests performed.
   - Communicate the findings to the healthcare provider responsible for the patient's care to guide diagnosis and treatment decisions.

Performing a KOH preparation and examination for vaginal secretions is a valuable diagnostic tool that can aid in the identification of common vaginal infections, allowing for prompt and appropriate management of patients presenting with vaginal discharge or related symptoms. Proper technique, careful observation, and accurate interpretation of findings are essential for obtaining reliable results and facilitating optimal patient care.

9.3. Clinical Correlations

9.3.1. Bacterial Vaginosis

An overgrowth of normal vaginal flora is the cause of the condition known as bacterial vaginosis. Clinically, this most frequently manifests as increased, fishy-smelling vaginal discharge. The discharge itself is usually thin, white or gray in color. Following a diagnosis of bacterial vaginosis, women are more likely to contract other STIs, and pregnant women are more likely to give birth early. (Figure 9.6).

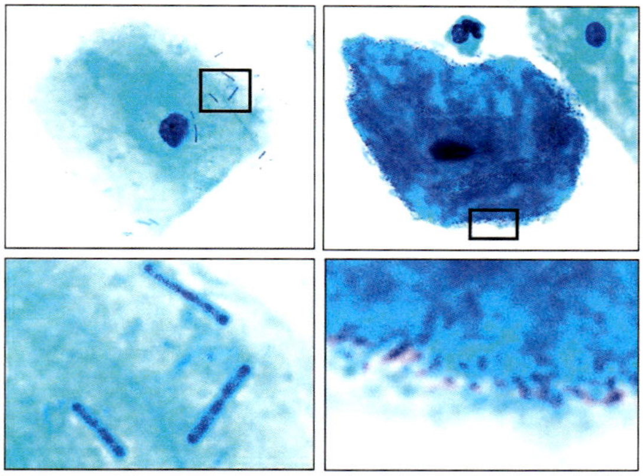

Figure 9.6. *Bacterial vaginosis.*

Source: By Mikael Häggström, M.D. Author info- Reusing images- Conflicts of interest: NoneMikael Häggström, M.D.Consent note: Consent from the patient or patient's relatives is regarded as redundant, because of absence of identifiable features (List of HIPAA identifiers) in the media and case information (See also HIPAA case reports guidance). - Own workSource pictures:Own work (Public Domain)Own work (Public Domain), CC0, https://commons.wikimedia.org/w/index.php?curid=122861127.

Etiology

Despite not being classified as a sexually transmitted infection, the role of transmissibility in bacterial vaginosis remains unclear. Sexual contact can spread bacteria between people, which can change the natural balance of bacterial flora in the vagina. Bacterial vaginosis seems to result from this imbalance. This illness is usually brought on by an overabundance of anaerobic bacteria and a decrease in the normal lactobacilli that produce hydrogen peroxide. When women have sex, Gardnerella vaginalis can spread through shared sex toys or direct contact of the mucous membranes.

Epidemiology

According to estimates, between 5 and 70% of women of reproductive age get bacterial vaginosis, the most common vaginal infection. It's interesting to note that this ailment is least common in Asia and Europe and most common in some regions of Africa globally. About 30% of American women between the ages of 14 and 49 are impacted. Although rates vary by ethnic group, non-white women (of whom 32% are Mexican Americans and 51% are African Americans) are the most likely to experience them.

Epidemiological data showed that women are more likely to report bacterial vaginosis if they have had multiple sexual partners, are unmarried, began to engage in intercourse at a young age, if they are commercial sex workers, or practice regularly douching.

Pathophysiology

Bacterial vaginosis is caused by an imbalance of the naturally occurring vaginal flora, characterized by both a change in the most common type of bacteria present as well as an increase in the total number of bacteria present. The *Lactobacilli* species dominate normal vaginal microbiota. Bacterial vaginosis is associated with a decline in the overall number of Lactobacilli. Although still uncertain, it is thought that most bacterial vaginosis infections start with *Gardnerella vaginalis,* creating a biofilm that then allows other opportunistic bacteria to grow within the vagina.

The association between BV and an increased risk for future STIs stems from the fact that BV allows the potential for other vaginal pathogens to gain access to the upper genital tract. BV is also responsible for the presence of enzymes that reduce the ability of host leukocytes to fight infection and for an increased release of endotoxins that stimulate cytokine and prostaglandin production within the vagina.

Histopathology

The hallmark of this diagnosis relies on the examination of vaginal fluid on a wet mount under a microscope. Bacterial vaginosis is characterized by the presence of clue cells, which are epithelial cells of the cervix that are embedded with rod-shaped bacteria.

History and Physical

Most women with bacterial vaginosis present with a complaint of malodorous vaginal discharge. Often this becomes more pronounced after sexual intercourse. Additional symptoms may include dysuria, dyspareunia, and vaginal pruritus; however, many affected women may be asymptomatic.

The clinician should elicit pertinent history regarding the risk factors for this disease, as well as a previous history of bacterial vaginosis infections. The risk factors for bacterial vaginosis include vaginal douching, multiple sexual partners, recent antibiotic use, cigarette smoking, and the use of an intrauterine device. For this reason, the U.S. Department of Health and Human Services strongly discourages the use of vaginal douching. Having a female sexual partner increases the risk of bacterial vaginosis by 60%; it is important to note that bacterial vaginosis is not an STI. By definition, an STI is caused by a source that is not endogenous to the vaginal flora. Since bacterial vaginosis is caused by an overgrowth of normal vaginal bacteria, it does not meet the definition of an STI. Furthermore, bacterial vaginosis can rarely be present in patients who have never had sexual intercourse.

A proper physical exam must include a pelvic exam to examine the characteristics of the vaginal discharge and to help exclude other similarly presenting diseases, including candidiasis, cervicitis, chlamydia, gonorrhea, herpes simplex virus, and trichomoniasis. In addition, bacterial vaginosis itself is a risk factor for pelvic inflammatory disease, HIV, STIs, and other obstetric disorders. Therefore, it is important to assess for cervical friability and cervical motion tenderness as well.

It is important to assess for fever, pelvic pain, and a history of sexually transmitted infections to rule out the more serious conditions that remain on the differential diagnosis. Cervical swabs may be sent to investigate the presence of chlamydia or gonorrhea infection.

Since clue cells are thought to be the most reliable diagnostic sign of bacterial vaginosis, it will be necessary to examine the vaginal fluid under a microscope. This diagnostic step can also help to rule out the presence of yeast or trichomonads. It is important to note that many of these diseases can occur concomitantly, so it is necessary to scan the entire specimen for the presence of clue cells even if another pathology is identified. Testing the vaginal fluid pH can also assist in the diagnosis of bacterial vaginosis. (Holmes, 1984; Rein and Muller, 1984)

Evaluation

Diagnosis of bacterial vaginosis is typically suggested clinically and confirmed by obtaining a vaginal swab of the cervical region or discharge and creating a wet mount slide to review under a microscope. The swab may contain a higher than normal vaginal pH (greater than 4.5), the presence of clue cells on wet mount, and a positive whiff test. To determine the vaginal pH, pH paper can be utilized and compared to color controls. To identify clue cells, a drop of sodium chloride solution is placed on the wet mount slide, and the slide is examined under the microscope for visualization of the characteristic clue cells. The whiff test is performed by adding a small amount of potassium hydroxide to the microscopic slide containing the vaginal discharge and is considered to be positive if a characteristic fishy odor is revealed. Typically, two of these positive tests, in addition to the presence of the characteristic discharge, are enough to confirm the diagnosis of bacterial vaginosis. If no discharge is present, then all three of these criteria are needed to make the diagnosis.

In clinical practice, bacterial vaginosis is often diagnosed by the Amsel criteria. At least three of the four criteria are needed to confirm the diagnosis. The Amsel criteria include a thin white, a yellow, homogenous discharge, clue cells on microscopy, pH of vaginal fluid more than 4.5, and the release of a fishy odor after adding an alkali solution (10% KOH) to the specimen. The modified Amsel criteria accept the presence of just two of the above factors, and research has shown that this is equally diagnostic. The sensitivity and specificity of the Amsel criteria are 70% and 94%, respectively.

Alternatively, a gram-stain of the vaginal fluid can be done to examine the predominant strain of bacteria. This technique is referred to as the Nugent process. Data have shown that this technique has a sensitivity and specificity of 89% and 83%, respectively, but it rarely is used in clinical practice.

Risk Factors

Several factors have been associated with an

increased risk of developing bacterial vaginosis, including:

- **Sexual Activity:** BV is more common among sexually active women, particularly those with multiple sexual partners or a new sexual partner.
- **Douching:** Vaginal douching disrupts the natural balance of vaginal bacteria and has been linked to an increased risk of BV.
- **Hormonal Factors:** Hormonal fluctuations, such as those occurring during menstruation, pregnancy, or menopause, can predispose women to BV.
- **Smoking:** Cigarette smoking has been identified as a risk factor for bacterial vaginosis, possibly due to its effects on vaginal immunity and inflammation.
- **Use of Intrauterine Devices (IUDs):** Women who use intrauterine devices for contraception may have a higher risk of developing BV, although the reasons for this association are not fully understood.
- **Race and Ethnicity:** Studies have found differences in the prevalence of BV among different racial and ethnic groups, with higher rates observed among African American and Hispanic women compared to white women.

Symptoms

Bacterial vaginosis can manifest with a variety of symptoms, although many women with BV remain asymptomatic. When symptoms do occur, they may include:

- **Vaginal Discharge:** Women with BV often experience a thin, grayish-white vaginal discharge with a characteristic "fishy" odor, particularly after sexual intercourse or during menstruation.
- **Vaginal Odor:** The characteristic odor associated with bacterial vaginosis is often described as "fishy" and may become more pronounced after sexual activity or when the vaginal discharge mixes with semen or menstrual blood.
- **Vaginal Itching or Irritation:** Some women with BV may experience itching, redness, or discomfort in the vaginal area, although these symptoms are less common than vaginal discharge and odor.

It's important to note that bacterial vaginosis can be asymptomatic in many cases, making it essential for sexually active women to undergo regular gynecological examinations and STI screenings.

Diagnosis

Diagnosing bacterial vaginosis typically involves a combination of clinical evaluation, laboratory testing, and diagnostic criteria. Key aspects of the diagnostic process may include:

- **Medical History:** The healthcare provider will inquire about symptoms, sexual activity, and potential risk factors for BV.
- **Pelvic Examination:** A pelvic examination allows the healthcare provider to assess the appearance of the vaginal discharge, vaginal pH, and the presence of other signs of inflammation or infection.

- **Amsel Criteria:** The Amsel criteria are a set of clinical criteria used to diagnose bacterial vaginosis based on the presence of specific signs and symptoms, including vaginal discharge, vaginal pH >4.5, characteristic odor (whiff test), and the presence of clue cells on microscopic examination of vaginal fluid.
- **Laboratory testing:** Various laboratory tests can be used to confirm the diagnosis of bacterial vaginosis and identify the presence of specific bacteria associated with BV. These tests include:
  - **Wet Mount Microscopy:** A sample of vaginal discharge is examined under a microscope for the presence of clue cells (epithelial cells covered with bacteria) and other signs of BV.
  - **Gram stain:** Gram staining of vaginal fluid can reveal the presence of "clue cells" and changes in the vaginal microbiota consistent with BV.
  - **Nucleic Acid Amplification Tests (NAATs):** Polymerase chain reaction (PCR) and other NAATs can detect specific bacterial DNA associated with BV, providing a more sensitive and specific diagnostic method.

Treatment

Bacterial vaginosis is typically treated with antimicrobial medications aimed at restoring the balance of vaginal bacteria. The recommended first-line treatment for BV is oral or intravaginal antibiotics, such as metronidazole or clindamycin. Treatment regimens may vary depending on factors such as the severity of symptoms, medical history, and medication availability. Women need to complete the full course of antibiotics as prescribed, even if symptoms improve before the medication is finished. Sexual partners of women with BV do not routinely require treatment unless they have symptoms of BV or other STIs.

Complications

Untreated bacterial vaginosis can lead to various complications, particularly in pregnant women. Some potential complications of BV include:

- **Increased Risk of Other STIs:** Bacterial vaginosis has been associated with an increased risk of acquiring other sexually transmitted infections (STIs), including HIV, herpes simplex virus (HSV), chlamydia, and gonorrhea. The inflammation and disruption of the vaginal microbiota associated with BV may facilitate the transmission and acquisition of other STIs.
- **Pelvic Inflammatory Disease (PID):** Bacterial vaginosis has been linked to an increased risk of developing pelvic inflammatory disease (PID), a serious infection of the female reproductive organs. PID can cause chronic pelvic pain, infertility, ectopic pregnancy, and other complications.
- **Pregnancy Complications:** Bacterial vaginosis during pregnancy has been associated with adverse pregnancy outcomes, including preterm birth, low birth weight, premature rupture of membranes, and postpartum endometritis. Pregnant women with BV may require treatment to

reduce the risk of complications for themselves and their babies.

Prevention

Preventing bacterial vaginosis involves adopting healthy behaviors and minimizing risk factors that can disrupt the natural balance of vaginal bacteria. Some preventive measures include:

- **Practice Safe Sex:** Using condoms consistently and correctly during vaginal, anal, and oral sex can reduce the risk of BV and other STIs. Condoms provide a barrier that helps prevent the exchange of genital fluids and reduces the transmission of infectious agents.
- **Limit Vaginal Douching:** Avoiding vaginal douching and other intravaginal hygiene practices can help preserve the natural balance of vaginal bacteria and reduce the risk of BV. Douching can disrupt the normal pH and microbial composition of the vagina, making it more susceptible to infections.
- **Avoid Smoking:** Cigarette smoking has been identified as a risk factor for bacterial vaginosis and other reproductive health issues. Quitting smoking or avoiding exposure to secondhand smoke can help reduce the risk of BV and improve overall health.
- **Attend Regular Gynecological Check-ups:** Undergoing regular pelvic examinations and STI screenings can help detect bacterial vaginosis and other reproductive health issues early, allowing for prompt treatment and management.

Public Health Implications

Bacterial vaginosis poses significant public health challenges due to its high prevalence, association with adverse reproductive outcomes, and potential for transmission to sexual partners. Efforts to control bacterial vaginosis and reduce its impact on women's health require a multifaceted approach that includes:

- **Increasing awareness:** Education campaigns aimed at healthcare providers and the general public can help raise awareness about bacterial vaginosis, its risk factors, symptoms, and prevention strategies. Providing accurate information and dispelling myths and misconceptions about BV can empower women to seek timely medical care and adopt healthy behaviors.
- **Screening and Treatment Programs:** Implementing routine screening programs for bacterial vaginosis in high-risk populations, such as pregnant women, can help identify and treat infections early, reducing the risk of adverse pregnancy outcomes and other complications. Ensuring access to affordable and culturally sensitive healthcare services, including STI testing and treatment, is essential for addressing disparities in BV prevalence and outcomes.
- **Research and Surveillance:** Continued research into the epidemiology, pathogenesis, and treatment of bacterial vaginosis is needed to inform evidence-based interventions and public health policies. Surveillance systems for monitoring BV prevalence and trends can help guide resource

allocation and intervention strategies, ultimately improving women's health outcomes and reducing the burden of BV-related complications.

9.3.2. Candidiasis

Vulvovaginitis, most commonly occurs in reproductive-aged women and is caused by several underlying etiologies. Candidiasis is a fungal infection caused by *Candida albicans*, a polymorphic opportunistic fungus; vulvovaginitis secondary to candidiasis is also known as vaginal candidiasis. Candidal vulvovaginitis is responsible for about one-third of vulvovaginitis occurrences. Typical clinical features include vulvar and vaginal erythema, excoriations, thick white adherent discharge, and swelling. The condition is primarily diagnosed by clinical examination and diagnostic studies, including vaginal wet prep, pH testing, and cultures to exclude other etiologies of vaginal discharge and infection (eg, bacterial vaginosis and gonococcal and chlamydial disease). This activity for healthcare professionals is designed to enhance the learner's competence when managing vaginal candidiasis, equipping them with updated knowledge, skills, and strategies for timely identification, effective interventions, and improved coordination of care, leading to better outcomes for patients.

- **Etiology:** Candidal vulvovaginitis is caused by inflammatory changes in the vaginal and vulvar epithelium secondary to infection with *Candida* species, most commonly *Candida albicans*. However, *Candida* is part of the normal flora in many women, identified in 10% of asymptomatic women. Therefore, candidal vulvovaginitis requires both the presence of *Candida* in the vagina and associated symptoms (e.g., irritation, itching, dysuria, or inflammation).
- **Epidemiology:** Candidal vulvovaginitis is a common condition responsible for a third of all cases of vulvovaginitis in reproductive-aged women. Approximately 70% of women report having had candidal vulvovaginitis in their lifetime, and an estimated 8% of women suffer recurrent candidal vulvovaginitis. The most common responsible pathogen is *C. albicans,* accounting for 90% of cases, with most of the remaining cases caused by *Candida glabrata*. Because over-the-counter treatments are widely available, candidal vulvovaginitis is under-reported; therefore, detailed epidemiological data for this disease process is unavailable. Furthermore, diagnosis is based on both clinical and ancillary evaluation. As a result, epidemiologic reports based on culture alone, in which 10% of asymptomatic women have positive candidal cultures, overestimate the disease incidence. Furthermore, studies demonstrate that because self-diagnosis is inaccurate, data derived from a patient query is also imprecise.

Recognized risk factors for acute candidal vulvovaginitis include estrogen use, elevated endogenous estrogens (e.g., pregnancy or obesity), diabetes mellitus, immunosuppression (i.e., chemotherapy or antimetabolite medications, HIV infection, or transplant patients), and broad-spectrum antibiotic use. Although candidal vulvovaginitis is more common in sexually active women, evidence that candidal infection is sexually transmitted is lacking. Patients with recurrent candidal vulvovaginitis, defined as 4 or more episodes of culture-proven candidal vulvovaginitis, have predisposing genetic factors that cause them to be susceptible to recurrent fungal infections. These factors may also cause a predisposition to *Candida* hypersensitivity reactions.

- **Pathophysiology:** Candidal vulvovaginitis occurs when *Candida* species superficially penetrate the mucosal lining of the vagina and cause an inflammatory response. The dominant inflammatory cells are typically polymorphonuclear cells and macrophages. The inflammatory response results in copious thick discharge and vaginal irritation, excoriations, dysuria, itching, burning, dyspareunia, or swelling.
- **History and Physical:** Characteristic clinical symptoms of vaginal candidiasis include vaginal and vulvar irritation, itching, and burning. Symptoms are often prominent just before the patient's menstrual period. Many patients have a history of similar symptoms and report attempting over-the-counter treatment with topical agents or alternative therapies.

  On pelvic exam, common findings include vulvar and vaginal erythema, excoriations, thick white adherent discharge, and swelling. In some patients, little to no discharge is noted. In patients with candidal vulvovaginitis, inflammation is evident during a pelvic exam. However, the cervix is typically normal and not inflamed. The patient should not have cervical motion tenderness, and there should be no abnormal discharge from the cervical OS. Ulcers, asymmetric swelling or masses, or foreign bodies should prompt consideration of differential diagnoses. The degree of irritation is typically severe in patients with acute vulvovaginal candidiasis. Conversely, patients with *Candida glabrata* infections usually have mild symptoms. Various vulvovaginitis etiologies have similar presentations, and therefore, further diagnostic studies, including wet mount, whiff testing, and pH testing, should be considered for uncertain diagnoses.
- **Evaluation:** Diagnostic studies utilized to confirm the presence of *Candida* include 10% potassium hydroxide (KOH) and wet mount smears of the vaginal discharge for microscopy, pH testing, and potentially fungal culture or commercial polymerase chain reaction (PCR) tests. In patients with vulvovaginal candidiasis, the vaginal pH is typically below 5. [ACOG Practice bulletin 215 Vaginitis in Nonpregnant] Characteristic findings of vaginal candidiasis include the prominence of lactobacillus bacteria and inflammatory cells on wet prep, a negative Whiff test (i.e., no fishy odor with the application of KOH to the slide), and budding yeast, hyphae, or pseudohyphae on microscopy, which are typically seen most

easily on the KOH prep. Microscopy and pH testing can also identify clue cells, indicating bacterial vaginosis, and trichomonads, indicating trichomoniasis, which should be ruled out (or diagnosed) concurrently.

Most infections are secondary to *Candida albicans;* therefore, consistent microscopy findings in the clinical setting of a reproductive-age woman with vulvovaginitis, confirmatory cultures for *Candida* are unnecessary. Cultures should be considered in patients with recurrent disease and patients with a negative work-up in the setting of symptoms consistent with vulvovaginal candidiasis. However, if cultures cannot be performed, empiric treatment is reasonable.

Because *Candida* species are part of normal vaginal flora in many women, routine cultures in asymptomatic women are discouraged.

- **Treatment / Management:** Acute candidal vulvovaginitis is treated with antifungal agents. Since most candidal vulvovaginitis cases are secondary to *C albicans* species, and *C albicans* does not demonstrate resistance to azole antifungals, these are the agents of choice. Antifungals may be administered through several methods, including a single dose of fluconazole 150 mg orally or terconazole applied intravaginally once or in multiple dose regimens ranging from 3 to 7 days available over the counter. These options are equally efficacious in patients with uncomplicated disease (e.g., immunocompetent status or nonrecurrent candidal vulvovaginitis). Therefore, treatment decisions may be based on cost, patient preference, and drug interactions. In unresponsive patients, cultures may be warranted to look for other *Candida* species, often resistant to standard therapy.

  For complicated candidal vulvovaginitis, including patients who are immunosuppressed or have a recurrent infection, extended treatment regimens are commonly utilized, such as intravaginal azole therapy for at least 1 week or oral treatment with fluconazole 150 mg (renally adjusted for CrCl <50 ml/min) once every 3 days for 3 doses. Patients with recurrent candidal vulvovaginitis may benefit from suppressive therapy with weekly oral fluconazole for 6 months. However, pregnant patients should not be given oral antifungals. In these patients, a 7-day course of intravaginal treatment is recommended. Fluconazole is considered safe in breastfeeding women. Nonpharmacologic therapies (e.g., intravaginal or oral yogurt therapy, intravaginal garlic, or douching) have not been found to be effective.

- **Differential Diagnosis:** Differential diagnoses that should also be considered include:
  - Allergic reaction
  - Atopic dermatitis
  - Lichen sclerosis
  - Lichen simplex chronicus

- Neoplasm
- Paget disease
- Physiologic leukorrhea
- Psoriasis
- Sexual abuse
- Vulvodynia

- **Prognosis:** Despite appropriate treatment, recurrence is relatively common and is estimated to range from 14% to 28% in otherwise healthy individuals. Most often, recurrent disease arises from persistent vaginal organisms or endogenous reinfection with an identical strain of *Candida*. Less commonly, the disease may result from a new strain of *Candida*. Recurrent disease may be triggered by antibiotic use, sexual activity, or dietary factors. Genetic susceptibility may also affect a person's risk for recurrent disease.

  Topical imidazole and oral fluconazole are less likely to be effective in patients with non-*albicans* species of *Candida*. Therefore, fungal culture is indicated in patients with persistent symptoms after standard treatment for uncomplicated vulvovaginal candidiasis. Boric acid (600 mg vaginally for at least 14 days) is often effective against *C glabrata* and other atypical species. Note that boric acid can be fatal if orally ingested, so patients must be well-counseled on its use.

- **Complications:** Complications secondary to vaginal candidiasis are rare but, in severe cases, may cause extensive vulvar erythema, edema, excoriation, and vaginal or vulvar fissures. Adverse events that may occur with antifungal treatment include abdominal pain, nausea and vomiting, diarrhea, flatulence, headache, central nervous system disorder, musculoskeletal disorder, rash, allergic reaction, menstrual disorder, and alopecia.

- **Deterrence and Patient Education:** Patients should be instructed only to use recommended vaginal candidiasis treatments as inappropriate use of over-the-counter preparations can result in treatment delay and the development of other vulvovaginitis etiologies. Clinicians should also counsel patients that there is little evidence supporting the use of probiotics or homeopathic medications for vaginal candidiasis treatment. Individuals with persistent symptoms should be instructed to return for follow-up visits. General recommendations to help prevent recurrent episodes of *Candida* infection include keeping the vaginal area dry by changing out of wet clothes immediately after swimming or exercising, avoiding soap in the vulvovaginal area, wearing breathable fabrics, avoiding douches, and considering preventative antifungal treatment while taking antibiotics.

- **Pearls and Other Issues:** Although vaginitis is not a dangerous disease, symptoms are often irritating and, in severe cases, disabling. Therefore, clinicians should address social issues and sexual dysfunction in addition to the infection itself. A broad differential diagnosis should always be considered. Trauma, abuse, foreign body, malignancy, immune diseases, inflammatory bowel disease, and sexually transmitted infections can all present with vaginal discomfort. Clinicians should always perform a careful and complete physical exam, appropriate ancillary testing, and further diagnostic studies if treatment failure occurs.

- **Enhancing Healthcare Team Outcomes:** Candida vulvovaginitis is usually managed by a gynecologist, nurse practitioner, primary care clinician, or internist. The condition has been clinically diagnosed and managed with antifungal medications. Most simple cases are resolved within days. Patients with complicated candidal vulvovaginitis require more extended therapy. Pharmacists and pharmacy technicians can help direct patients toward appropriate therapy. Pregnant patients should not be given oral antifungals. In these patients, a 7-day course of intravaginal treatment is appropriate. Fluconazole is considered safe in breastfeeding women. There is inadequate evidence to recommend intravaginal or oral yogurt therapy, intravaginal garlic, or douching.

  At the same time, patient education is essential. The condition is not life-threatening but can be associated with embarrassment and withdrawal from sexual activities. It is also vital to maintain a broad differential diagnosis. Trauma, abuse, foreign body, malignancy, immune diseases, inflammatory bowel disease, and sexually transmitted infections can all present with vaginal discomfort. If treatment failure occurs, clinicians should always perform a careful and complete physical exam, appropriate ancillary testing, and further testing (Verstraelen and Verhelst, 2009; Donders et al., 2017; Yudin and Money, 2017; Denning et al., 2018; Coleman and Gaydos, 2018; Verstraelen and Swidsinski, 2018; Yano et al., 2019; Workowskie et al., 2021).

9.3.3. Atrophic Vaginitis

Atrophic vaginitis, also known as vaginal atrophy, is a common condition characterized by inflammation, thinning, and dryness of the vaginal walls due to decreased estrogen levels.

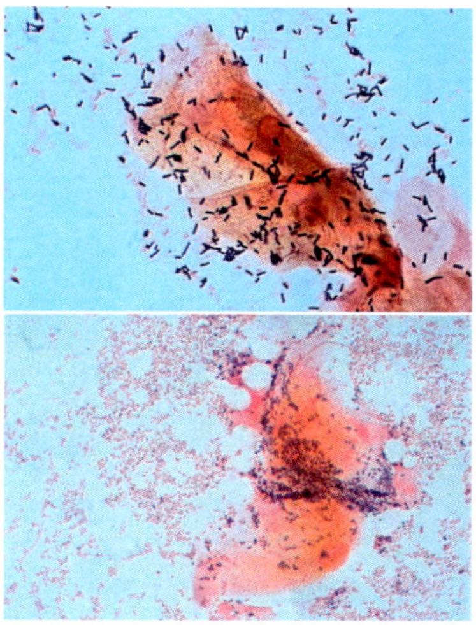

Figure 9.7. *Gram stain of cells from the vagina (the same magnification) with normal bacterial flora (top) and the bacteria that cause vaginosis (bottom).*

It primarily affects postmenopausal women but can also occur in women during perimenopause, after childbirth, during breastfeeding, or in those who have undergone cancer treatments like chemotherapy or radiation therapy. This comprehensive discussion of atrophic vaginitis covers its causes, symptoms, diagnosis, treatment options, and strategies for prevention and management (Figure 9.7).

9.3.3.1. Causes and Risk Factors

Atrophic vaginitis primarily results from declining estrogen levels, which can occur due to natural menopause or as a result of surgical removal of the ovaries (oophorectomy), chemotherapy, or radiation therapy for cancer treatment. Estrogen plays a crucial role in maintaining the health and elasticity of vaginal tissues, lubrication, and maintaining the acidity of the vaginal environment. When estrogen levels decrease, the vaginal walls become thinner, drier, and less elastic, leading to symptoms of atrophic vaginitis.

Risk factors for developing atrophic vaginitis include:

- **Menopause:** Natural decline in estrogen levels during menopause is the most common cause.
- **Surgical Menopause:** Removal of both ovaries (bilateral oophorectomy) leads to an abrupt decrease in estrogen levels.
- **Breastfeeding:** Estrogen levels are lower during breastfeeding, which can contribute to vaginal dryness.
- **Cancer Treatments:** Chemotherapy, radiation therapy, or hormonal therapies for breast or gynecological cancers can cause a decline in estrogen levels, leading to vaginal atrophy.
- **Certain Medications:** Some medications, such as GnRH agonists used to treat endometriosis or prostate cancer, can induce a menopause-like state with low estrogen levels.
- **Smoking:** Smoking has been associated with an increased risk of developing vaginal atrophy, possibly due to its negative effects on blood circulation and hormone levels.

9.3.3.2. Symptoms

The symptoms of atrophic vaginitis can vary in severity and may include:

- **Vaginal Dryness:** This is one of the hallmark symptoms of atrophic vaginitis. Women may experience a persistent sensation of dryness or discomfort in the vaginal area, especially during sexual activity.
- **Vaginal Itching or Burning:** Irritation and itching in the vaginal area can occur due to the thinning and inflammation of the vaginal tissues.
- **Dyspareunia (Painful Intercourse):** Vaginal dryness and thinning of the vaginal walls can cause discomfort or pain during sexual intercourse.
- **Vaginal Discharge:** Some women may experience a decrease in vaginal lubrication, leading to a decrease in vaginal discharge.
- **Urinary Symptoms:** Atrophic changes in the urinary tract can lead to symptoms such as urinary urgency, frequency, or recurrent urinary tract infections (UTIs).
- **Bleeding:** Thinning of the vaginal tissues can make them more prone

to bleeding, especially after sexual intercourse.

It's essential for women experiencing these symptoms to seek medical evaluation to determine the underlying cause and receive appropriate treatment.

9.3.3.3. Diagnosis

Diagnosing atrophic vaginitis typically involves a thorough medical history, physical examination, and may include additional tests or procedures to rule out other conditions. Key aspects of the diagnostic process may include:

- **Medical History:** The healthcare provider will inquire about symptoms, menopausal status, medical history, medications, and any previous treatments for gynecological conditions.
- **Pelvic Examination:** A pelvic examination allows the healthcare provider to assess the vaginal walls for signs of thinning, dryness, inflammation, or other abnormalities.
- **Vaginal pH Testing:** Measurement of the vaginal pH can help differentiate atrophic vaginitis from other causes of vaginal irritation or infection. Vaginal pH is typically higher (>4.5) in women with bacterial vaginosis or trichomoniasis but lower in atrophic vaginitis.
- **Laboratory Tests:** In some cases, additional tests such as vaginal swabs or cultures may be performed to rule out other infections or conditions that may present with similar symptoms.
- **Biopsy:** In rare cases where the diagnosis is unclear or there are concerns about other underlying conditions, a biopsy of the vaginal tissues may be recommended (Verstraelen and Verhelst, 2009; Donders et al., 2017; Yudin and Money, 2017; Denning et al., 2018; Coleman and Gaydos, 2018; Verstraelen and Swidsinski, 2018; Yano et al., 2019; Workowskie et al., 2021).

9.3.3.4. Treatment Options

Treatment for atrophic vaginitis aims to alleviate symptoms, improve vaginal health, and enhance quality of life. Several treatment options are available, and the choice of treatment depends on factors such as the severity of symptoms, underlying health conditions, and personal preferences. Treatment modalities for atrophic vaginitis may include:

- **Hormone Therapy (HT):** Estrogen therapy, in the form of vaginal estrogen creams, tablets, rings, or patches, is the most effective treatment for atrophic vaginitis. These products deliver estrogen directly to the vaginal tissues, helping to restore moisture, thickness, and elasticity of the vaginal walls. Estrogen therapy is available in various formulations and dosages, and the healthcare provider will prescribe the most appropriate option based on individual needs and preferences. Systemic estrogen therapy, such as oral hormone replacement therapy (HRT), may also be used for women with severe symptoms or additional menopausal symptoms.
- **Non-hormonal Moisturizers and Lubricants:** Over-the-counter

vaginal moisturizers and lubricants can provide temporary relief from vaginal dryness and discomfort. These products help to hydrate the vaginal tissues and reduce friction during sexual activity. Non-hormonal moisturizers are suitable for women who prefer not to use estrogen therapy or have contraindications to hormonal treatments.

- **Vaginal Dilators:** Vaginal dilators are medical devices used to gently stretch and expand the vaginal tissues. Regular use of vaginal dilators can help maintain vaginal elasticity, reduce discomfort during intercourse, and prevent vaginal stenosis (narrowing of the vagina). Vaginal dilators are often recommended as part of a comprehensive treatment plan for women with atrophic vaginitis, especially those experiencing dyspareunia.
- **Pelvic Floor Physical Therapy:** Pelvic floor physical therapy involves exercises, manual techniques, and other interventions designed to improve pelvic floor muscle function and alleviate symptoms of pelvic floor dysfunction, including pelvic pain and sexual dysfunction. Pelvic floor physical therapy may be beneficial for women with atrophic vaginitis who experience pelvic floor muscle tension or weakness contributing to their symptoms.

9.3.3.5. Prevention and Management

While atrophic vaginitis cannot always be prevented, certain lifestyle modifications and strategies can help reduce the risk of developing symptoms or manage existing symptoms more effectively. Some preventive measures and management strategies for atrophic vaginitis include:

- **Maintain Optimal Overall Health:** Eating a balanced diet, engaging in regular physical activity, and avoiding smoking can help support overall health and hormonal balance.
- **Stay Hydrated:** Drinking an adequate amount of water can help maintain hydration levels in the body, including the vaginal tissues.
- **Use Lubricants During Sexual Activity:** Using water-based or silicone-based lubricants during sexual intercourse can help reduce friction and discomfort associated with vaginal dryness.
- **Practice Safe Sex:** Using condoms during sexual activity can help reduce the risk of sexually transmitted infections (STIs), which can exacerbate symptoms of atrophic vaginitis.
- **Attend Regular Gynecological Check-ups:** Regular visits to the healthcare provider for pelvic examinations and screenings can help detect any changes in vaginal health and address them promptly.

9.3.4. Trichomoniasis

Trichomoniasis is a sexually transmitted infection (STI) caused by the protozoan parasite Trichomonas vaginalis. It is one of the most common curable STIs worldwide, affecting millions of people annually. Trichomoniasis can have significant implications for reproductive and overall health, yet it often goes undiagnosed and untreated due to its asymptomatic nature in many cases. This comprehensive discussion of trichomoniasis covers its etiology, transmission, symptoms, diagnosis, treatment, complications, prevention, and public health implications (Figure 9.8).

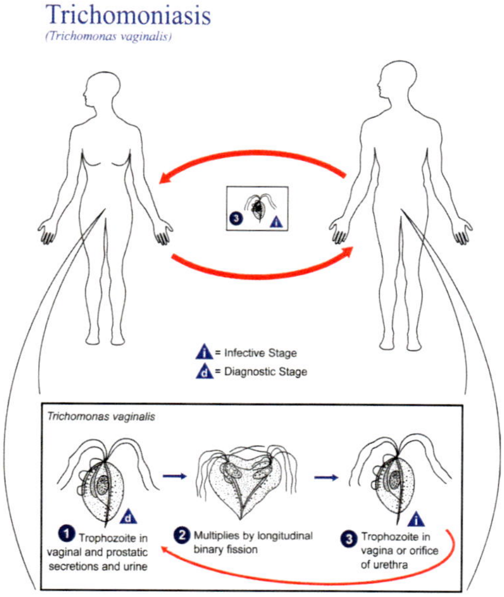

Figure 9.8. *Trichomoniasis is an infection that mainly affects females at birth. It spreads through sexual intercourse and doesn't typically cause symptoms.*

Source: Public Domain, https://commons.wikimedia.org/w/index.php?curid=2740683.

- **Etiology:** Trichomoniasis is caused by Trichomonas vaginalis, a single-celled protozoan parasite that primarily infects the urogenital tract. T. vaginalis is pear-shaped and has flagella, which it uses for movement. The parasite primarily colonizes the vagina and urethra in women and the urethra in men. Transmission typically occurs through sexual contact, including vaginal intercourse, anal intercourse, and genital-to-genital contact. However, it can also be transmitted through non-sexual means, such as sharing contaminated objects or from mother to child during childbirth.
- **Epidemiology:** Trichomoniasis occurs more frequently in people with multiple sexual partners who also have other sexually transmitted infections. In one study with 4057 participants, *T. vaginalis* infection was found in 0.5% of males and 1.8% of females in the study population. They found prevalence among Black study participants to be higher, with 4.2% and 8.9% infection rates noted in males and females, respectively.

  According to another article, the estimated infection rate of *Trichomoniasis vaginalis* is 3.2%. *T. vaginalis* infection rates in the United States are higher than those of *Neisseria gonorrhoeae* and *Chlamydia trachomatis* infection rates combined. Trichomoniasis is most prevalent amongst women ages 40 to 49, which is starkly different from the rate of chlamydia infections, which peaks in the 19 to 24-year-old age group.
- **Pathophysiology:** Trichomonas is a motile organism with a size comparable to a white blood cell. It has at least 4 flagella that provide undulating motility. The organism resides in the lumen of the urogenital tract. The organism releases cytotoxic proteins that destroy the epithelial lining. During an infection, the vaginal pH usually increases.

  In women, *T. vaginalis* has an incubation period of five to twenty-eight days. Women with trichomoniasis often complain of a foul-smelling yellow or green vaginal discharge, dyspareunia, urinary frequency, dysuria, and/or vulvar pruritus or erythema. In men, it often does not cause symptoms. If a male is symptomatic, the most common symptom is urethritis. Less commonly, men may also develop prostatitis and epididymitis.

- **History and Physical:** Women will often present with a chief complaint similar to other sexually transmitted infections, including vaginal discharge, painful intercourse, urinary tract infection symptoms, vaginal itching, or pelvic pain. Men may be asymptomatic, or on occasion, they may present with symptoms including penile discharge, testicular pain, dysuria, urinary frequency, or cloudy urine. Trichomoniasis can cause urethritis in men and occasionally epididymitis or prostatitis.
    - Critical questions to ask when gathering a history include past treatment for STIs, condom use with intercourse, and the presence of foul-smelling discharge.
    - A physical exam will often include a pelvic exam for women and a urethral swab for men.
    - A vaginal discharge is common in women; the discharge is thin, frothy, and has an abnormal odor. The genitals are often red and edematous. A strawberry cervix is seen in about 40% of patients. Palpation of the pelvis may reveal mild tenderness.
- **Evaluation:** The most common diagnostic testing performed is wet prep microscopy. Trichomonads are motile organisms with flagella and can be seen moving in the preparation when viewed with a microscope. This test has been shown to be only 40% to 60% sensitive but is typically the most common testing method used due to convenience and low cost.

  Nucleic acid amplification tests (NAATs) are gaining favor when testing for *Trichomonas vaginalis*. They have become the gold standard when testing for gonorrhea and chlamydia. Many of the NAATs available have been shown to have greater than 90% sensitivity and specificity when testing for *Trichomonas vaginalis*.

  Before NAATs and other point-of-care options were developed, the gold standard was a culture when testing for *Trichomonas vaginalis* with a negative wet prep and a symptomatic patient.

  The vaginal pH is usually more than 4.5 in the presence of trichomoniasis, but this is not a specific finding. The whiff test is done by adding drops of potassium hydroxide to a sample of vaginal discharge. This generates a fishy smell.
- **Transmission:** Trichomoniasis is primarily transmitted through sexual contact with an infected partner. Individuals who engage in unprotected sex with multiple partners, have a history of STIs, or

have a partner with a history of STIs are at increased risk of acquiring trichomoniasis. The infection can be transmitted from an infected person even if they do not have symptoms, making it important for sexually active individuals to practice safe sex and undergo regular STI screenings.

- **Symptoms:** Trichomoniasis can manifest with a wide range of symptoms, although many individuals infected with *T. vaginalis* remain asymptomatic. When symptoms do occur, they typically appear within 5 to 28 days after exposure and may include:
  - **Vaginal Discharge:** Women may experience a frothy, yellow-green, or gray vaginal discharge with a foul odor.
  - **Genital Itching or Irritation:** Itching, redness, and discomfort in the genital area may occur due to inflammation and irritation of the vaginal and urethral tissues.
  - **Dysuria (Painful Urination):** Burning or pain during urination can occur due to inflammation of the urethra.
  - **Dyspareunia (Painful Intercourse):** Sexual intercourse may be uncomfortable or painful due to inflammation and irritation of the genital tissues.

  In men, symptoms of trichomoniasis are typically milder and may include urethral discharge, itching or irritation of the penis, and discomfort during urination or ejaculation. However, many men with trichomoniasis remain asymptomatic.
- **Diagnosis:** Diagnosing trichomoniasis typically involves a combination of clinical evaluation, laboratory testing, and diagnostic procedures. Key aspects of the diagnostic process may include:
  - **Medical History:** The healthcare provider will inquire about symptoms, sexual activity, and potential risk factors for STIs.
  - **Physical Examination:** A pelvic examination in women or a genital examination in men may reveal signs of inflammation or discharge.
- **Laboratory testing:** Various laboratory tests can be used to detect *T. vaginalis* in genital specimens. These include:
  - **Wet Mount Microscopy:** A sample of vaginal or urethral discharge is examined under a microscope for the presence of motile trichomonads.
  - **Nucleic Acid Amplification Tests (NAATs):** Polymerase chain reaction (PCR) and other NAATs can detect *T. vaginalis* DNA in genital specimens with high sensitivity and specificity.
  - **Culture:** Trichomonas culture involves growing the parasite in a special medium under laboratory conditions. Although less commonly used than wet mount microscopy or NAATs, culture can provide definitive confirmation of trichomoniasis.
- **Treatment:** Trichomoniasis is

typically treated with antimicrobial medications that are effective against T. vaginalis. The recommended first-line treatment for uncomplicated trichomoniasis is oral metronidazole or tinidazole. These medications work by disrupting the DNA and metabolic processes of the parasite, leading to its death. Treatment regimens may vary depending on factors such as the severity of symptoms, medical history, and medication availability. It's important for both sexual partners to receive treatment simultaneously to prevent reinfection.

- **Complications:** Untreated trichomoniasis can lead to various complications, particularly in women. Some potential complications of trichomoniasis include:
  - **Increased Risk of HIV Transmission:** Trichomoniasis has been associated with an increased risk of HIV acquisition and transmission. The inflammation and ulceration caused by *T. vaginalis* infection can facilitate the entry and spread of HIV in the genital tract.
  - **Pelvic Inflammatory Disease (PID):** Trichomoniasis can ascend from the lower to the upper genital tract, leading to inflammation and infection of the uterus, fallopian tubes, and surrounding tissues. PID can cause chronic pelvic pain, infertility, and ectopic pregnancy.
  - **Pregnancy Complications:** Trichomoniasis during pregnancy has been linked to adverse pregnancy outcomes, including preterm birth, low birth weight, and premature rupture of membranes.
  - **Urethritis and Prostatitis:** Men with trichomoniasis may develop inflammation of the urethra (urethritis) or prostate gland (prostatitis), leading to symptoms such as dysuria, urethral discharge, and pelvic pain.
- **Prevention:** Preventing trichomoniasis involves practicing safe sex and reducing the risk of exposure to the parasite. Some preventive measures include:
  - **Abstaining From Sexual Activity:** Abstinence from sexual intercourse is the most effective way to prevent trichomoniasis and other STIs.
  - **Using Condoms:** Consistent and correct use of latex or polyurethane condoms can reduce the risk of trichomoniasis transmission during vaginal or anal intercourse. However, condoms may not provide complete protection, as the parasite can infect areas not covered by the condom.
  - **Limiting Sexual Partners:** Having fewer sexual partners and choosing partners who have been tested for STIs can reduce the risk of trichomoniasis and other STIs.
  - **Screening and Treatment:** Undergoing regular STI

screenings, including tests for trichomoniasis, can help detect and treat infections early, reducing the risk of transmission to sexual partners.

- **Public Health Implications:** Trichomoniasis poses significant public health challenges due to its high prevalence, asymptomatic nature, and potential for adverse health outcomes. Efforts to control trichomoniasis require a comprehensive approach that includes:
    - **Increasing Awareness:** Education campaigns aimed at raising awareness about trichomoniasis, its transmission, symptoms, and prevention strategies can help reduce stigma, promote testing, and encourage treatment-seeking behavior.
    - **Screening Programs:** Implementing routine screening programs for trichomoniasis in high-risk populations, such as sexually active individuals and pregnant women, can help identify and treat infections early, reducing the burden of disease.
    - **Access to Healthcare:** Ensuring access to affordable and culturally sensitive healthcare services, including STI testing and treatment, is essential for addressing trichomoniasis disparities and improving health outcomes.
    - **Research and Surveillance:** Continued research into the epidemiology, transmission dynamics, and treatment of trichomoniasis is needed to inform evidence-based interventions and public health policies. Surveillance systems for monitoring trichomoniasis prevalence and trends can help guide resource allocation and intervention strategies (Verstraelen and Verhelst, 2009; Donders et al., 2017; Yudin and Money, 2017; Denning et al., 2018; Coleman and Gaydos, 2018; Verstraelen and Swidsinski, 2018; Yano et al., 2019; Workowskie et al., 2021)

A Closer Look

Vulvovaginitis

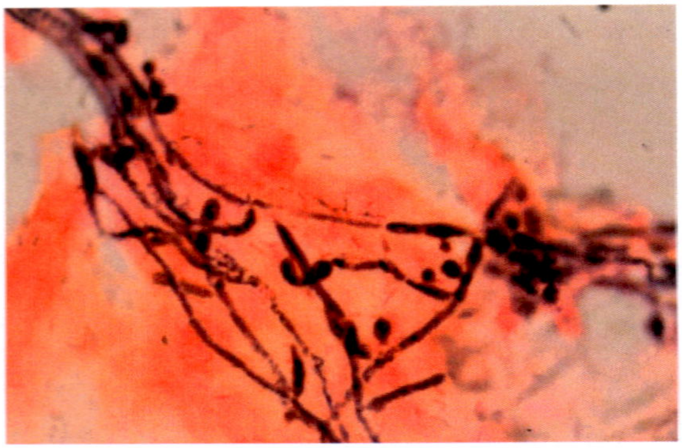

Candida-caused vulvovaginitis: By Dr Graham Beards – Own work, CC BY-SA 4.0, https://commons.wikimedia.org/w/index.php?curid=123445682.

Vulvovaginitis is a common gynecological condition with various causes and presentations. This condition can affect women of all ages, from prepubertal girls to postmenopausal women. The most common symptoms of vulvovaginitis include vaginal itching, burning, irritation, abnormal vaginal discharge, and discomfort during sexual intercourse or urination.

Numerous factors can contribute to the development of vulvovaginitis, including infections, allergic reactions, hormonal changes, and irritants. Infectious causes, such as bacterial vaginosis, candidiasis (yeast infection), and trichomoniasis (a sexually transmitted infection), account for a significant proportion of cases. These infections often result from an imbalance in the vaginal microbiota, allowing pathogenic organisms to proliferate.

Non-infectious causes of vulvovaginitis may include allergic reactions to soaps, detergents, perfumes, or other personal hygiene products, as well as irritants like chemicals found in contraceptives or lubricants. Hormonal changes, such as those occurring during pregnancy or menopause, can also predispose women to vulvovaginal irritation and inflammation due to alterations in vaginal pH and moisture levels.

Diagnosis of vulvovaginitis involves a comprehensive medical history, pelvic examination, and laboratory tests, including vaginal swabs and cultures, to identify the underlying cause. Treatment strategies vary depending on the specific etiology but often include antifungal medications for yeast infections, antibiotics for bacterial infections, and antimicrobial agents for sexually transmitted infections. Non-infectious vulvovaginitis may require avoidance of allergens or irritants and symptomatic relief with topical corticosteroids or soothing emollients.

Preventive measures for vulvovaginitis include practicing good hygiene, avoiding irritants, wearing breathable cotton underwear, and maintaining a healthy lifestyle. Additionally, practicing safe sex and using barrier protection can help prevent sexually transmitted infections associated with vulvovaginitis. Overall, early recognition, accurate diagnosis, and appropriate management are essential for effectively treating vulvovaginitis and preventing recurrence, improving the quality of life for affected individuals.

Summary

- Analyzing vaginal secretions involves a comprehensive assessment of these characteristics. Consistency provides insights into hormonal status, with thinner, clearer discharge often indicating ovulation. Changes in color, such as pinkish or brownish tinges, may signal the presence of blood, possibly related to menstruation or abnormalities.
- The pH of vaginal secretions must be determined at the time of specimen collection by the healthcare provider. Commercial pH paper can be placed directly on the lateral wall of the vagina for about 1 minute to absorb the secretions.
- Microscopic examinations should be performed as soon as possible on vaginal secretion specimens, particularly for detection of *T. vaginalis*, for which identification depends solely on observing actively motile organisms. The vaginal swab is placed into a tube containing approximately 1.0 mL of sterile physiologic saline (0.9% NaCl) and is agitated or twirled for a few seconds to release the secretions from the swab.
- Bacterial vaginosis is a condition caused by an overgrowth of normal vaginal flora. Most commonly, this presents clinically with increased vaginal discharge that has a fish-like odor. The discharge itself is typically thin and either gray or white. After being diagnosed with bacterial vaginosis, women have an increased risk of acquiring other sexually transmitted infections (STI), and pregnant women have an increased risk of early delivery.
- Vulvovaginitis, or inflammation of the vulva and vagina, most commonly occurs in reproductive-aged women and is caused by several underlying etiologies. Candidiasis is a fungal infection caused by Candida albicans, a polymorphic opportunistic fungus; vulvovaginitis secondary to candidiasis is also known as vaginal candidiasis.
- Atrophic vaginitis is an inflammatory process that occurs in clients experiencing vaginal atrophy. Vaginal atrophy develops secondary to a lack of estrogen due to menopause. Diagnosis is made clinically based on symptoms. This activity reviews the anatomic and histopathologic changes contributing to vaginal atrophy and the role of the interprofessional team in the evaluation and management of atrophic vaginitis.
- Trichomoniasis (trich) is a common, but curable, sexually transmitted infection (STI). A parasite causes trich. Most people who have trich don't have symptoms. Treatment for trich involves taking antibiotics.

References

1. Achkar, J. M., & Fries, B. C. (2010). Candida infections of the genitourinary tract. *Clinical Microbiology Reviews, 23*(2), 253–273.
2. Aguirre-Quiñonero, A., Castillo-Sedano, I. S., Calvo-Muro, F., & Canut-Blasco, A. (2019). Accuracy of the BD MAX™ vaginal panel in the diagnosis of infectious vaginitis. *European Journal of Clinical Microbiology & Infectious Diseases, 38*(5), 877–882.
3. Barnes, P., Vieira, R., Harwood, J., & Chauhan, M. (2017). Self-taken vaginal swabs versus

clinician-taken for detection of candida and bacterial vaginosis: a case-control study in primary care. *British Journal of General Practice, 67*(665), e824–e829.

4. Bayigga, L., Kateete, D. P., Anderson, D. J., Sekikubo, M., & Nakanjako, D. (2019). Diversity of vaginal microbiota in sub-Saharan Africa and its effects on HIV transmission and prevention. *American Journal of Obstetrics & Gynecology, 220*(2), 155–166.
5. Blostein, F., Levin-Sparenberg, E., Wagner, J., & Foxman, B. (2017). Recurrent vulvovaginal candidiasis. *Annals of Epidemiology, 27*(9), 575–582.e3.
6. Brunham, R. C., Paavonen, J., Stevens, C. E., et al. (1984). Mucopurulent cervicitis—the ignored counterpart in women of urethritis in men. *New England Journal of Medicine, 311*, 1–6.
7. Buggio, L., Somigliana, E., Borghi, A., & Vercellini, P. (2019). Probiotics and vaginal microecology: fact or fancy? *BMC Women's Health, 19*(1), 25.
8. Coleman, J. S., & Gaydos, C. A. (2018). Molecular Diagnosis of Bacterial Vaginosis: an Update. *Journal of Clinical Microbiology, 2018 Aug 27;56(9):e00342-18.*.
9. Cooke, G., Watson, C., Deckx, L., Pirotta, M., Smith, J., & van Driel, M. L. (2022). Treatment for recurrent vulvovaginal candidiasis (thrush). *Cochrane Database of Systematic Reviews, 1*(1), CD009151.
10. Coughlin, G., & Secor, M. (2010). Bacterial vaginosis: update on evidence-based care. *Advances in Nurse Practice, 18*(1), 41–4, 53.
11. Crouss, T., Sobel, J. D., Smith, K., & Nyirjesy, P. (2018). Long-Term Outcomes of Women with Recurrent Vulvovaginal Candidiasis After a Course of Maintenance Antifungal Therapy. *Journal of Lower Genital Tract Disease, 22*(4), 382–386.
12. Deese, J., Pradhan, S., Goetz, H., & Morrison, C. (2018). Contraceptive use and the risk of sexually transmitted infection: systematic review and current perspectives. *Open Access Journal of Contraception, 9*, 91–112.
13. Denning, D. W., Kneale, M., Sobel, J. D., & Rautemaa-Richardson, R. (2018). Global burden of recurrent vulvovaginal candidiasis: a systematic review. *The Lancet Infectious Diseases, 18*(11), e339–e347.
14. Donders, G. G. G., Ravel, J., Vitali, B., Netea, M. G., Salumets, A., & Unemo, M. (2017). Role of Molecular Biology in Diagnosis and Characterization of Vulvo-Vaginitis in Clinical Practice. *Gynecologic & Obstetric Investigation, 82*(6), 607–616.
15. Eastment, M. C., & McClelland, R. S. (2018). Vaginal microbiota and susceptibility to HIV. *AIDS, 32*(6), 687–698.
16. Eschenbach, D. A. (1983). Vulvovaginal discharge. In B. M. Peckham & S. S. Shario (Eds.), *Signs and Symptoms in Gynecology* (pp. 254–261). Philadelphia: JB Lippincott.
17. Farhan, M. A., Moharram, A. M., Salah, T., & Shaaban, O. M. (2019). Types of yeasts that cause vulvovaginal candidiasis in chronic users of corticosteroids. *Medical Mycology, 57*(6), 681–687.
18. Fleury, F. J. (1981). Adult vaginitis. *Clinical Obstetrics and Gynecology, 24*, 407–38.
19. Greenbaum, S., Greenbaum, G., Moran-Gilad, J., & Weintraub, A. Y. (2019). Ecological dynamics of the vaginal microbiome in relation to health and disease. *American Journal of Obstetrics & Gynecology, 220*(4), 324–335.
20. Han, C., Li, H., Han, L., Wang, C., Yan, Y., Qi, W., & Xue, F. (2019). Aerobic vaginitis in late

pregnancy and outcomes of pregnancy. *European Journal of Clinical Microbiology & Infectious Diseases, 38*(2), 233–239.

21. Holmes, K. K. (1984). Lower genital tract infections in women: cystitis/urethritis, vulvovaginitis, and cervicitis. In K. K. Holmes, P. A. Mardh, P. F. Sparling, et al. (Eds.), *Sexually Transmitted Diseases* (pp. 557–89). New York: McGraw-Hill.

22. Jain, J. P., Bristow, C. C., Pines, H. A., Harvey-Vera, A., Rangel, G., Staines, H., & Strathdee, S. A. (2018). Factors in the HIV risk environment associated with bacterial vaginosis among HIV-negative female sex workers who inject drugs in the Mexico-United States border region. *BMC Public Health, 18*(1), 1032.

23. Javed, A., Parvaiz, F., & Manzoor, S. (2019). Bacterial vaginosis: An insight into the prevalence, alternative treatments regimen and its associated resistance patterns. *Microbial Pathogenesis, 127*, 21–30.

24. Lamont, R. F., Keelan, J. A., Larsson, P. G., & Jørgensen, J. S. (2017). The treatment of bacterial vaginosis in pregnancy with clindamycin to reduce the risk of infection-related preterm birth: a response to the Danish Society of Obstetrics and Gynecology guideline group's clinical recommendations. *Acta. Obstetricia. et Gynecologica. Scandinavica., 96*(2), 139–143.

25. Makanjuola, O., Bongomin, F., & Fayemiwo, S. A. (2018). An Update on the Roles of Non-albicans Candida Species in Vulvovaginitis. *Journal of Fungi (Basel), 2018 Oct 31;4(4):121.*

26. McLellan, R., Spence, M. R., Brockman, M., et al. (1982). The clinical diagnosis of trichomoniasis. *Obstetrics & Gynecology, 60*, 30–34.

27. Paavonen, J. (1983). Physiology and ecology of the vagina. *Scandinavian Journal of Infectious Diseases. Supplementum, 40*, 31–35.

28. Paavonen, J. A., & Brunham, R. C. (2020). Vaginitis in Nonpregnant Patients: ACOG Practice Bulletin Number 215. *Obstetrics & Gynecology, 135*(5), 1229–1230.

29. Piot, P., & Vanderheyden, J. (1984). Gardnerella vaginalis and non-specific vaginitis. In K. K. Holmes, P. A. Mardh, P. F. Sparling, et al. (Eds.), *Sexually Transmitted Diseases* (pp. 421–27). New York: McGraw-Hill.

30. Rein, M. F., & Muller, M. (1984). Trichomonas vaginalis. In K. K. Holmes, P. A. Mardh, P. F. Sparling, et al. (Eds.), *Sexually Transmitted Diseases* (pp. 525–536). New York: McGraw-Hill.

31. Risser, W. L., Risser, J. M., & Risser, A. L. (2017). Current perspectives in the USA on the diagnosis and treatment of pelvic inflammatory disease in adolescents. *Adolescent Health, Medicine and Therapeutics, 8*, 87–94.

32. Russo, R., Karadja, E., & De Seta, F. (2019). Evidence-based mixture containing Lactobacillus strains and lactoferrin to prevent recurrent bacterial vaginosis: a double blind, placebo controlled, randomised clinical trial. *Beneficial Microbes, 10*(1), 19–26.

33. Sobel, J. D., & Sobel, R. (2018). Current treatment options for vulvovaginal candidiasis caused by azole-resistant Candida species. *Expert Opinion on Pharmacotherapy, 19*(9), 971–977.

34. Stamm, W. E., Hamson, R., Alexander, E. R., et al. (1984). Diagnosis of Chlamydia trachomatis infections by direct immunofluorescence staining of genital secretions. *Annals of Internal Medicine, 101*, 638–41.

35. Tam, M. R., Stamm, W. E., Hundsfield, H. H., et al. (1984). Culture. Independent diagnosis of

Chlamydia trachomatis using monoclonal antibodies. *New England Journal of Medicine, 310*, 1146–50.

36. van der Meijden, W. I., Boffa, M. J., Ter Harmsel, B., Kirtschig, G., Lewis, F., Moyal-Barracco, M., & Sherrard, J. (2022). 2021 European guideline for the management of vulval conditions. *Journal of the European Academy of Dermatology and Venereology, 36*(7), 952–972.
37. van der Meijden, W. I., Boffa, M. J., Ter Harmsel, W. A., Kirtschig, G., Lewis, F. M., Moyal-Barracco, M., & Sherrard, J. (2017). 2016 European guideline for the management of vulval conditions. *Journal of the European Academy of Dermatology and Venereology, 31*(6), 925–941.
38. van Schalkwyk, J., & Yudin, M. H. (2015). Vulvovaginitis: screening for and management of trichomoniasis, vulvovaginal candidiasis, and bacterial vaginosis. *Journal of Obstetrics and Gynaecology Canada, 37*(3), 266–274.
39. Verstraelen, H., & Swidsinski, A. (2019). The biofilm in bacterial vaginosis: implications for epidemiology, diagnosis and treatment: 2018 update. *Current Opinion in Infectious Diseases, 32*(1), 38–42.
40. Verstraelen, H., & Verhelst, R. (2009). Bacterial vaginosis: an update on diagnosis and treatment. *Expert Review of Anti-infective Therapy, 7*(9), 1109–1124.
41. Workowski, K. A., Bachmann, L. H., Chan, P. A., Johnston, C. M., Muzny, C. A., Park, I., & Bolan, G. A. (2021). Sexually Transmitted Infections Treatment Guidelines, 2021. *MMWR. Recommendations and Reports, 70*(4), 1–187.
42. Yano, J., Sobel, J. D., Nyirjesy, P., Sobel, R., Williams, V. L., Yu, Q., & Fidel, P. L. (2019). Current patient perspectives of vulvovaginal candidiasis: incidence, symptoms, management and post-treatment outcomes. *BMC Women's Health, 19*(1), 48.
43. Yudin, M. H., & Money, D. M. (2017). No. 211-Screening and Management of Bacterial Vaginosis in Pregnancy. *Journal of Obstetrics and Gynaecology Canada, 39*(8), e184–e191.

Chapter 10

FECAL ANALYSIS

Contents

Introduction

Feces can reveal vital information that helps with the differential diagnosis of a number of gastrointestinal tract conditions, from bleeding or infection by bacteria, viruses, or parasites to maldigestion and malabsorption. Fecal analysis can also be used to identify pancreatic diseases that result in insufficient digestive enzymes and hepatic and biliary conditions that cause decreased bile secretion. The chemical test for occult, or hidden, blood is currently the test that is done on feces the most often. The earliest and most common initial symptom of colorectal cancer is known to be occult blood. Regular fecal blood testing is advised for all individuals 50 years of age and above. A positive fecal blood test can be caused by bleeding anywhere in the gastrointestinal tract, from the mouth to the anus; further testing is necessary to determine the precise cause of the bleeding, though. Fecal analysis is helpful in the differential diagnosis of diarrhea as well as in identifying the presence of elevated fecal lipids (steatorrhea).

Orientation and Directional Terms

Term	Definition	Illustration
Malabsorption	Malabsorption is a condition that occurs when the body has difficulty absorbing nutrients from food.	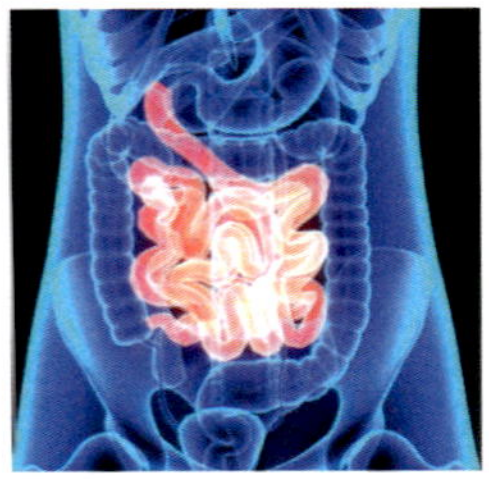
Fecal occult blood test	A fecal occult blood test (FOBT) is a lab test that looks for hidden blood in stool samples. The test is often used to screen for colorectal cancer, especially in developed countries. Blood in the stool can be a sign of: colorectal cancer, polyps, ulcers, and hemorrhoids.	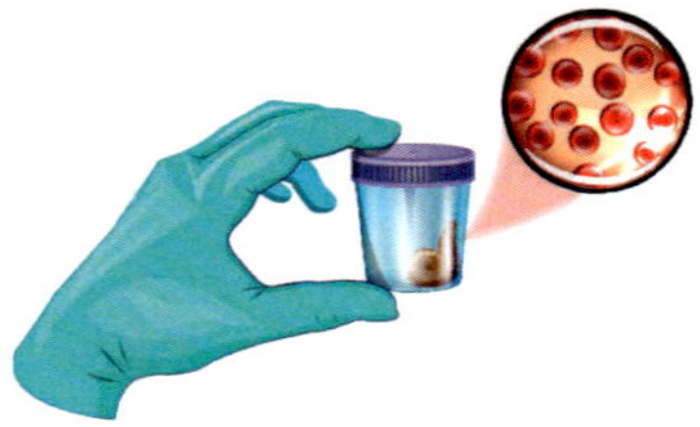
Pseudomembranous enterocolitis	Pseudomembranous enterocolitis (PMC) is a severe inflammation of the colon caused by an overgrowth of the bacterium Clostridioides difficile (C. diff). It's often associated with antibiotic use, and can be diagnosed with a blood test, imaging tests, or stool sample test.	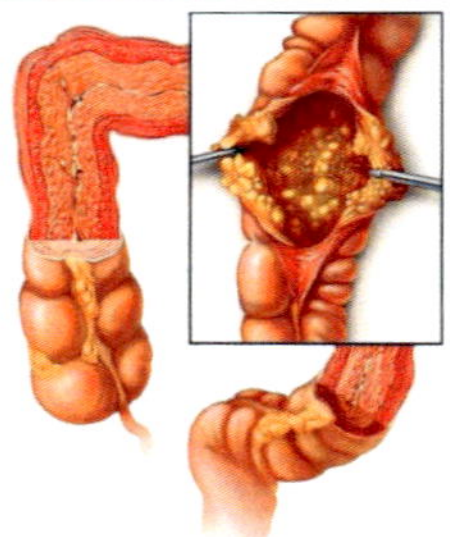
Pancreatic secretions	Pancreatic secretion is the production and release of digestive enzymes and hormones by the pancreas.	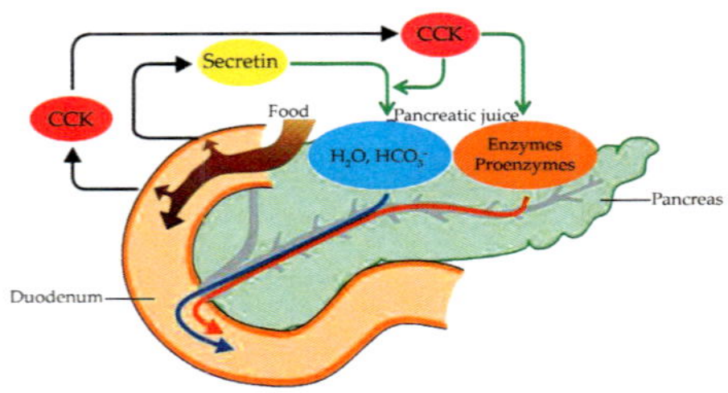
Steatorrhea	Feces is the solid organic refuse of the human body, composed of about 80% water and 20% dry material.	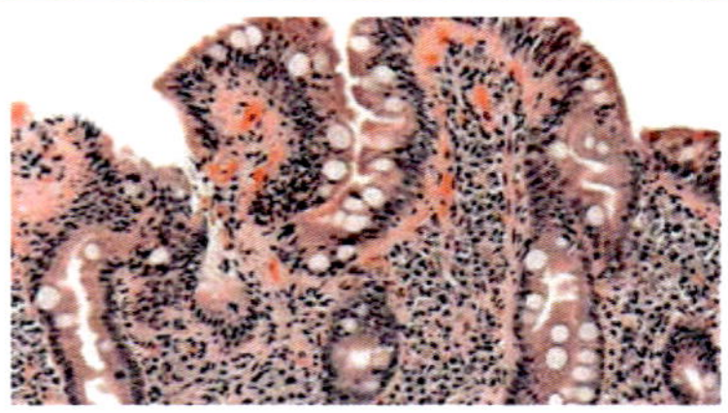

10.1. Fecal Analysis (Stool Analysis)

Fecal analysis is a non-invasive laboratory test that can be used to diagnose digestive tract issues. These conditions can include cancer, bacterial, viral, or fungal infections, inflammation, and malabsorption. It is carried out in conjunction with endoscopy, x-ray imaging, physical examination, and blood work to confirm these conditions. The most popular test performed on a stool is known as the fecal occult blood test (FOBT), which can identify blood traces in the stool.

During the defecation process, solid waste from the large intestine is eliminated through the anus. This waste is called feces. It is composed of water, bacteria, cellulose, and other indigestible food materials. Additionally, bile pigments in the form of urobilinogen, pancreatic and GI secretions, trypsin, small amounts of fats, and epithelial cells shed from the gastrointestinal tract are all commonly found in feces. The pancreas produces the proteolytic enzyme trypsin.

An average adult excretes 100 to 300 grams of fecal material every day, which is the leftover material from the 10 liters of liquid that enters the GI tract every day. Macroscopic examination (volume, odor, shape, color, consistency, and presence of mucus), microscopic examination (leukocytes, epithelial cells, and meat fibers), and chemical tests for particular substances (occult blood, trypsin, estimation of carbohydrates) are all included in the laboratory analysis of feces.

The nurses' responsibilities during a stool collection and fecal analysis include handling specimens properly, accurately identifying samples, making sure all supplies are suitable for collection, and promptly transporting specimens to the lab.

10.1.1. Indications of Fecal Analysis

Stool analysis is used to:

- Aid in diagnosing disorders related to gastrointestinal (GI) bleeding or medication therapy that results in bleeding
- Assist in the diagnosis of pseudomembranous enterocolitis following the use of broad-spectrum antibiotic therapy
- Help diagnose suspected inflammatory bowel syndrome (IBS)
- Identify the cause of diarrhea of unknown origin
- Investigate disorders of protein digestion
- Screen for colorectal cancer
- Screen for cystic fibrosis
- Determine intestinal parasitic infestation, as indicated by diarrhea of unknown cause
- Evaluate the effectiveness of therapeutic regimen for intestinal malabsorption or pancreatic insufficiency

10.1.2. Interfering Factors

These are factors or conditions that may affect the outcome of the study:

- Medications that irritate the gastric mucosa such as non-steroidal anti-inflammatory medicines (NSAIDs), anticoagulants, colchicine, corticosteroids, phenylbutazone, and iron preparations can cause positive results for occult blood
- High doses of vitamin C (more than 250 mg per day) can cause false negative occult blood

- Dietary intake of high in red meat, certain vegetables (radishes, turnips, cauliflower, broccoli), and fruits (bananas, apples, cantaloupe) can cause false-positive results for occult blood
- Constipated stools may not show any trypsin activity due to prolonged exposure to intestinal bacteria

10.1.3. Procedure for Stool analysis

The following are the steps in collecting a stool specimen:

1. **Collect a Fecal Sample:** Wear clean gloves and collect a stool specimen and put it directly in a leak-proof container with a tight-fitting lid. If the patient is bedridden, collect the specimen in a clean, dry bedpan, and then, using a tongue blade, transfer into a properly labeled container. If doing a rectal swab, insert the swab 2-3 cm through the rectal sphincter, rotate gently, and remove. Transfer the swab to the container.
2. **Fill Out the Test Request form Completely:** Note on the laboratory request the patient's demographics, stool consistency, and date and time of collection. Indicate previous or present antibiotic therapy and any pertinent history
3. **Transport the Specimen to the Laboratory:** Send the specimen to the laboratory immediately for processing and analysis. If a liquid or soft stool sample can't be processed within 30 minutes of passage, place it in a preservative; If a formed stool specimen can't be studied immediately, place it in a preservative or refrigerator.

10.1.4. Nursing Responsibility for Stool Analysis

The following are the nursing interventions and nursing care considerations for the patient

- **Before the Procedure:** The following are the nursing interventions before a stool analysis.
  - o **Assess the Patient's Level of Comfort:** Collecting stool specimen may produce a feeling of embarrassment and discomfort to the patient.
  - o **Encourage the Patient to Urinate:** Allow the patient to urinate before collecting to avoid contaminating the stool with urine.
  - o **Avoid Laxatives:** Advise patient that laxatives, enemas, or suppositories are avoided three days prior to collection.
  - o **Instruct a Red-meat Free and High Residue Diet:** The patient is indicated for an occult blood test, must follow a special diet that includes generous amounts of chicken, turkey, and tuna, raw and uncooked vegetables and fruits such as spinach, celery, prunes and bran containing cereal for two (2) days before the test.
- **After the Procedure:** The nurse should note the following nursing interventions after fecal analysis:
  - o **Instruct Patient to Do Handwashing:** Allow the patient to thoroughly clean his or her hands and perianal area.

- o **Resume activities:** The patient may resume his or her normal diet and medication therapy unless otherwise specified.
- o **Recommend Regular Screening:** The American Cancer Society recommends yearly occult blood test as part of the screening for colorectal cancer starting at the age of 45 years old for people with average risk.

10.1.5. Normal Results

There are two methods where stool can be examined:

- **Macroscopic Examination:** for appearance and color
- **Microscopic Examination:** for cell count and presence of meat fibers; leukocyte esterase, for leukocytes; Benedict's solution (copper sulfate) for reducing substances; guaiac, for occult blood; x-ray paper, for trypsin (Table 10.1)

Table 10.1. Performance of the Novodiag® Stool Parasites Assay (NSP) and microscopy (Micro) (*n* = 156) for Detecting Pathogens in Stool

Targets	Number of Samples with				Se (%)	Sp (%)	Concordance (%)	Coef. Kappa
	Micro (+) NSP (+)	Micro (−) NSP (−)	Micro (+) NSP (−)	Micro (−) NSP (+)				
Giardia intestinalis	23	126	4	3	85.2%	97.7%	95.5%	0.84
Blastocystis hominis	29	98	1	28	96.7%	77.8%	81.4%	0.55
Entamoeba histolytica [a]	3	147	0	6	100%	96.1%	96.1%	0.48
Dientamoeba fragilis	1	132	1	22	50%	85.7%	85.3%	0.06
Cyclospora cayetanensis	2	154	0	0	100%	100%	100%	1
Cystoisospora belli	0	155	1	0	0%	100%	99.4%	NC

[a]—E. histolytica species was confirmed by Amplidiag® Stool Parasites real-time PCR kit. Se—Sensitivity; Sp—Specificity; NC—Cohen's kappa not calculable (zero values).

Source: Chauvin P, Barba F, Guemas E, Charpentier E, Cottrel C, Fillaux J, Valentin A, Baklouti S, Cassaing S, Ménard S, et al. Evaluation of the Performance of the Novodiag® Stool Parasites Assay for the Detection of Intestinal Protozoa and Microsporidia. Pathogens. 2023; 12(7):889. https://doi.org/10.3390/pathogens12070889.

10.1.6. Abnormal Results

Abnormal findings in a stool exam may reveal the potential medical diagnosis. These includes:

- **Unusual Appearance:**
  - **Mucous:** Intestinal wall inflammation
  - **Bloody:** Excessive intestinal wall irritation or malignancy
  - **Frothy or bulky:** Malabsorption
  - **Ribbonlike or Slender:** Obstruction
- **Unusual Color:**
  - **Red:** Beets and food coloring, lower GI bleed, phenazopyridine hydrochloride compounds, rifampicin
  - **Black:** Bismuth (antacid) or charcoal ingestion, iron therapy, upper GI bleeding
  - **Yellow:** Rhubarb
  - **Green:** Antibiotics, biliverdin, green vegetables
  - **Grayish White:** Barium ingestion, bile duct obstruction
- **Increased:**
  - **Blood:** related to GI bleeding
  - **Occult blood:** Diverticular disease, esophagitis, gastritis, esophageal varices, anal fissure, hemorrhoids, infectious diarrhea, inflammatory bowel disease, polyps, tumors, ulcers, Mallory-Weiss tears
  - **Leukocytes:** Inflammation of the intestines related to bacterial infections of the intestinal wall, ulcerative colitis, shigellosis, or salmonellosis
  - **Epithelial cells:** Inflammatory bowel disorders
  - **Carbohydrates/Reducing Substances:** Inability to digest some sugar, malabsorption syndromes
  - **Fats:** Sprue (celiac disease), cystic fibrosis related to malabsorption, pancreatitis
  - **pH:** Related to inflammation in the intestine from colitis, cancer, or antibiotic use
  - **Meat Fibers:** Pancreatitis, impaired protein digestion
- **Decreased:**
  - **Leukocytes:** Disorders resulting from toxins, cholera, viral diarrhea, amebic colitis, parasites
  - **Carbohydrates/Reducing Substances:** Cystic fibrosis, sprue, malnutrition, medications such as colchicine or birth control pills
  - **pH:** Related to poor absorption of carbohydrate or fat
  - **Trypsin:** Malabsorption syndrome, pancreatic deficiency, cystic fibrosis

10.2. Fecal Formation

An average person passes between 100 and 200 g of feces every day. The excrement contains partially digested food items (e.g., cellulose), loosely adhered intestinal epithelium, intestinal microorganisms, and digestive secretions (e.g., digestive enzymes), water, electrolytes, and bile pigments. The large intestine typically takes 18 to 24 hours to expel the contents that the small intestine presents to it in the form of feces due to the slow movement of fecal material in that organ.

While food digestion and absorption are functions of the small intestine, water, sodium, and chloride absorption are the main functions of the large intestine. Food, water, saliva, gastric secretions, bile, pancreatic secretions, and small intestinal secretions all contribute to the approximately 9000 mL of fluid that enters the digestive tract. However, only 500–1500 mL really pass through to the large intestine per day, and normal feces excrete approximately 150 mL of fluid. The large intestine can only absorb a maximum of 2700 mL of liquid at a time, so any volume of fluid that is given to it beyond this limit results in watery stools, or diarrhea. Similar to this, diarrhea happens when water absorption is impeded or when the absorption process is given insufficient time. Constipation, on the other hand, is caused by stationary bowel contents (or decreased intestinal motility) that allow increased water absorption. Constipated people usually have small, hard, frequently spherical masses in their feces called scybala, which are difficult and painful to pass.

Flatus, also known as intestinal gas, is typically produced at a rate of 400 to 700 mL per day by intestinal bacteria fermenting food in the large intestine. Intestinal enzymes are not always able to fully break down certain carbohydrates like brown beans and are easily broken down by gut microbes to release copious amounts of gas. Stools that are foamy and float can be the result of increased gas production and its absorption into the feces. These stools can be normal, but patients with steatorrhea and lactose intolerance frequently produce them.

10.3. Diarrhea

An increase in the volume, liquidity, and frequency of bowel movements relative to a person's typical bowel movement pattern is referred to as diarrhea. There are three different types of diarrhea: diarrhea brought on by intestinal hypermotility, osmotic diarrhea, and secretory diarrhea (Figure 10.1). Water is drawn into and held in the intestinal lumen by the presence of an unabsorbed solute in cases of secretory and osmotic diarrhea. This osmotically active solute has a different source. Increased intestinal secretion of a solute causes secretory diarrhea, whereas consumption of an osmotically active solute (e.g., lactose).

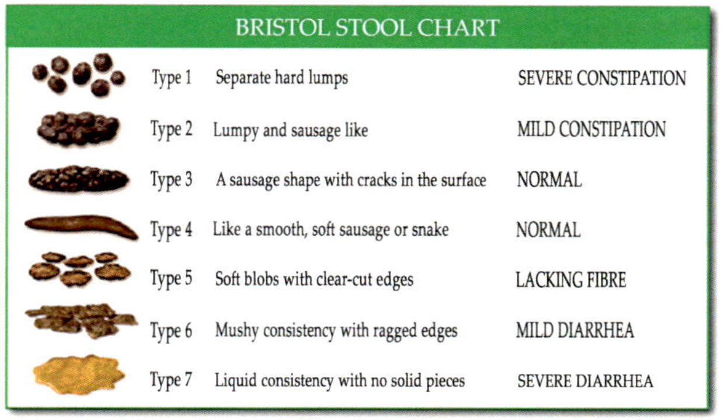

Figure 10.1. *Classification of diarrhea.*

Source: By Cabot Health, Bristol Stool Chart - http://cdn.intechopen.com/pdfs-wm/46082.pdf, CC BY-SA 3.0, https://commons.wikimedia.org/w/index.php?curid=41761316.

Determining the levels of fecal osmolality, fecal sodium, and fecal potassium is necessary to distinguish between these two conditions. Equation 1 is used to calculate a "calculated" fecal osmolality based on the potassium and sodium levels in the feces.

$$\text{Calculated fecal osmolality} = 2 \times (Na^{+}_{fecal} + K^{+}_{fecal}) \quad (1)$$

If the variation (i.e., The patient is suffering from osmotic diarrhea when the difference (osmotic gap) between the calculated and measured fecal osmolality is greater than 20 mOsm/kg. The patient has secretory diarrhea if the measured and calculated fecal osmolalities agree by 10 to 20 mOsm/kg.

A variety of organisms that produce enterotoxins can cause secretory diarrhea. These microorganisms secrete chemicals that increase intestinal secretions that are electrolytrichous. Similarly, secretory diarrhea may also result from illness or medication-induced damage to the intestinal mucosa.

Maldigestion or malabsorption are conditions that are associated with osmotic diarrhea. The incapacity to break down food into easily absorbed substances, or maldigestion, is primarily caused by a number of hepatic and pancreatic disorders. The bile salts or pancreatic digestive enzymes required for lipase activation and fat emulsification are absent or insufficient in patients with these disorders. The lack of additional digestive enzymes, like disaccharidases (e.g., maldigestion can also be brought on by lactase buildup in the small intestine. On the other hand, intestinal malabsorption is defined by normal digestive capacity but insufficient intestinal absorption of foods that have already undergone processing. Certain parasite infestations, illnesses of the mucosa (e.g., ulcerative colitis, tropical sprue, celiac sprue), inherited illnesses (e.g., disaccharidase deficiency), medical treatments, and medications can result in osmotic diarrhea and malabsorption. In summary, an abnormally high amount of food is presented to the large intestine by maldigestion and malabsorption. These compounds that exhibit osmoticism (i.e., the foods) result in the excretion of a watery stool or diarrhea and the retention of significant amounts of water and electrolytes in the intestinal lumen.

When intestinal contents transit too quickly for proper intestinal absorption to take place, intestinal hypermotility leads to diarrhea. Intestinal distention typically stimulates intestinal motility. Bulky foods, including dietary fiber, naturally cause intestinal distention, which has the laxative effect. Emotions, hormones, nerves, and chemicals can all affect intestinal motility. Intestinal motility is increased by parasympathetic nerve activity and castor oil, while intestinal motility is decreased by sympathetic nerve activity. The increased lumen fluid in secretory and osmotic diarrhea leads to intestinal distention, which in turn increases intestinal motility and exacerbates the diarrheal illness.

When diarrhea is severe, the body's acid-base balance is upset and blood volume is decreased (hypovolemia). Metabolic acidosis may arise from significant fluid loss and the ensuing electrolyte depletion (especially of sodium, bicarbonate, and potassium).

10.4. Steatorrhea

The average amount of fat excreted in the feces each day is less than 7 g. The diet, gastrointestinal secretions, bacterial byproducts of metabolism, and shed intestinal epithelium are the main sources of this fat. Keep in mind that the total amount of lipids excreted in the feces (fatty acid salts, neutral fat) can differ significantly from the amount of dietary fat consumed. Additionally, the amount of dietary fat consumed has a negligible impact on this total amount (Figure 10.2).

Patients with malabsorption syndromes frequently experience steatorrhea, or the excretion of fecal fat exceeding 7 g per day. Steatorrheal fecal specimens are characterized by their extreme foul smell and their pale, greasy, bulky, spongy, or pasty appearance. Because they contain a lot of gas, they have varying degrees of fluidity and can float or foam. Gas can also be found in normal stools, so this latter feature is not very important.

Clinically, separating steatorrhea from diarrhea is crucial. Even though a macroscopic examination of the feces can strongly suggest steatorrhea, differentiation can be challenging in certain diarrheal conditions. Therefore, a fecal fat determination is done to diagnose steatorrhea. Steatorrhea is a symptom of any condition that affects the digestion or absorption of fat. Steatorrhea-causing conditions can happen concurrently with diarrhea. Finding the source of either the steatorrhea, the diarrhea, or both is necessary before starting appropriate patient management. This is typically accomplished by adhering to an algorithm like the one shown in Figure 10.1. A thorough patient history is crucial because a conclusive diagnosis might not be obvious right away. Information directly related to the cause of the patient's condition can be found in the patient history (e.g., diet, surroundings, recent interactions, or exposure). For instance, applying the algorithm shown above to a negative stool culture eliminates some bacteria but leaves viruses, parasites, and other inflammatory conditions unchecked. A thorough review of the patient's medical history can provide important details, such as travel history, exposure to tainted water sources, use of cathartic herbs, or recent consumption of fresh oysters.

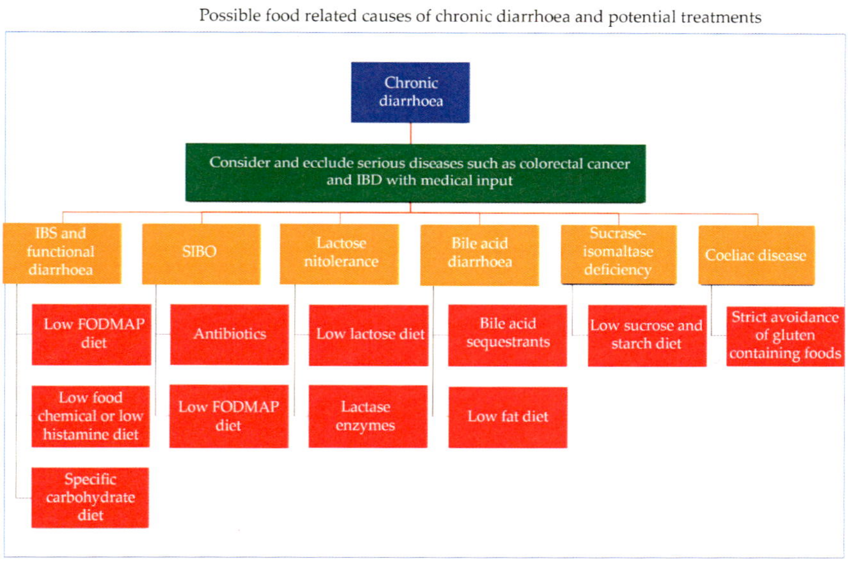

Figure 10.2. *Evidence-based approaches for the management of chronic diarrhea.*

Source: O'Brien L, Wall CL, Wilkinson TJ, Gearry RB. What Are the Pearls and Pitfalls of the Dietary Management for Chronic Diarrhea? Nutrients. 2021; 13(5):1393. https://doi.org/10.3390/nu13051393.

10.5. Specimen Collection

10.5.1. Patient Education

People can't really control when they urinate, but they can control when they excrete. Furthermore, most people find it extremely unpleasant to collect fecal specimens, which is thought to be at least partly the cause of the high noncompliance rate (50–90%) in fecal specimen collection for occult blood testing seen in colorectal cancer studies. Given these details, it is crucial to properly collect fecal specimens and educate patients on the significance of testing. Patients should be given written and verbal instructions as well as a suitable specimen container (Table 10.2).

Table 10.2. Common Causes of Chronic Diarrhea—Pharmaceutical and Dietary Responsive

Common Causes of Chronic Diarrhea	Mechanism	Dietary Management
Predominantly Pharmaceutical Responsive		
Pancreatic insufficiency	Insufficient secretion of pancreatic digestive enzymes into the small intestine	Teaching patients sources of fat so they are able to titrate digestive enzymes effectively
Microscopic colitis	Inflammation occurring at a microscopic level in the lining of the large intestine	N/A
Combination of Pharmaceutical and Dietary Responsive		
Short-bowel syndrome	Reduced mucosal surface due to removal or damage of part of the small intestine	Dietary manipulation to enhance absorption such as small frequent meals, higher protein and less refined sugar
Inflammatory bowel diseases	Chronic intestinal inflammation occurring throughout the gastrointestinal tract	Dietary and nutrition therapies to manage inflammation and promote maintenance of remission
Small intestinal bacterial overgrowth	Overgrowth of colonic bacteria in the small intestine	Restriction of fermentable carbohydrates (the low FODMAP diet) or an elemental diet may reduce overgrowth if antibiotics have not been responsive
Bile acid diarrhea	Excess bile acids entering the large intestine	A low-fat diet may reduce the production of bile acids
Predominantly Dietary Responsive		
Irritable bowel syndrome	Mechanisms are not clearly understood but could be due to increased gut transit, visceral hypersensitivity or altered gut microbiome	Dietary strategies could include: reducing portion sizes, regular eating, reducing fermentable carbohydrates or reducing natural food chemicals
Lactose intolerance	Reduced lactase enzyme activity in the small intestine	Limiting lactose-containing milk and milk products
Sucrase-isomaltase intolerance	Reduced enzyme activity of sucrase and or isomaltase in the small intestine	Reducing dietary intake of foods containing sucrose, isomaltose and maltose
Coeliac disease	Genetic condition resulting in damage to the lining of the small intestine when gluten is consumed	A strict lifelong gluten-free diet resolves symptoms and results in healing the lining of the small intestine

Source: O'Brien L, Wall CL, Wilkinson TJ, Gearry RB. What Are the Pearls and Pitfalls of the Dietary Management for Chronic Diarrhoea? Nutrients. 2021; 13(5):1393. https://doi.org/10.3390/nu13051393.

10.5.2. Specimen Containers

Containers for fecal specimens differ based on the volume of specimens to be gathered. Basically, anything that is leakproof, sealable, and nonbreakable can be used as long as it is clean. It is common practice to collect specimens over several days in large containers like paint cans. Urine collection cups or other appropriate containers can be used for single, random collections. The patient needs to be advised on which portion of the stool to sample or bring to the lab because not all stool samples are needed for all tests. For recovering feces after they are passed into the toilet onto a sheet of floating tissue paper, there are certain commercial fecal collection kits available. Patients' ability to collect feces has been considerably aided by these kits. The patient can flush the remainder of the feces after sampling some of it.

10.5.3. Type and Amount Collected

Depending on the test to be conducted, different specimen types and quantities are collected. Fecal analysis only needs a small portion of a randomly selected specimen to detect occult blood, white blood cells, or qualitative fecal fat. On the other hand, two or three days of fecal collection are typically needed for quantitative testing for the daily fecal excretion of any substance. The need for multiple day collections arises from the fact that the patient's daily fecal excretion does not closely match the quantity of food consumed within a 24-hour period. Furthermore, dietary restrictions might be required prior to the collection to guarantee the best possible fecal specimen (e.g., tests for quantitative fecal fat and occult blood).

10.5.4. Contaminants to Avoid

It is imperative to prevent the fecal specimen from becoming contaminated with urine, toilet paper, or toilet water. Urine contamination can negatively impact protozoa detection, and potent cleaning or deodorizing products in restrooms can cause problems for chemical testing. Additionally, patients need to be taught not to: (1) contaminate the outside of collection containers; and (2) apply an excessive amount of sample to a slide or collection device.

10.5.5. Gas Formation

Both in vivo and in vitro bacterial fermentation causes gas production in fecal specimens. As a result, closed fecal specimen containers should be carefully opened and covered with a disposable tissue or towel. In the unlikely event that gas buildup results in the abrupt release of fecal contents upon container opening, this covering prevents fecal matter from spattering.

10.6. Macroscopic Examination

10.6.1. Color

The macroscopic analysis of feces entails a visual evaluation of form, consistency, and color. Mucus and undigested material are two other noteworthy components of the feces. Bile pigments give feces their typical brown color. Conjugated bilirubin hydrolyzes back to its unconjugated form when it is secreted into the small intestine as bile. The three colorless tetrapyrroles known as the urobilinogens—stercobilinogen, mesobilinogen, and urobilinogen—are the result of subsequent reduction by intestinal anaerobic bacteria. In the intestine, these urobilinogens spontaneously oxidize to form the orange-brown urobilins, mesobilin, and stercobilin, which give the excrement its color (Table 10.3). The color of the feces changes under circumstances where the small intestine's ability to secrete bile is partially or totally blocked. These posthepatic obstructions are characterized by stools that are pale or clay-colored, commonly referred to as acholic stools. Note that fecal specimens of the same color resulting from contamination with barium sulfate can be obtained after a diagnostic procedure to assess gastrointestinal function (e.g., barium enema). It is also possible to experience unusual fecal colors after consuming specific foods or medications, or when there is blood present.

Table 10.3. The Pearls and Pitfalls of Dietary Therapies for the Management of Chronic Diarrhea

Disease	Dietary Therapy	Pearls	Pitfalls
Irritable bowel syndrome (IBS)	Low FODMAP diet	The most studied dietary intervention across all age groups.	The long length of time to establish likely trigger foods.
		There are multiple resources; designated websites, apps, recipes, Facebook pages, books, magazines.	Obsolete and outdated information is likely; resources need regular review by qualified health professionals.
		Comprehensive dietitian training is available.	FODMAP content differs by country. Individual tolerance may differ.
		Commercial product FODMAP testing is available increases consumer choice.	Phase 1 may restrict prebiotic food intake.
		A modified version can be used with those at high risk.	Restrictive diets may contribute to disordered eating patterns.
		Small amounts of wheat are allowed so a gluten-free diet is not required.	Phase 1 may reduce abundance of multiple bacterial species.
		High-lactose dairy is avoided. A dairy free diet is not required.	
	Specific-carbohydrate diet	*Breaking the Vicious Cycle* book provides detailed instruction.	Limited evidence of mechanisms, food composition and efficacy.
		Online support is available.	Long length of time to achieve improvements.
			No evidence of impact on diet adequacy, quality of life and mental health.
			Limited and conflicting guidance on use of the diet and reintroducing foods.
			Restrictive diets may contribute to disordered eating patterns.
			Likely restricts prebiotic food intake and nutrient intake.
	The low-food chemical/low-histamine diet	The Royal Prince Alfred Hospital provides detailed instruction for the low-food chemical diet.	Limited evidence of efficacy.

		There are multiple resources; designated websites, apps, recipes, Facebook pages, books.	Limited and conflicting food chemical content data.
		Relatively short elimination period.	Triggers may be non-diet related.
		A modified version can be used with those at high risk.	Likely restricts prebiotic and nutrient intake.
		May address a wider range of intolerances.	Restrictive diets may contribute to disordered eating patterns.
Small intestinal bacteria overgrowth (SIBO)	Low FODMAP diet	Excellent support information available.	Online information is prevalence, but given the lack of evidence in this field, it is likely to lack any validity.
Dietary changes may not be needed if antibiotics are effective			Reoccurrence of SIBO is common, risking nutritional deficiencies if repeated dietary restriction is conducted.
	Elemental diet	Nutritional complete	Provides no fibre and restricts prebiotics.
		Patients may not require any dietary restrictions.	May not be palatable and therefore poorly tolerated.
Lactose intolerance	Low-lactose diet	Credible methods for diagnosing are available.	Lactose-free products or lactase enzymes may not be easily available or affordable for all.
		Suitable alternatives are available providing nutrition in similar amounts.	Risk of low intake of calcium and vitamin D.
		High-lactose dairy is avoided. A dairy free diet is not required.	
Bile acid diarrhoea	Low-fFat diet	May be better tolerated than bile acid sequestrants.	Risk of inadequate intake of fat-soluble vitamins and reduction in overall energy intake leading to unintended weight loss.
Dietary changes may not be needed if bile acid sequestrants are effective		A variety of low-fat products are readily available at same cost to the full fat varieties.	
Sucrase-isomaltase deficiency (SID)	Low-sucrose/starch diet	There are multiple resources; designated websites, apps, recipes, Facebook pages, books.	Limited research on the long-term management of dietary changes.
		Oral enzymes are available to allowing for a broader range of foods to be eaten.	Sucrose enzymes are not available in all countries.
		With good planning the diet can still provide adequate fiber.	May restrict prebiotic food intake.

			Limited research on the long-term management of dietary changes.
Coeliac disease	Gluten-free diet	Gold standards for diagnosis.	Lifelong avoidance of all gluten-containing food is required.
		Gluten-free food alternatives are readily available.	Cross contamination can occur.
		There are multiple resources; designated websites, apps, recipes, Facebook pages, books.	Gluten-free alternatives can be more expensive, reducing diet compliance for some.

Source: O'Brien L, Wall CL, Wilkinson TJ, Gearry RB. What are the pearls and pitfalls of the dietary management for chronic diarrhoea? Nutrients. 2021; 13(5):1393. https://doi.org/10.3390/nu13051393.

10.6.2. Consistency and Form

Feces can vary in consistency from small, hard masses (constipation) to loose, watery stools (diarrhea). Normally, feces form into masses; soft stools are a sign of increased fecal water content. The latter may be associated with gastrointestinal disorders, be normal, or be related to laxatives. The medical professional can ascertain whether the patient has observed a change in the consistency of his stools by reviewing the patient's medical history. Foods that have not fully digested or an increase in gas in the stool can cause constipation.

It may also be possible to see undigested materials like proglottids from intestinal parasites, vegetable skins, or seed casings. The excretion of long, ribbon-like stools, on the other hand, may indicate intestinal obstruction or lumen narrowing due to strictures. Normal stools are formed, cylindrical masses.

10.6.3. Mucus

The translucent, gelatinous material known as mucus is absent from typical feces. When mucus is present, it can range widely, from a tiny amount to the large amounts linked to a colon tumor called a villous adenoma. Mucus has been linked to gastrointestinal disorders like colitis, intestinal tuberculosis, ulcerative diverticulitis, bacillary dysentery, neoplasms, and rectal inflammation, as well as benign conditions like straining during bowel movements or constipation.

10.6.4. Odor

The metabolic byproducts of the intestinal bacterial flora give feces their typical smell. Fecal odor can shift if the regular flora is disturbed or if the foods fed to the flora significantly alter. For instance, the bacterial breakdown of undigested lipids in steatorrhea causes distinctly foul-smelling feces.

10.7. Microscopic Examination

A sample of a stool suspension is subjected to microscopic examination, which can help distinguish between different causes of diarrhea or identify steatorrhea. White blood cells and undigested food items like fats, meat fibers, and vegetable fibers can be distinguished under a microscope. This examination is simple to conduct and can yield information that is helpful for diagnosis, despite being solely qualitative.

10.7.1. Fecal Leukocytes

The differential diagnosis of diarrhea is aided by the presence of pus, an exudate containing white blood cells, or fecal leukocytes, which are white blood cells. Fecal leukocytes are typically found in an inflammatory exudate when the intestinal wall is infected or irritated. Conversely, fecal leukocytes are typically absent if the mucosal wall is intact. Several disorders like bacillary dysentry can be differentiated from diarrhea by looking for fecal leukocytes under a microscope.

Leukocytes are normally absent from feces, so their presence—even in small amounts—one to three per high-power field suggests an inflammatory and invasive condition. Wet preparations can be stained with Wright's or methylene blue stain to improve the identification of leukocytes in feces.

10.7.2. Fecal Fat, Qualitative

It is possible to detect an increase in fat in feces macroscopically and to confirm it microscopically and chemically. Fecal fat excretion exceeding 7 g/day, or starvation, is a common sign of malabsorption or maldigestion. The definitive diagnosis of steatorrhea is established by quantitative measurements of fecal fat, even though a qualitative assessment can be made under a microscope.

To identify elevated fat in feces, a straightforward two-slide qualitative method can be employed. The evaluation is based on the distinctive orange to red hue of neutral fat (triglycerides) when a fecal suspension is stained with Oil Red O, Sudan III, or Sudan IV. This process involves adding multiple drops of 95% ethanol to a feces suspension on a microscope slide to identify neutral fats. After that, stain is added, a coverslip is placed on, and the wet preparation is examined under a microscope to check for the presence of fat globules that are characteristically stained. Less than 60 globules of neutral fat per high-power field are found in healthy feces.

An additional aliquot of the fecal suspension is heated and acidified with acetic acid on a second slide. An estimate of the total fat content in feces is given on this slide, which includes neutral fats, fatty acids, and fatty acid salts (soaps). Soaps are hydrolyzed to their respective fatty acids by acidification, and the stain is then absorbed by the fatty acids through heating (Figure 10.3).

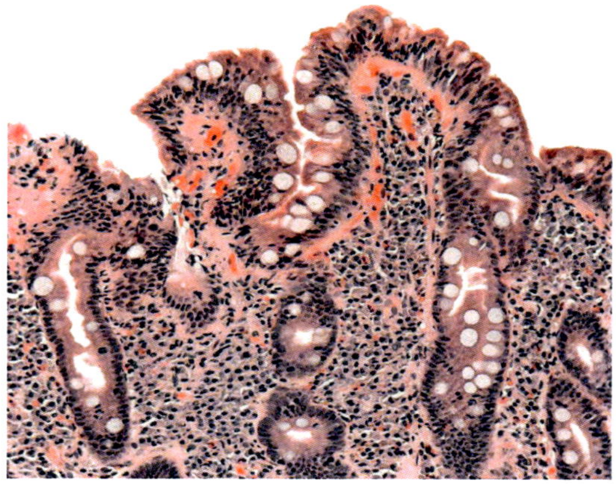

Figure 10.3. *Celiac disease.*

Source: By Samir, CC BY-SA 3.0, https://commons.wikimedia.org/w/index.php?curid=2007909.

Fatty acids and their salts, or soaps, are found in normal feces, which is why the second slide has more orange-red-staining fat globules than the first. Both the quantity and diameter of the fat globules are significant. Less than 100 globules per high-power field are typically seen, and their diameter shouldn't be larger than 4 mm, or roughly half the size of a red blood cell. Both an increase in globule count and abnormally large globules (i.e., are typical in cases of steatorrhea (40–80 mm). By comparing the data from the two slides, maldigestion and malabsorption can frequently be distinguished from one another. When intestinal malabsorption is observed, it is indicated by a normal amount of neutral fat in the feces (on the first slide) and an increased amount of total fat (on the second slide). Stated differently, the increased fat content is mainly made up of fatty acids and soaps that the small intestine was unable to absorb. On the first slide, however, there is more neutral fat, which indicates maldigestion.

10.7.3. Meat Fibers

Feces can be used to identify foods that have not been digested, such as vegetable and meat fibers, under a microscope. Rectangular in shape, meat fibers have distinctive cross-striations. A qualitative examination of the fecal fat is frequently combined with identification and a qualitative assessment of the quantity of meat fibers present. Meat fiber content is estimated while the first fecal fat slide is screened for neutral fat globules. Applying a few drops of fecal suspension to a slide and staining it with an eosin in 10% alcohol solution is an alternate method. A higher quantity of meat fibers in the feces (creatorrhea) is associated with faster intestinal transit and poorer digestion (Van de Kamer et al., 1977).

10.8. Chemical Examination

10.8.1. Fecal Blood

Blood can be seen in the feces if there is bleeding anywhere in the gastrointestinal (GI) tract, from the mouth (bleeding gums) to the anus (hemorrhoids). The American Cancer Society recommends annual screening for anyone over 50 because fecal blood is a common and early indicator of colorectal cancer. More than half of all GI tract cancers are colorectal, and a favorable prognosis is directly correlated with early detection and treatment. 4 Apart from cancer, esophageal varices, ulcers, hemorrhoids, bleeding gums, inflammatory diseases, and different medications that irritate the intestinal mucosa (e.g., aspirin, and iron supplements) can result in feces containing blood. Fecal blood can be seen macroscopically when it is present in large quantities. Bright red blood may cover the surface of stools when there is bleeding in the lower GI tract; in contrast, darker or mahogany-colored stools are frequently the result of bleeding in the upper GI tract. Melena is the term for the dark or black stools that are excreted due to high fecal blood content (50 to 100 mL/day). Heme oxidation, or the breakdown of hemoglobin by intestinal and bacterial enzymes, is the cause of the dark coloration of feces (Figure 10.4).

Less than 2.5 milliliters of blood (or about 2 milligrams of hemoglobin per gram of stool) are lost in the feces every day in healthy individuals. Any increase in fecal blood is noteworthy, and its cause needs to be looked into further. Occult blood is the term for a tiny amount of blood found in feces that is frequently invisible to the naked eye. The fact that (1) GI bleeding is typically sporadic and (2) patients are reluctant to have a fecal sample taken are additional complicating factors in the detection of fecal occult blood. Note that whichever test is used, the results could be negative if bleeding is not present at the time of sample collection.

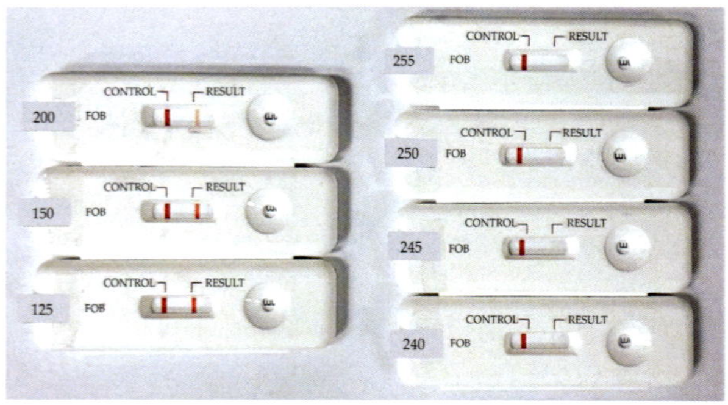

Figure 10.4. *Fecal occult blood testing: An example kit.*

Source: Lin K-W, Chang Y-C. Embedded Immunodetection System for Fecal Occult Blood. Biosensors. 2021; 11(4):106. https://doi.org/10.3390/bios11040106.

To optimize the detection of fecal blood and accurately identify those who require additional testing (e.g., colonoscopy), sample collection needs to be simple to improve patient compliance, and the occult blood test that is employed needs to be accurate and precise. The two most common techniques for identifying fecal occult blood are immunochemical assays and guaiac-based tests. The main purpose of these tests is to check for colorectal cancers that result in lower gastrointestinal bleeding (i.e., colon). Less frequently performed, a third fluorescence-based test is mainly used to identify upper gastrointestinal bleeding. The basis for guaiac-based fecal occult blood tests (gFOBTs) is the heme moiety of hemoglobin's pseudoperoxidase activity. Equation 2 states that the heme moiety catalyzes the oxidation of the indicator in the presence of hydrogen peroxide, causing a change in color.

$$H_2O_2 + \underset{\text{(colorless)}}{\text{Guaiac}} \xrightarrow[\text{or peroxidase}]{\text{Pseudoperoxidase*}} \underset{\text{(colored)}}{\overset{\text{Oxidized}}{\text{Indicator}}} + H_2O \quad (2)$$

*Possible pseudoperoxidases and peroxidases: hemoglobin, myoglobin, bacterial peroxidases, and fruit and vegetable peroxidases.

The less sensitive indicator guaiac is only used for fecal testing because any substance with peroxidase or pseudoperoxidase activity can catalyze the reaction to produce positive results. Dietary restrictions are required to prevent the natural peroxidases found in consumed fruits and vegetables as well as the pseudoperoxidase activity of myoglobin and hemoglobin in meats and fish. False-positive results are still possible even though the sensitivity of these tests has been modified to take into consideration the typical volume of fecal blood and peroxidases from intestinal bacteria.

A standard gFOBT is made up of paper that has been impregnated with guaiac and is housed in a rigid cardboard holder or slide. To maximize test sensitivity when using these slide-based tests, it is standard practice to collect three fecal samples. Patients should ideally collect fecal material from stool samples taken on three separate days, or they should sample multiple portions of a single stool specimen. The patient opens the "front" of the slide, uses an applicator stick to apply fecal material to the exposed paper, closes the slide, and mails or returns it to the laboratory for analysis. In the lab, developer (hydrogen peroxide) is applied after the "back" of the slide is opened to reveal the guaiac-impregnated paper behind the fecal specimen. The indicator is oxidized and turns blue on the paper if hemoglobin or any other pseudoperoxidase or peroxidase is present in sufficient amounts. The amount of enzymatic activity present is correlated with the color's intensity. An internal positive and negative control section guarantees the correct execution of the test (Figure 10.5).

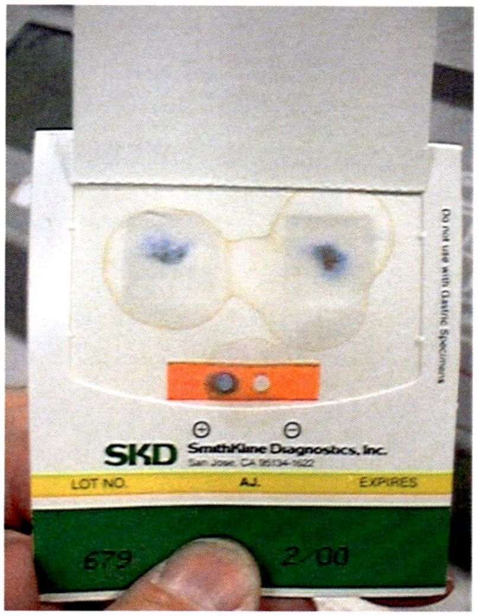

Figure 10.5. *Positive guaiac-based fecal occult blood test.*

Source: By Guaiac_test.jpg, Public Domain, https://commons.wikimedia.org/w/index.php?curid=8710881.

There are many things that can go wrong with a gFOBT. Applying too much or too little feces or using feces tainted with toilet water are examples of improper specimen collection techniques. Another source of interference is the presence of hemorrhoidal or menstrual blood in the specimen. Drugs may also cause problems. Medications that cause upper gastrointestinal tract bleeding, such as warfarin, aspirin, nonsteroidal anti-inflammatory drugs (NSAIDs), iron supplements, and antiplatelet agents, can result in a positive test. On the other hand, ascorbic acid, or vitamin C, and antacids can obstruct the chemical reaction on the test slide and potentially result in false-negative results. Falsenegative results can also arise from the following: (1) expired peroxide developer; (2) defective slides (e.g., expired), or (3) the prepared slide or fecal specimen is kept in storage for a long time prior to testing (e.g., >six days).

Hemoglobin that has been broken down is no longer detectable by a gFOBT and no longer has pseudoperoxidase activity. Keep in mind that heme degradation can happen in three different ways: (1) inside the digestive tract, (2) while the fecal specimen is being stored, or (3) after it has been placed on the gFOBT slide. Research has also demonstrated that if fecal specimens on the slides are hydrated with water prior to testing, false-positive results may be obtained. As a result, the American Cancer Society advises against rehydrating slides prior to testing and instead suggests testing them within six days of collection. Finally, some research has shown that patients do not always follow dietary guidelines or provide multiple fecal samples.

10.8.1.1. Immunochemical Fecal Occult Blood Tests

Polyclonal antihuman antibodies that are directed against the globin component of undegraded human hemoglobin are used in immunochemical tests for fecal occult blood. These techniques are very focused and unaffected by dietary items or drugs that could negatively impact a gFOBT. Immunochemical fecal occult blood tests (iFOBTs) typically do not detect blood from an upper GI bleed (esophageal, gastric) because digestive and bacterial enzymes break down hemoglobin as it travels through the GI tract. Because of this, these tests are more specific for lower gastrointestinal bleeding (i.e., colon, rectum, and cecum).

There are many iFOBT tests available globally, and each manufacturer has a different collection device for their product. The Hemoccult ICT test, for instance, uses a collection card that resembles a gFOBT (Beckman Coulter Inc., Fullerton, California). In contrast, the OC FIT-Chek test (occult fecal immunochemical test; Polymedco, Inc.) uses a tiny collection bottle with an enclosed sample probe. New York's Cortlandt Manor. Patients apply excrement to the collection devices by scraping the surface of the stool until excrement covers the grooved portion of the sample probe (OC FIT) or applying it to the sample area of the card (Hemoccult ICT). After being closed, the collection devices are brought back to the lab for analysis.

Testing is done in the lab manually or with the aid of a fully automated system. Antihuman hemoglobin antibodies bind to the sample's undegraded hemoglobin in iFOBTs, and there are different ways to find hemoglobin-antibody complexes. The detection process can be either manual and visual, involving the observation of the test and control "lines" (Hemoccult ICT), or automated and photometric (OC FIT).

One major benefit of iFOBTs is that they don't require any kind of medication or diet restrictions. As a result, patients don't have to wait several days to start changing their diet or medication schedule before starting the specimen collection phase. It is thought that allowing patients to take a fecal sample right away after visiting their doctor improves patient compliance. The iFOBT's higher price when compared to the gFOBT is a drawback. Therefore, gFOBT currently dominates in colorectal cancer screening protocols even though iFOBT tests for GI bleeding have higher specificity (fewer falsepositive tests).

10.8.1.2. Porphyrin-Based Fecal Occult Blood Test

The HemoQuant test (SmithKline Diagnostics, Sunnyvale, CA) can be used to detect and quantify fecal blood. The chemical transformation of heme into highly fluorescent porphyrins serves as the basis for this test. The test makes it possible to identify and measure the entire amount of hemoglobin in feces, including the amount that has been converted to porphyrins in the intestine and the portion that remains intact. It should be noted that the majority of fecal hemoglobin in a specimen may take the form of heme-derived porphyrins in cases of upper gastrointestinal bleeding or prolonged specimen storage. HemoQuant is unaffected by many of the factors that interfere with other FOBTs because it measures only heme and heme-derived porphyrins. Red meats and other non-human sources of hemoglobin, however, may result in a false-positive test result. When compared to other FOBTs, the HemoQuant test is more costly, labor-intensive, and time-consuming. It is currently mostly carried out by reference laboratories and has limited clinical utility.

10.8.2. Fetal Hemoglobin in Feces (Apt Test)

Investigating a newborn infant's emesis, gastric aspirate, or stool containing blood is necessary. This blood might have come from the newborn's gastrointestinal tract or might have been mother blood that was consumed during childbirth. It's critical to distinguish between these two sources.

A fresh, bloody stool sample or a soiled, bloody diaper would both qualify as fresh, "red" blood specimens. Stools that are tarry or black are not acceptable as they signify the breakdown of hemoglobin into hematin. When using the Apt test, the specimen is suspended (e.g., feces, emesis, and gastric aspirate) is prepared with water and centrifuged to remove any particles from the pink supernatant. The resulting pink supernatant is aliquoted in five milliliters and placed into two tubes. When assessing color changes in the second, or "alkaline," tube, one tube serves as a "reference." One milliliter of sodium hydroxide (0.25 mol/L) is added to the "alkaline" tube, the tube is mixed, and the liquid's color is watched for at least two minutes. Within two minutes, if the specimen's initial pink hue turns yellow or brown, the hemoglobin type found in it is maternal hemoglobin (Hb A). Fetal hemoglobin (Hb F) is the type of hemoglobin that is present if the pink color persists. Keep in mind that every time a specimen is tested, control specimens need to be examined. Baby peripheral or cord blood can be used to create positive controls, and an adult blood sample can be used to create negative controls.

10.8.3. Quantitative Fecal Fat

The gold standard for diagnosing steatorrhea is a quantitative measurement of fecal fat. This chemical test does not determine the cause of the increased excretion, but it does confirm that abnormal amounts of dietary lipids are being eliminated. Patients are required to restrict their fat intake to 100–150 grams per day for three days prior to specimen collection and during the collection period. Furthermore, they are prohibited from using laxatives, artificial fat substitutes (e.g., Olestra), or dietary supplements that block fat. Patients must be careful not to contaminate the specimen during collection with creams, lubricants, or mineral oils as this could result in false-positive results.

The patient gathers all excreted feces for two to three days in sizable, preweighed collection containers (e.g., paint cans). The complete fecal collection is weighed and homogenized in the lab (e.g., using a shaker that is mechanical). To perform a chemical analysis of the lipid content using nuclear magnetic resonance spectroscopy, titrimetry, or gravimetry, a portion of the homogenized fecal specimen is removed. Lipids are extracted from the fecal sample using a solvent in the gravimetric and titrimetric techniques. Fatty acids are created from neutral fats and soaps using the titrimetric method prior to extraction. After that, the fatty acid solution is extracted and titrated using sodium hydroxide. The titrimetric method measures about 80% of the total lipid content in feces because it cannot fully recover medium-chain fatty acids. The gravimetric approach, on the other hand, extracts and measures every fecal lipid that is present. The fecal sample is first microwave-dried in the nuclear magnetic resonance method before being subjected to hydrogen nuclear magnetic resonance spectroscopy (1 H NMR). This technique yields results that are comparable to those obtained using the gravimetric reference method, and it is quick and accurate.

$$\text{Percent fat retention} = \frac{\text{Dietary fat} - \text{Fecal fat}}{\text{Dietary fat}} \times 100 \quad (3)$$

In most cases, adults and children (3 years of age and up) absorb at least 95% of the fat that is consumed in food. Less than 95% of the values in these people suggest steatorrhea.

10.8.4. Fecal Carbohydrates

Disaccharides are not absorbed and instead pass into the large intestine when the enzymes (disaccharidases) required for the conversion of disaccharides into monosaccharides in the small intestine are insufficient or absent. Osmotic diarrhea is caused by the large amounts of water that are retained in the intestinal lumen as a result of these unhydrolyzed disaccharides, which are osmotically active. Even though hereditary disaccharidase deficiency is rare, it should be ruled out and taken into consideration in infants who have diarrhea but do not gain weight. disease-related deficiency of secondary disaccharidase (e.g., tropical sprue, celiac disease) or medication side effects (e.g., oral neomycin, kanamycin) is a transient, acquired condition that typically affects multiple disaccharides. Adults with lactose intolerance are not uncommon, especially in Asian and African populations. While these people could properly digest lactose as children, as they grew older, they gradually lost their ability to do so. As a result, when these people consume lactose, they experience gas, bloating, and violent diarrhea. The active fermentation of lactose in the intestinal lumen by intestinal bacteria is the cause of these clinical signs of disaccharidase deficiency. Large volumes of intestinal gas and diarrhoeal stools have a distinctively low pH (of roughly 5 to 6.) are produced as a result of this fermentation. Feces typically have a pH of greater than 7.0, which is alkaline due to intestinal secretions such as pancreatic secretions. By using pH paper to test the supernatant of a diarrheal stool, one can quickly determine the qualitative pH of feces. Another way to screen for the presence of carbohydrates (or reducing sugars) in diarrheal stools is to use the Siemens Healthcare Diagnostics Inc. Clinitest tablet test., Deerfield, Illinois. While the Clinitest's manufacturer does not recommend using it on fecal specimens, etc., U. S. Despite the lack of a request for Food and Drug Administration approval, its use in detecting fecal reducing substances is extensive and well-documented in the literature. A 1:3 dilution of the supernatant from a diarrheal stool is used to conduct the Clinitest on feces. Excretion of reducing substances in the feces exceeding 250 mg/dL is deemed abnormal. Although it cannot identify the substance being eliminated, a positive Clinitest suggests the presence of a reducing substance. Keep in mind that sucrose is not a reducing sugar, so this method cannot detect it. Chromatographic or particular chemical techniques must be applied to quantify or precisely identify the sugar(s) contained in fecal material.

The most accurate method of diagnosing an insufficient amount of an intestinal enzyme (e.g., lactase deficiency) entails a particular intestinal epithelium histochemical analysis. An oral tolerance test utilizing particular sugars (e.g., sucrose, lactose, etc.). To conduct an oral tolerance test, a predetermined dosage of a particular disaccharide like lactose, sucrose is taken by the patient.

Should the patient possess sufficient levels of the relevant intestinal disaccharidase (e.g., lactase), the sugar (e.g., lactose) is broken down into the appropriate monosaccharides (e. g., galactose, and glucose), which enter the patient's circulation and are absorbed. When blood glucose rises by more than 30 mg/dL above the patient's fasting glucose level, adequate enzyme activity is present (e.g., lactase); an elevation of less than 20 mg/dL over the patient's fasting glucose level signifies an enzyme deficit.

Inadequate intestinal absorption can also lead to the presence of carbohydrates in feces. A xylose absorption test is used to distinguish between maldigestion and malabsorption of carbohydrates.

Xylose is a pentose that is easily absorbed in the small intestine and does not require the liver or pancreas to be broken down. Normally, the body does not metabolize xylose and it is not found in the blood at significant levels. Furthermore, xylose is easily eliminated in the urine after passing through the glomerular filtration barrier. The xylose absorption test entails giving the patient a dose of xylose, after which a 2-hour blood sample and a 5-hour urine specimen are collected. Urine and blood are tested for xylose concentrations. Adults typically excrete 16–24% of the ingested dose of xylose, depending on the size of the initial oral dose.

10.9. The Importance of Stool Tests in the Diagnosis and Follow-up of Gastrointestinal Disorders

Stool examinations provide vital information about conditions affecting the gastrointestinal tract. Stool can be investigated using macro-, micro-, chemical, immunological, and microbiologic techniques. The stool samples that will be tested ought to be taken as soon as possible, stored in a clean container, or both.

10.9.1. Macroscopic Examination of the Stool

Macroscopically assessing stool samples for color, consistency, quantity, form, odor, and mucus presence is important. It's normal for stool to contain a tiny bit of mucus. On the other hand, excessive or bloody mucus production is abnormal. Because bilirubin and bile are present, the normal color is tawny. Stools in babies can have a pasty or watery consistency and may even be green. The color of stools varies a lot based on diet. Stool with a putty or clay color is seen in cases of biliary obstructions. Black, tarry stool is seen if the upper gastrointestinal tract loses more than 100 milliliters of blood. In addition to hemorrhaging, black stools could result from bismuth or iron therapy. When there is bleeding in the lower gastrointestinal tract, red stool is seen.

It has been demonstrated that assessing a newborn baby's stool color with a "stool color card" raises awareness of biliary atresia. It has been discovered that the Modified Bristol visual stool scale, which assesses stool consistency, is useful for tracking the effectiveness of treatment for functional constipation (Figure 10.6) (Chumpitazi et al., 2010).

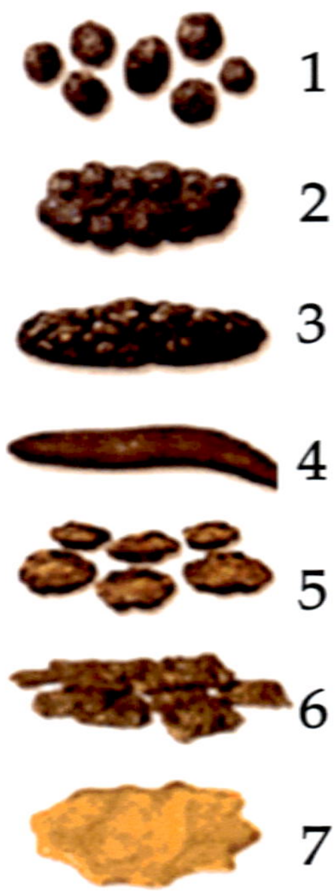

Figure 10.6. *The Bristol stool scale.*

Source: By Flominator (talk) - Own work based on: BristolStoolChart.png, CC BY-SA 4.0, https://commons.wikimedia.org/w/index.php?curid=55875092.

10.9.2. Microscopic Examination of the Stool

Microscopic examination of the stool is the most crucial step in the diagnosis of intestinal issues and stool abnormalities. Microscopic analysis is a diagnostic method used to identify helminths, protozoa, and fecal leukocytes. Leukocytes and erythrocytes are absent from normal stool. Stool samples taken from the mucous-producing area should be examined to look for leukocytes. Bacterial infections typically result in the observation of leukocytes. When parasites and viruses cause diarrhea, they are not seen. Since the capacity of leukocytes to identify inflammatory diarrhea varies widely, their presence in the stool is not a sensitive test for the condition.

It is possible to examine fresh stool right away for moving organisms. To check for helminths and protozoa, the stool may be preserved in 10% formalin if examination is not possible right away. Two to five grams of stool is the minimum amount needed for testing. To examine parasites, at least three consecutive stool samples are needed. Urine contamination of stool ought to be prevented. In 50–70% of cases, giardia can be found in a single sample; in 90% of cases, it can be found in a third sample. Entamoeba histolytica cysts and trophozoites are used in the diagnosis of intestinal amoebiasis. Histolytica) are studied by means of microscopy analyses. But the individual conducting the examination needs to be an authority in this field. Furthermore, microscopy analyses are unable to distinguish Entamoeba dispar strains of histolytica (*E. dispar*) as well as strains of *Entamoeba moshkovskii*. Due to the variable excretion of cysts and trophozoites, it may be necessary to send three samples on different days to detect infection. To find cysts, the samples are brightened and stained with iodine. To look for trophozoites, staining with iron hematoxylin and/or Wheatley trichrome should be done. Stool samples from patients with invasive intestinal amoebiasis typically contain blood. It is not possible to diagnose *E. coli* by looking for phagocyted erythrocytes. infection with histolytica. With *E. coli*, phagocyted erythrocytes can also be observed. discrepancy. Because parasitic organisms have the ability to break down leukocytes, it is possible that they are not always visible in the stool. When diagnosing Giardia, Cryptosporidium, and Entamoeba infections, a quick antigen test is more helpful than microscopy analyses.

10.9.3. Occult Blood in the Stool

Hematin and/or hemoglobin's peroxidase-like activity turns the catalyst blue in peroxidase-based assays. It might not be necessary to follow a strict diet during the exam. Following a restricted diet did not lower the rate of occult blood positivity, as a systematic review showed. Oral iron preparations do not result in a positive hemoccult test result. Large vitamin C intakes can lead to false-negative results, so it's best to keep vitamin C intake under 250 mg per day for three days or longer prior to sampling. Stool samples shouldn't be diluted once more prior to examination. Although dilution raises the test's sensitivity, it also raises the number of false-positive findings. Because aspirin and non-steroidal anti-inflammatory drugs cause minor bleeding in the mucosa of the gastrointestinal tract, they may result in false positive results. To improve the test's accuracy, it should also be run again using two samples each day for three days. In the intestines, a daily blood loss of roughly 2-4 mL is typical. The hemoccult test can identify hemorrhages that exceed this threshold. Using monoclonal or polyclonal antibodies against the globin portion of human hemoglobin, immunohistochemical occult blood tests were created to measure hemoglobin in the stool directly. When it comes to identifying lower gastrointestinal hemorrhages, it has a high sensitivity and specificity. The sensitivity is reduced in upper gastrointestinal hemorrhages when the globin chain is broken down by proteases. Before the tests, there is no need for a special diet.

10.9.4. Detection of Fat in the Stool

Less than 6 g of fat is excreted daily in the stool by healthy humans, and this amount does not change even if they consume 100–125 g of fat per day. In patients without fat malabsorption who have diarrhea, there may be a slight increase in the excretion of fat in the stool. Patients whose stool weights exceeded 1000 g/day and volunteers whose diarrheas were brought on by laxatives both reported values as high as 14 g/day. Consequently, additional tests should be carried out to identify the cause of the diarrhea since a patient's moderate increase in fat excretion in the stool does not suggest that malabsorption is the main culprit.

It is possible to identify fat malabsorption (steatorrhea) using a variety of tests. Stool fat quantification is the gold standard for diagnosing steatorrhea. To achieve this goal, the patient is put on a daily diet containing 100 g of fat, and the stool is collected for 72 hours. However, because it is very challenging to collect stool for 72 hours, qualitative tests are also used as a screening tool for steatorrhea. Among these tests are the Sudan III stain and acid steatocrit tests. The 72-hour fecal fat test cannot be replaced by these tests, but they can be carried out more quickly and easily when compared to the 72-hour stool sample fat test.

10.9.4.1. Seventy-Two–Hour Fecal Fat Test

This protocol calls for collecting stool for 72 hours after a six-day, high-fat diet. It is best to collect stool over a 3-day period as this will reduce errors and variability that may occur from using a shorter time frame. Estimating daily fecal weight is also possible with a longer stool collection period. This is typically greater than 200 g per day in steatorrhea patients. For a precise estimate, patients should consume 70–120 g of fat per day. Stool fat exceeding 6 grams per day is considered pathological. On the other hand, patients with steatorrhea typically have daily stools containing more than 20 g of fat. If less than 60 grams of fat are ingested each day, the test yields an inaccurate result.

Once the mean daily fat intake has been established, the fractional fat absorption, or percentage of absorbed fat, can be computed. The formula below is used to calculate fractional fat absorption.

(Fat intake - fat excreted)/fat intake x 100.

Normal fractional fat absorption has an absorption rate of 94%. Differentiating between the causes of steatorrhea cannot be accomplished by quantitatively estimating the amount of fat in the stool.

10.9.4.2. Detection of Fecal Fat using Sudan III Staining

In clinical practice, qualitative tests like the Sudan III stain are still employed because it is challenging to collect stool for 72 hours. When used correctly, Sudan III staining can identify over 90% of patients with steatorrhea that is clinically significant. General sensitivity and reliability are constrained by variation in the test's execution and interpretation. Examining objects under a microscope is not sensitive enough, especially when done by a novice. According to reports, the Sudan III test has a sensitivity of 77% and a specificity of 98%.

Fatty acids and neutral fats can be identified after Sudan III staining stool samples. A tiny piece of stool is placed on a microscope slide, and two drops each of water and 95% ethyl alcohol are added to the slide to detect neutral fats. Add three or four drops of Sudan III dye. It is looked into whether soaps and free triglycerides are present. Seldom are these seen as globules or crystals, but more often as bundles or plaques. It is a dark orange stain. Two to three drops of 36% glacial acetic acid are splattered onto the preparation to detect fatty acids. Add three or four drops of Sudan III dye. Heating with flame is done. A microscopy analysis is carried out. Fatty acid concentrations are measured and documented as orange-colored fat drop globules. Generally, there should be less than fifty neutral fat particles and less than one hundred fatty acid particles. The Sudan III method of separating neutral fat and fatty acids cannot distinguish between an absorption disorder and a digestive disorder. A method for measuring the dimensions of fat globules on fecal fat microscopic examination (fecal qualitative fat microscopic examination) using Sudan III dye has been demonstrated to have a high diagnostic accuracy and a close relationship with chemically measured fetal fat excretion. Accordingly, globules observed to have a diameter of 10 μm or more are classified as (+), globules observed to have a diameter of 20–100 μm are classified as (++), and globules with a diameter of more than 100 globules that are fat and have large diameters are classified as (+++).

10.9.4.3. Acid Steatocrit Test

A small stool sample is examined, and the examination is based on weight measurement. It's an easy, quick, affordable, and dependable method. Its sensitivity is 100%, its specificity is 95%, and its positive predictive value is 90% when compared to the gold standard, the 72-hour fat collection test.

$$\text{Acid steatocrit }\% = \text{fat layer}/(\text{fat layer}+\text{solid layer}) \times 100$$

The fat content in the stool can be measured in the following way:

$$\text{Fecal fat} = -0.43+[0.45\ (\text{acid steatocrit }\%)]\ \text{g/24 hours}$$

10.9.4.4. Near-infrared Reflectance Analysis: NIRA

With the help of this analysis, it is possible to measure fat, nitrogen, and carbohydrates all at once in a single stool sample. It has the same accuracy as the fecal fat test after 72 hours. It is an easy, quick, and accurate way to measure steatorrhea. It only takes a small fecal sample. Fecal samples ought to be examined as soon as they are collected or, at most, preserved for a few days.

10.9.5. Fecal pH, Electrolytes, and Reducing Substances

Following homogenization and centrifugation, the pH and electrolyte intensities in the watery portion of the feces are measured. Nitrazine paper is used to measure the pH of feces in a newly sampled feces. The typical pH range for feces is 7.0 to 7.5. Excrement with a pH of less than 5.5 is considered acidic. Fecal pH in infants that are breastfed is slightly acidic. The osmolarity of feces is the same as that of serum (290 mosmol/kg). The fecal osmolarity is subtracted from the osmotic gap (osmotic gap= 290 – (Na + K) x 2), which is calculated by multiplying the total of the Na and K values in the fecal water by two. For patients suffering from osmotic diarrhea, it is crucial to specify the osmotic gap in the stool. When there is secretory diarrhea (>125 mosmol/kg), the osmotic gap is small, whereas it is high in osmotic diarrhea (>125 mosmol/kg). Because bacterial fermentation or the contamination of fecal samples with concentrated urine after the stool is collected can result in an artificially high osmolarity, this formula is preferred over direct measurement of fecal osmolarity.

If there is a suspicion of carbohydrate malabsorption, the Benedict or Fehling test should be used to look for a reducing substance in the stool. Sugars that reduce include glucose, lactose, and fructose; sucrose does not. Colonic bacteria have the ability to convert unabsorbed sucrose to glucose and fructose, which results in a positive reducing substance test result. In a test tube, the Benedict solution (Clinitest) is combined with an equal volume of stool and heated. A reducing substance is present (the test is positive) if the supernatant fluid turns green-brown. Should the quantity of reducing agent in the stool be.<0.25 mg/dL, the test result is normal. If it is 0.25–0.5 mg/dL, the test result is suspicious. If it is > 0.05 mg/dL, the test result is out of the ordinary.

Because lactose and other sugars that are left in the stool by enzymes continue to break down for two to fourteen hours, the fecal sample for the reducing substance test needs to be fresh and arrive at the lab no later than one and a half hours. If the test is not conducted promptly, sugars like lactose break down and lead to a false positive. There should be no contact between the stool and diapers, water, toilet paper, or urine. Due to the fact that most toilet paper contains sugar, the outcome will be untrue. diapers and cellulose both absorb moisture.

10.9.6. Fecal Sugar Chromatography

When a reducing substance is discovered in the stool, this test is used. It makes fecal sugar evaluation possible. When diagnosing lactose intolerance, fructosuria/hereditary fructose intolerance, sucrose malabsorption, or classic galactosemia, it might be useful. Lactose, galactose, and glucose can all be found in cases of lactase deficiency. Only glucose and galactose are found in congenital glucose-galactose malabsorption.

10.9.7. Fecal Alpha-1 Antitrypsin Test

The primary constituent of alpha-1 globulins is the glycoprotein known as alpha-1 antitrypsin, or alpha-1 AT, which is produced in the liver. Because alpha-1 AT is resistant to proteolysis and disintegration in the intestinal lumen, it has a higher molecular weight than albumin and is eliminated in the feces without degrading. Alpha-1 AT excretion from the feces occurs at a rate of less than 2 points-6 mg/day, and intestinal clearance is less than 13 mL/day. Increased enteral protein loss is suggested by an increase in alpha-1 AT clearance. For the alpha-1 AT clearance test to measure alpha-1 AT in the plasma simultaneously, a 24-hour fecal sample and serum sample are needed.

Alpha-1 AT clearance = (fecal volume) x (fecal alpha-1 AT) / (serum alpha-1 AT)

Diarrhea may increase alpha-1 AT clearance in the absence of protein losing enteropathy.

In patients without diarrhea, the alpha-1 AT clearance value is greater than 27 mL/day, and in patients with diarrhea, it is greater than 56 mL/day. These values are consistent with protein-losing enteropathy. Because alpha-1 AT is disintegrated when the pH of the gastric acid falls below 3 points5, alpha-1 AT clearance should be measured while acid suppression (omeprazole 40 mg/day) is administered in individuals who have been found to have normal alpha-1 AT clearance despite known gastrointestinal protein loss.

10.9.8. Indirect Pancreatic Function Tests

The effects of exocrine pancreatic insufficiency are measured by indirect tests. When compared to direct pancreatic function tests, indirect tests are less complicated, more affordable, and easier to perform. These tests' primary purpose is to diagnose advanced exocrine pancreatic insufficiency. When compared to direct tests, they are significantly less sensitive in identifying the early stages of exocrine pancreatic insufficiency. False-positive results in gastrointestinal disorders other than pancreatic diseases and the requirement for stool collection are additional drawbacks.

10.9.8.1. Fecal Elastase-1 Test

Fecal elastase is the most specific and sensitive indirect test for pancreatic function. Unlike other pancreatic enzymes, elsastase-1 is a pancreas-specific proteolytic enzyme that binds to bile salts and does not break down during intestinal transit. It makes up roughly 6% of all the enzymes secreted by the pancreas. The measurement of fecal elastase-1 exhibits a strong correlation with the pancreatic production of trypsin, amylase, lipase, and elastase-1. A level of fecal elastase-1 less than 200 mcg/g is deemed abnormal. It is advisable to repeat measurements that fall between 200 and 250 mcg/g as they may represent a threshold. Its sensitivity is 63%, 100%, and 100%, respectively, for mild, moderate, and severe exocrine pancreatic insufficiency in patients with chronic pancreatitis. In patients with exocrine pancreatic insufficiency, its specificity is 93%. Fecal samples may be diluted by watery diarrhea brought on by non-pancreatic illnesses or medications, potentially producing false-positive results. Fecal samples can be lyophilized to solve this issue.

10.9.8.2. Fecal Chymotrypsin Test

One enzymatic byproduct of pancreatic secretion that can be used to identify pancreatic insufficiency is fecal chymotrypsin. In contrast to fecal elastase-1, chymotrypsin exhibits a lower sensitivity and specificity for exocrine pancreatic insufficiency. Fecal chymotrypsin sensitivity for mild and moderate-to-advanced pancreatic insufficiency is 49% and 85%, respectively. When diarrhea is present, chymotrypsin may be diluted as it passes through the intestines, where it is affected in different ways. Patients should stop taking exogenous enzymes two days prior to the test because chymotrypsin can also be present in enzyme preparations sold in stores.

10.9.9. Fecal Calprotectin

A cytosolic protein with antimicrobial, antiproliferative, and immunomodulatory properties is called calprotectin. Calprotectin levels rise in response to infections, inflammation, and cancer. It's a calcium- and zinc-binding protein that neutrophils and monocytes typically release. By breaking down zinc-dependent enzymes, it uses a zinc-binding mechanism to carry out its antimicrobial activity. It can be discovered in bodily fluids, stool, and tissue samples. As a result, it is a useful indicator of neutrophil efficiency. Fecal calprotectin levels rise in cases of intestinal inflammation. Thus, distinguishing between inflammatory and non-inflammatory causes of chronic diarrhea may be helpful. In inflammatory bowel diseases, fecal calprotectin levels rise (IBD). There is a correlation between the amount of fecal calprotectin and polymorphonuclear leukocyte infiltration of the intestinal mucosa.

In IBDs, there is a significant correlation between calprotectin and both clinical and histopathologic activity. Fecal calprotectin sensitivity and specificity in adults with IBD have been reported to be 93% and 96% in adults, and 92% and 76% in children. It has been suggested that calprotectin may be more helpful in diagnosing IBD in patients who visit gastroenterology clinics (where the prevalence is high) and in primary care settings (where the prevalence is low) when patients present with diarrhea or abdominal pain. Therefore, a negative fecal calprotectin result could help primary care doctors rule out IBD. More than 80% of patients with positive fecal calprotectin results in a primary care context did not have a significant abnormality revealed by colonoscopy. Indicating a colonoscopy with a calprotectin threshold of 250 µg/d reduces the sensitivity for diagnosing inflammatory bowel disease. Another test that could be useful in the differential diagnosis of persistent diarrheas is fecal calprotectin. It might be useful for monitoring clinical activity in IBD and screening for colorectal cancer, among other things. As of yet, these indications are not part of standard clinical practice.

The amount of fecal calprotectin varies with age. During the first year of life, the threshold values are higher (<350 µg/d) than in childhood (<275 µg/d) or adulthood (<50 µg/d). Various threshold values for fecal calprotectin have been used in studies involving children (Degraeuwe et al., 2015; Manceau et al., 2017; Conroy et al., 2018). Figure 10.7 displays the implications fecal calprotectin.

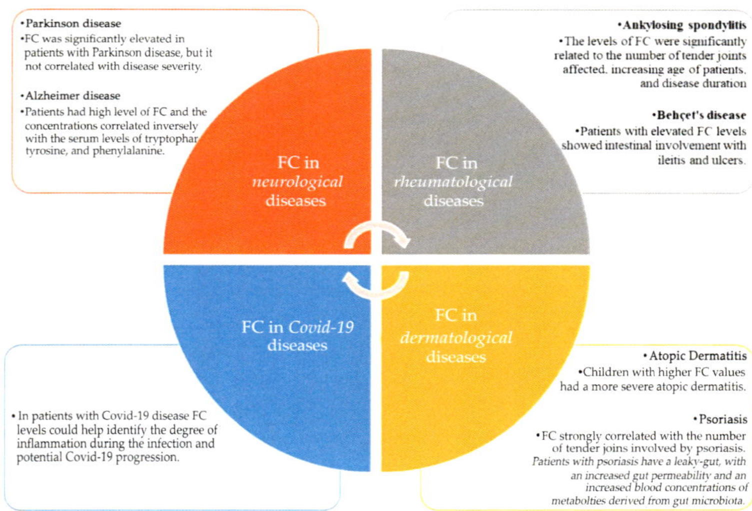

Figure 10.7. *Fecal calprotectin in extra gastro-intestinal diseases.*

Source: Saviano A, Candelli M, Zanza C, Piccioni A, Migneco A, Ojetti V. Gastrointestinal Involvement in Extra-Digestive Disease: Which Is the Role of Fecal Calprotectin? Medicina. 2022; 58(10):1384. https://doi.org/10.3390/medicina58101384.

10.9.10. Fecal Antigen Tests

1. **Helicobacter Pylori (H. pylori) Stool Antigen Test:** Finding H. stool contains the pylori antigen, which suggests a persistent infection. For this reason, a stool antigen test could be employed to diagnose *H. pylori* infection as well as to verify its eradication. In regions where *H. pylori* is prevalent, the stool antigen test is the most economical diagnostic procedure. The incidence of *H. pylori* is low to moderate. Similar to the urea breath test, monoclonal immunoassays (EIA) carried out in laboratories have high sensitivity (94%) and specificity (97%) rates. Proton pump inhibitors (PPI), antibiotics, and bismuth compounds have all been used recently and have an impact on the stool antigen test. In spite of data that suggests the stool antigen test can predict eradication as early as 7 days after treatment is finished, patients should avoid using PPIs for 1-2 weeks and antibiotics for 4 weeks before the test to prevent false-negative results.

   The stool antigen test's specificity may be reduced by active bleeding brought on by peptic ulcers. Nonetheless, monoclonal EIA sensitivity is still high in patients who have recently experienced a peptic ulcer hemorrhage. Due to its low sensitivity, the polyclonal EIA stool antigen test is not currently in use. Rapid monoclonal immunochromatographic stool antigen tests for use in offices have a low sensitivity of 50% and a high specificity of 96%. Remembering that the *H. pylori* is sensitive and specific. The type of commercial test used, the threshold selected, and how weak-positive results are interpreted all affect the pylori stool antigen test (Joint ESPGHAN/NASPGHAN Guidelines for the Management of *Helicobacter pylori* in Children and Adolescents, Update 2016).

2. **Rotavirus Stool Antigen Test:** Immune-based tests, such as the polymerase chain reaction (PCR) and the enzyme-linked immunosorbent assay (ELISA), as well as nucleic acid tests like latex agglutination tests, are used to identify rotavirus in the stool. The two most often used tests are latex agglutination and ELISA. The most sensitive test is the polymerase chain reaction. Using the ELISA test, the virus can be identified 1-2 days before the onset of clinical illness. The detection rate of rotavirus is 94% 1-4 days after the onset of the disease and 76% 4-6-8 days after the onset of the disease. It can occasionally be found even two weeks after the illness has healed.

3. **Adenovirus Stool Antigen Test:** When compared to rotavirus, enteric adenoviruses (type 40 or 41) can cause diarrhea for a longer period of time. For ELISA analysis specific to adenoviruses, stool samples are utilized. This diagnostic test is appropriate for use in primary care environments. The sensitivity and specificity of ELISA are 78% and 100%, respectively.

4. **Giardia Stool Antigen Test:**

For stool analysis, many immunoserological techniques have been developed that employ antibodies against cysts or trophozoite antigens. In general, these techniques are more sensitive than non-traditional microscopy tests. The specificity and cost are relatively comparable. The direct immunofluorescence antigen test has the highest sensitivity. Immunoserologic methods have a limited area of use after the treatment of infection. The disappearance of stool antigens after treatment suggests that the treatment was effective, but the detection of antigens in the stool may be caused by excretion of dead parasites.

5. **Entamoeba Stool Antigen Test:** Entamoeba antigens can be found in stool, which makes it a sensitive, specific, quick, and practical method for differentiating *E. histolytica* as well as E. discrepancy. There are commercial stool and serum antigen tests for *E. histolytica* infection that bind to the pathogenic epitopes using monoclonal antibodies. strains of histolytica. Non-pathogenic *E. coli* does not contain these epitopes. different strains. Antigen test kits have been developed using techniques such as immunofluorescence, radioimmunoassay, and ELISA.

10.9.11. Measurement of Clostridium Difficile (C. Difficile) Toxin in the Stool

Only patients with diarrhea should have their stool samples examined, and no follow-up testing should be done once treatment has ended. Some *C. difficile* strains only produce A or B toxins, but other strains produce both A and B toxins. It has not been reported that A toxin alone causes difficile-related illness. On the other hand, an EIA test that looks at both toxins is more sensitive than one that looks only at toxin B. When it comes to A and B toxins, EIA has a sensitivity of roughly 75% and a specificity of 99%. The test has a high false-negative rate because it requires the presence of 100–1000 pg of toxins to be positive.

It has a 64% positive predictive value in children. There is a higher incidence of false negativity for EIA in younger children. Particularly in younger kids, the identification of *C. difficile* in the stool does not always mean that it is the source of the diarrhea.

10.9.12. Multiplex Molecular Panels

This technique was created to use PCR to identify gastrointestinal pathogens in stool samples. It makes it possible to quickly (one hour) detect a large number of pathogens, including more than 20 bacteria, viruses, and parasites. Infectious diarrheas can be diagnosed with it quickly and accurately. This approach helps distinguish between acute graft-versus-host reactions and infectious etiologies, particularly in immunocompromised patients who have received organ transplants and are presenting with diarrhea. Clinical diagnoses can be completed quickly with this approach (Vernon, 1997; Veijola et al., 2005; Vandenberg et al., 2006).

A Closer Look

Maldigestion

Maldigestion refers to the incomplete or inadequate breakdown of food in the digestive tract, leading to the malabsorption of nutrients and subsequent abnormalities in fecal analysis.

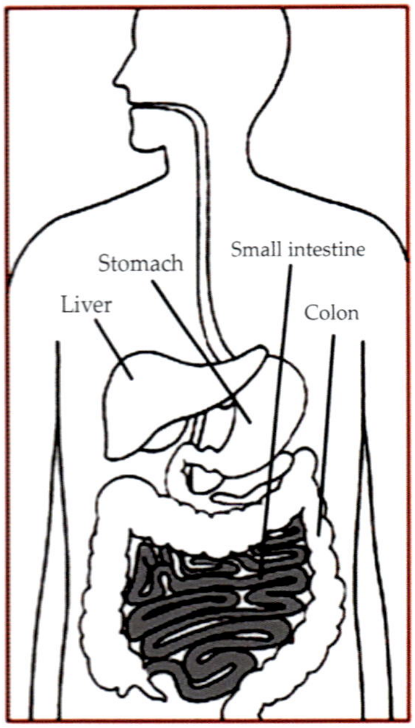

Source: By US gov - US gov, Public Domain, https://commons.wikimedia.org/w/index.php?curid=2141337.

Maldigestion can result from deficiencies in digestive enzymes produced by the pancreas, such as amylase, lipase, and proteases. Without adequate enzyme activity, carbohydrates, fats, and proteins are not properly broken down, leading to their presence in the feces.

Fecal analysis may reveal abnormal characteristics such as increased fat content (steatorrhea), undigested food particles, or oily, greasy stools. These findings indicate impaired digestion and absorption of dietary nutrients.

Maldigestion can lead to malabsorption of nutrients, including carbohydrates, fats, proteins, vitamins, and minerals. As a result, deficiencies in essential nutrients may develop, leading to nutritional imbalances and related health issues.

Patients with maldigestion may experience symptoms such as diarrhea, abdominal bloating, flatulence, weight loss, and nutritional deficiencies. These symptoms are often chronic and may vary in severity depending on the underlying cause of maldigestion.

Fecal analysis, including stool microscopy, fecal fat quantification, and fecal elastase testing, can help diagnose maldigestion by identifying abnormalities in fecal composition and nutrient content. Additional diagnostic tests, such as blood tests, imaging studies, and endoscopic procedures, may be necessary to identify the underlying cause of maldigestion.

Treatment of maldigestion focuses on addressing the underlying cause and managing symptoms. This may involve enzyme replacement therapy, dietary modifications (such as a low-fat or low-fiber diet), nutritional supplementation, and treatment of any underlying gastrointestinal disorders contributing to maldigestion.

Maldigestion can lead to abnormalities in fecal analysis, including increased fat content, undigested food particles, and malabsorption of nutrients. Proper diagnosis and management of maldigestion are essential to prevent nutritional deficiencies and improve gastrointestinal health.

Summary

- Fecal analysis is a noninvasive laboratory test useful in identifying disorders of the digestive tract. These disorders may include malabsorption, inflammation, infection (bacteria, viruses, or fungi), or cancer.
- The function of the small intestine includes the digestion and absorption of foodstuffs, whereas the principal function of the large intestine is the absorption of water, sodium, and chloride.
- Diarrhea is defined as an increase in the volume, liquidity, and frequency of bowel movements compared with an individual's normal bowel movement pattern.
- Normally, fecal excretion of fat consists of less than 7 g per day. This fat originates from several sources: the diet, gastrointestinal secretions, bacterial by-products of metabolism, and sloughed intestinal epithelium.
- Fecal specimen containers vary depending on the amount of specimen to be collected. Essentially any clean, nonbreakable container that is sealable and leakproof is acceptable.
- The macroscopic examination of feces involves visual assessment of color, consistency, and form. Other notable substances within the feces include mucus and undigested matter.
- Mucus, a translucent gelatinous substance, is not present in normal feces. When present, mucus can vary dramatically from a small amount to the massive quantities associated with a villous adenoma (a tumor of the colon).
- Bleeding anywhere in the gastrointestinal (GI) tract from the mouth (bleeding gums) to the anus (hemorrhoids) can result in detectable blood in the feces.

References

1. Ahlquist, D. A., McGill, D. B., Schwartz, S., et al. (1984). HemoQuant: a new quantitative assay for fecal hemoglobin. *Annals of Internal Medicine, 101*(3), 297.
2. Alejo-Cancho, I., Fernández Avilés, F., Capón, A., et al. (2017). Evaluation of a multiplex panel for the diagnosis of acute infectious diarrhea in immunocompromised hematologic patients. *PLoS One, 12*(11), e0187458.
3. Amann, S. T., Josephson, S. A., & Toskes, P. P. (1997). Acid steatocrit: a simple, rapid gravimetric method to determine steatorrhea. *The American Journal of Gastroenterology, 92*(12), 2280–2284.
4. Apt, L., & Downey, W. S. (1955). Melena neonatorum: swallowed blood syndrome—a simple test for the differentiation of adult and fetal hemoglobin in bloody stools. *The Journal of Pediatrics, 47*(1), 5.
5. Assiri, A., Saeed, A., Alnimri, A., et al. (2013). Five Arab children with glucose-galactose malabsorption. *Paediatrics & International Child Health, 33*(2), 108–110.
6. Benini, L., Caliari, S., Guidi, G. C., et al. (1989). Near infrared spectrometry for faecal fat measurement: comparison with conventional gravimetric and titrimetric methods. *Gut, 30*(10), 1344–1347.

7. Beşer, O. F., Sancak, S., Erkan, T., et al. (2014). Can Fecal Calprotectin Level Be Used as a Marker of Inflammation in the Diagnosis and Follow-Up of Cow's Milk Protein Allergy? *Allergy, Asthma & Immunology Research, 6*(1), 33–38.
8. Bijoor, A. R., Geetha, S., & Venkatesh, T. (2004). Faecal fat content in healthy adults by the 'acid steatocrit method'. *Indian Journal of Clinical Biochemistry, 19*(1), 20–22.
9. Binnicker, M. J. (2015). Multiplex Molecular Panels for Diagnosis of Gastrointestinal Infection: Performance, Result Interpretation, and Cost-Effectiveness. *Journal of Clinical Microbiology, 53*(12), 3723–3728.
10. Caballero, B., Solomons, N. W., & Torún, B. (1983). Fecal reducing substances and breath hydrogen excretion as indicators of carbohydrate malabsorption. *Journal of Pediatric Gastroenterology and Nutrition, 2*(3), 487–490.
11. Chumpitazi, B. P., Lane, M. M., Czyzewski, D. I., et al. (2010). Creation and initial evaluation of a Stool Form Scale for children. *The Journal of Pediatrics, 157*(4), 594–597.
12. Conroy, S., Hale, M. F., Cross, S. S., et al. (2018). Unrestricted faecal calprotectin testing performs poorly in the diagnosis of inflammatory bowel disease in patients in primary care. *Journal of Clinical Pathology, 71*(4), 316–322.
13. Degraeuwe, P. L., Beld, M. P., Ashorn, M., et al. (2015). Faecal calprotectin in suspected paediatric inflammatory bowel disease. *Journal of Pediatric Gastroenterology and Nutrition, 60*(3), 339–346.
14. Deshpande, A., Pasupuleti, V., Patel, P., et al. (2011). Repeat stool testing to diagnose Clostridium difficile infection using enzyme immunoassay does not increase diagnostic yield. *Clinical Gastroenterology and Hepatology, 9*(8), 665–669.
15. Drummey, G. D., Benson, J. A., & Jones, G. M. (1961). Microscopical examination of the stool for steatorrhea. *The New England Journal of Medicine, 264*(2), 85.
16. Eherer, A. J., & Fordtran, J. S. (1992). Fecal osmotic gap and pH in experimental diarrhea of various causes. *Gastroenterology, 103*(2), 545–551.
17. Fine, K. D., & Fordtran, J. S. (1992). The effect of diarrhea on fecal fat excretion. *Gastroenterology, 102*(6), 1936–1939.
18. Fine, K. D., & Ogunji, F. (2000). A new method of quantitative fecal fat microscopy and its correlation with chemically measured fecal fat output. *American Journal of Clinical Pathology, 113*(4), 528–534.
19. Gill, C. J., Lau, J., Gorbach, S. L., et al. (2003). Diagnostic accuracy of stool assays for inflammatory bacterial gastroenteritis in developed and resource-poor countries. *Clinical Infectious Diseases, 37*(5), 365–375.
20. Holtman, G. A., Lisman-van Leeuwen, Y., Kollen, B. J., et al. (2016). Diagnostic Accuracy of Fecal Calprotectin for Pediatric Inflammatory Bowel Disease in Primary Care: A Prospective Cohort Study. *Annals of Family Medicine, 14*(5), 437–445.
21. Jones, N. L., Koletzko, S., Goodman, K., et al. (2017). Joint Espghan/Naspghan Guidelines for the Management of Helicobacter pylori in Children and Adolescents (Update 2016). *Journal of Pediatric Gastroenterology and Nutrition, 64*(6), 991–1003.
22. Khouri, M. R., Huang, G., & Shiau, Y. F. (1989). Sudan stain of fecal fat: new insight into an old test. *Gastroenterology, 96*(2), 421–427.

23. Korpi-Steiner, N., Ward, J. N., Kumar, V., & McConnell, J. P. (2009). Comparative analysis of fecal fat quantitation via nuclear magnetic resonance spectroscopy (1H NMR) and gravimetry. *Clinical Chemistry and Laboratory Medicine, 47*(12), 33.

24. Leeds, J. S., Oppong, K., & Sanders, D. S. (2011). The role of fecal elastase-1 in detecting exocrine pancreatic disease. *Nature Reviews Gastroenterology & Hepatology, 8*(7), 405–415.

25. Lewis, S. J., & Heaton, K. W. (1997). Stool form scale as a useful guide to intestinal transit time. *Scandinavian Journal of Gastroenterology, 32*(9), 920–924.

26. Li, F., Ma, J., Geng, S., et al. (2015). Fecal calprotectin concentrations in healthy children aged 1-18 months. *PLoS One, 10*(4), e0119574.

27. Lien, T. H., Chang, M. H., Wu, J. F., et al. (2011). Effects of the infant stool color card screening program on 5-year outcome of biliary atresia in Taiwan. *Hepatology, 53*(1), 202–208.

28. Liesman, R. M., & Binnicker, M. J. (2016). The role of multiplex molecular panels for the diagnosis of gastrointestinal infections in immunocompromised patients. *Current Opinion in Infectious Diseases, 29*(4), 359–365.

29. Manceau, H., Chicha-Cattoir, V., Puy, H., et al. (2017). Fecal calprotectin in inflammatory bowel diseases: update and perspectives. *Clinical Chemistry and Laboratory Medicine, 55*(4), 474–483.

30. Mandel, J. S., Church, T. R., Bond, J. H., et al. (2000). The effect of fecal occult-blood screening on the incidence of colorectal cancer. *New England Journal of Medicine, 343*(22), 1603.

31. Martin, A. L., & Kudesia, G. (1990). Enzyme linked immunosorbent assay for detecting adenoviruses in stool specimens: Comparison with electron microscopy and isolation. *Journal of Clinical Pathology, 43*(6), 514–515.

32. Meurman, O., Ruuskanen, O., & Sarkkinen, H. (1983). Immunoassay diagnosis of adenovirus infections in children. *Journal of Clinical Microbiology, 18*(6), 1190–1195.

33. Neumeister, V., Henker, J., Kaltenborn, G., et al. (1997). Simultaneous determination of fecal fat, nitrogen, and water by near-infrared reflectance spectroscopy. *Journal of Pediatric Gastroenterology and Nutrition, 25*(4), 388–393.

34. Robertson, D. J., Lee, J. K., Boland, C. R., et al. (2017). Recommendations on Fecal Immunochemical Testing to Screen for Colorectal Neoplasia: A Consensus Statement by the US Multi-Society Task Force on Colorectal Cancer. *Gastroenterology, 152*(5), 1217–1237.

35. Rosenthal, P., & Jennings, M. T. (1992). Comparison of fecal occult blood tests for detection of gastrointestinal bleeding in pediatric patients. *American Journal of Gastroenterology, 87*(11), 1575–1579.

36. Shim, J. O. (2014). Clostridium difficile in Children: To Treat or Not to Treat? *Pediatric Gastroenterology, Hepatology & Nutrition, 17*(2), 80–84.

37. Shimoyama, T. (2013). Stool antigen tests for the management of Helicobacter pylori infection. *World Journal of Gastroenterology, 19*(46), 8188–8191.

38. Simko, V. (1981). Fecal fat microscopy. Acceptable predictive value in screening for steatorrhea. *The American Journal of Gastroenterology, 75*(3), 204–208.

39. Stein, J., Purschian, B., Zeuzem, S., et al. (1996). Quantification of fecal carbohydrates by near-infrared reflectance analysis. *Clinical Chemistry, 42*(2), 309–312.

40. Strygler, B., Nicar, M. J., Santangelo, W. C., et al. (1990). Alpha 1-antitrypsin excretion in stool in normal subjects and in patients with gastrointestinal disorders. *Gastroenterology, 99*(5), 1380–1387.

41. Thomas, E. E., Puterman, M. L., Kawano, E., et al. (1988). Evaluation of seven immunoassays for detection of rotavirus in pediatric stool samples. *Journal of Clinical Microbiology, 26*(6), 1189–1193.

42. Uyar, Y., & Taylan Ozkan, A. (2009). [Antigen detection methods in diagnosis of amebiasis, giardiasis and cryptosporidiosis] [Article in Turkish]. *Turkiye Parazitoloji Dergisi, 33*(2), 140–150.

43. Van de Kamer, J. H., Ten Bokel Huinink, H., & Weyers, H. W. (1949). Rapid method for the determination of fat in feces. *Journal of Biological Chemistry, 177*(1), 347.

44. Vandenberg, O., Van Laethem, Y., Souayah, H., et al. (2006). Improvement of routine diagnosis of intestinal parasites with multiple sampling and SAF-fixative in the triple-faeces-test. *Acta. Gastroenterologica. Belgica., 69*(4), 361–366.

45. Veijola, L., Myllyluoma, E., Korpela, R., et al. (2005). Stool antigen tests in the diagnosis of Helicobacter pylori infection before and after eradication therapy. *World Journal of Gastroenterology, 11*(47), 7340–7344.

46. Vernon, S. W. (1997). Participation in colorectal cancer screening: a review. *Journal of the National Cancer Institute, 89*(19), 1406.

INDEX

C

D

E

F

G

H

I

J

K

L

M

N

O

P

R

S

FSC
www.fsc.org
MIX
Papier | Fördert gute Waldnutzung
FSC® C083411

Kolibri 360 GmbH
Ferdinand-Jühlke-Straße 7
99095 Erfurt, Deutschland
produktsicherheit@kolibri360.de